Extracranial Stereotactic Radiotherapy and Radiosurgery

Extracranial Stereotactic Radiotherapy and Radiosurgery

Edited by

Ben J. Slotman
Department of Radiation Oncology, VU University Medical Center
Amsterdam, The Netherlands

Timothy D. Solberg
Department of Radiation Oncology, University of Nebraska
Omaha, Nebraska, U.S.A.

Dirk Verellen
Department of Radiotherapy, AZ-VUB
Brussels, Belgium

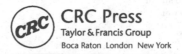

CRC Press
Taylor & Francis Group
Boca Raton London New York

CRC Press is an imprint of the
Taylor & Francis Group, an **informa** business

CRC Press
Taylor & Francis Group
6000 Broken Sound Parkway NW, Suite 300
Boca Raton, FL 33487-2742

First issued in paperback 2019

ISBN-13: 978-0-8247-2697-3 (hbk)
ISBN-13: 978-0-367-39187-4 (pbk)

This book contains information obtained from authentic and highly regarded sources. While all reasonable efforts have been made to publish reliable data and information, neither the author[s] nor the publisher can accept any legal responsibility or liability for any errors or omissions that may be made. The publishers wish to make clear that any views or opinions expressed in this book by individual editors, authors or contributors are personal to them and do not necessarily reflect the views/opinions of the publishers. The information or guidance contained in this book is intended for use by medical, scientific or health-care professionals and is provided strictly as a supplement to the medical or other professional's own judgement, their knowledge of the patient's medical history, relevant manufacturer's instructions and the appropriate best practice guidelines. Because of the rapid advances in medical science, any information or advice on dosages, procedures or diagnoses should be independently verified. The reader is strongly urged to consult the relevant national drug formulary and the drug companies' and device or material manufacturers' printed instructions, and their websites, before administering or utilizing any of the drugs, devices or materials mentioned in this book. This book does not indicate whether a particular treatment is appropriate or suitable for a particular individual. Ultimately it is the sole responsibility of the medical professional to make his or her own professional judgements, so as to advise and treat patients appropriately. The authors and publishers have also attempted to trace the copyright holders of all material reproduced in this publication and apologize to copyright holders if permission to publish in this form has not been obtained. If any copyright material has not been acknowledged please write and let us know so we may rectify in any future reprint.

A CIP record for this book is available from the British Library.

Library of Congress Cataloging-in-Publication Data available on application

Visit the Taylor & Francis Web site at
http://www.taylorandfrancis.com

and the CRC Press Web site at
http://www.crcpress.com

Preface

A few years ago, out of common interest in the emerging field of extracranial body radiosurgery, the editors considered it worthwhile to summarize the on-going efforts by different research centers. An added benefit was that the editors themselves have different backgrounds illustrating the truly multidisciplinary character of radiation oncology. Moreover, as the editors live and work in either Europe or the United States the subtle differences in approaching clinical issues will be represented in the work creating a bridge between both continents. As always the subject of this work is not new, yet technological evolution often creates new possibilities, and innovative centers have put large efforts in finding individualized solutions to these common challenges. Inevitably, a myriad of treatment strategies can be found in the literature; the current work aims at being a comprehensive overview of emerging developments in this sub-specialty in radiation oncology, as well as illustrating possible clinical applications of these new and challenging technologies and approaches. As the basic concept was to generate a general, objective, and comprehensive overview without overlooking any possible strategy, great care has been taken to invite specialists in their respective fields to act as contributing authors. In retrospect the editors believe this objective has been reached and hope the reader will find this book to be a truly practical reference work on the topic.

Enjoy reading

Ben J. Slotman
Timothy Solberg
Dirk Verellen

Contents

Contributors

John R. Adler   Stanford University Medical Center, Stanford, California, U.S.A.

Lluis Escudé   Servei de Radio-oncologia, Instituto Oncológico Teknon, Barcelona, Spain

Jack F. Fowler   Department of Human Oncology, University Hospital, Madison, Wisconsin, U.S.A.

Martin Fuss   Department of Radiation Oncology, The University of Texas Health Science Center, San Antonio, Texas, U.S.A.

Klaus K. Herfarth   Department of Radiation Oncology, University of Heidelberg, Germany

Frank J. Lagerwaard   Department of Radiation Oncology, VU University Medical Center, Amsterdam, The Netherlands

Steve P. Lee   Department of Radiation Oncology, UCLA Medical Center, Los Angeles, California, U.S.A.

Paul Medin   Department of Radiation Oncology, UCLA Medical Center Los Angeles, California, U.S.A.

Raymond Miralbell   Servei de Radio-oncologia, Instituto Oncológico Teknon, Barcelona, Spain and Service de Radio-oncologie, Hôpitaux Universitaires, Geneva, Switerland

Meritxell Mollà   Servei de Radio-oncologia, Instituto Oncológico Teknon, Barcelona, Spain

Samuel Ryu   Department of Radiation Oncology and Neurosurgery, Henry Ford Hospital, Detroit, Michigan, U.S.A.

Bill Salter   Department of Radiation Oncology, The University of Texas Health Science Center, and Cancer Therapy and Research Center, San Antonio, Texas, U.S.A.

Achim Schweikard   Luebeck University, Luebeck, Germany

Suresh Senan   Department of Radiation Oncology, VU University Medical Center, Amsterdam, The Netherlands

Hiroya Shiomi   Osaka University Hospital, Osaka, Japan

Ben J. Slotman   Department of Radiation Oncology, VU University Medical Center, Amsterdam, The Netherlands

Robert Smee   Department of Radiation Oncology, Prince of Wales Hospital, Randwick, New South Wales, Australia

Guy Soete   Department of Radiotherapy, AZV-UB, Brussels, Belgium

Timothy Solberg   Department of Radiation Oncology, University of Nebraska, Omaha, Nebroska, U.S.A.

Guy Storme   Department of Radiotherapy, AZV-UB, Brussels, Belgium

Robert D. Timmerman   Department of Radiation Oncology, Indiana University School of Medicine, Bloomington, Indiana, U.S.A.

Minaro Uchida   Stanford University Medical Center, Stanford, California, U.S.A.

Dirk Verellen   Department of Radiotherapy, AZV-UB, Brussels, Belgium

H. Rodney Withers   Department of Radiation Oncology, UCLA Medical Center, Los Angeles, California, U.S.A.

Jörn Wulf   Department of Radiotherapy, University of Würzburg, Würzburg, Germany

Reinhard Würm   Abteilung Strahlentherapie, Universität Klinikum, Charite, Berlin, Germany

Fang-Fang Yin   Department of Radiation Oncology, Duke Medical Center, Detroit, Michigan, U.S.A.

1

Introduction

Ben J. Slotman

*Department of Radiation Oncology, VU University Medical Center,
Amsterdam, The Netherlands*

Timothy Solberg

*Department of Radiation Oncology, University of Nebraska, Omaha,
Nebraska, U.S.A.*

Reinhard Würm

Abteilung Strahlentherapie, Universität Klinikum, Charite, Berlin, Germany

Dirk Verellen

Department of Radiotherapy, AZ-VUB Brussels, Brussels, Belgium

The concept of stereotactic radiosurgery was first described by Lars Leksell in 1951, as a single-fraction irradiation of intracranial targets, which, in selected patients, would replace surgery. Stereotactic radiosurgery (SRS) is characterized by the delivery of a high radiation dose to a small volume in a short time with high accuracy and high conformality. This is performed using a stereotactic technique, in which the location of a target is related to a three dimensional Cartesian coordinate system. Based on this concept, any intracranial localization can easily be identified in relation to the frame, which is fixed to the head.

Following the first use of an orthovoltage dental X-ray tube in 1951 and the investigation of protons and early-generation linear accelerators (linacs), Leksell and Larsson started their clinical work in 1967 with the gamma knife. The latter in its current version consists of 201 cobalt-60 sources focused at one locus. The clinical usefulness of the GammaKnife for the treatment of cranial base tumors and vascular malformations lead to further technical developments and the GammaKnife is presently in use in over 100 sites throughout the world. SRS using the GammaKnife carries, depending on the size, shape, and number of lesions, the need to use multiple isocenters with different beam diameters (collimator helmets), to produce dose plans that conform to irregular lesions. A derivative of the Gamma-Knife, the RGS system with 30 cobalt-60 radiation sources contained in a revolving hemispheric shell, was recently developed. The secondary collimator is a coaxial hemispheric shell with six groups of five collimator holes that are arranged in the same pattern as the radiation sources. By selection of which one of the groups of collimator holes is aligned with the radiation sources, different beam diameters can be produced avoiding the use of different collimator helmets to change beam diameters during treatments.

Protons for irradiation of deep-seated targets were first explored in the early 1950s. It was shown that larger proton beams may be beneficial for the treatment of malignant tumors, while narrow beams could be utilized for SRS of small circumscribed targets in the brain. However, the physical advantages of protons including the Bragg ionization peak, to reduce doses to the tissue beyond the target to a minimum, have not been substantiated by clinical data or in comparative trials. The high cost and limited number of facilities available are certainly factors that preclude the more widespread use of protons in SRS. Only a small percentage of patients currently treated with protons receive stereotactic proton-beam radiosurgery.

The widespread availability of linear accelerators (linacs) has lead to investigations on their use for SRS and stereotactic radiotherapy (SRT). The term SRS is generally reserved for single fraction stereotactic treatments, while the term SRT is reserved for fractionated stereotactic irradiation. Leksell first explored linac-based radiosurgery. In the early 1980s, following the description of the dosimetry of subcentimeter fields, Barcia-Salorio, Betti, Colombo, Sturm, and others developed radiosurgery equipment to adapt linacs to produce highly collimated narrow beams for SRS. Linac-based radiosurgical technologies were since then further advanced by incorporating improved stereotactic positioning devices and methods to measure the accuracy of various components. Over 500 such systems are thought to be presently in operation throughout the world. Most of these systems use circular collimators in combination with multiple isocenters techniques in which the patient couch is set at different angles and the radiation source describes an arc with the isocenter at its center, to deliver radiation that enters the cranium at many different points. More recently, different techniques have been developed to enhance the conformity of dose planning and delivery using linac-based systems. These include the use of micro-multileafcollimators for beam shaping and intensity modulation. Beam shaping involves modification of the traditionally circular contour of the radiosurgical collimators, so that the contour more accurately conforms to the beam's eye view of the target volume. Conformal blocks and micro-multileafcollimators can be used for static or dynamic beam shaping and require only a single isocenter. Using beam intensity modulation, the intensity can be varied across the beam and is weighted to be proportional to the target thickness, as assessed by the beam's eye view to obtain target conformity. The CyberKnife® (Accuray, Sunnyvale, California, U.S.A.) uses a 6-MeV linac attached to a six-axis robotic manipulator that positions the linac at different source positions, always aiming the center of the radiation beam at the target. During treatment, an image-processing system acquires X-ray images of the cranium of the patient and compares the actual images with images in a database, to determine the direction and amount of any head motion. This information is transferred to a robot, which corrects for this motion.

In linac radiosurgery, an invasive frame, which is attached to the head of the patient using pins, was used as reference frame for imaging, localization, and treatment. After placing this frame, or "headring," a localizer frame is attached to it. This localizer frame has a number of fiducials, which enable the transformation of image coordinates to stereotactic coordinates. The rigid system allows very accurate (re)positioning of the patient and targeting of the radiation beams. The disadvantages of this headring system are that it cannot easily be used for fractionated treatments over a longer period of time and that it can only be used for the treatment of intracranial lesions. For fractionated treatments of intracranial lesions, non-invasive systems have been developed making use of dental and occipital impressions, or fixation using ears and nose bridge. These fixation systems can be used as a frame of reference for imaging, treatment planning, and stereotactic treatment delivery.

The current growth of SRS is certainly connected to the tremendous advances in computer technologies and imaging in the past decade. Current dose-planning programs provide on-screen integration of (multimodality) images with the isodose curves, significantly reducing treatment-planning time. Recent versions facilitate the use of inverse planning, in which the target is three-dimensionally defined and the software, based on constraints and penalty-functions, generates a treatment plan, that can then be further adjusted and optimized. The advances in imaging techniques have improved long-term results due to better target definition and localization. Integrated use of magnetic resonance imaging (MRI) is now regarded standard because of its high-resolution and excellent tissue contrast providing improved anatomic detail. However, the reliability of MRI for stereotactic procedures is related to the stereotactic frame used and/or fusion of CT and MRI data. Techniques, such as positron emission tomography and magnetic resonance spectroscopy, provide important information for tumor localization and contouring and may enhance our understanding of the radiobiological effects of radiosurgery on different tissues even further.

The great success of stereotactic radiosurgery and stereotactic radiotherapy for intracranial lesions has led to an interest in the use of these techniques for the treatment of lesions outside the brain. The pioneering work in this area was done by the groups of Lax and Blomgren at Karolinska Hospital in Stockholm. Compared with intracranial SRS and SRT, extracranial SRS and SRT are more difficult, due to motion of targets and normal tissues. In the last decade, various approaches to deliver radiation to extracranial targets with stereotactic precision have been developed. These include the use of elaborate immobilization techniques and introduction of so-called image-guidance technology aiming at reducing patient set-up errors, and assessment of organ motion and organ changes during the course of treatment. Internal organ and tumor movement during treatment not only introduces an added risk of missing the target, but also introduces errors in the dose delivery, which in itself may have become variable in time for most intensity modulated techniques. With the introduction of intensity modulation not only the possibility of geographic miss will be a matter of concern, but also the possible interplay between target motion and the temporal dose delivery, and real-time knowledge of the target volume becomes of utmost importance. Stereotactic body frames emphasize on immobilization where the device is used for patient fixation, external reference system for determination and localization of the stereotactic coordinates, and a mechanical tool for reduction of breathing mobility. Image guidance in turn emphasizes on real time, 3D knowledge of target localization during treatment and guiding the dose delivery accordingly. These techniques include the use of optically-guided tracking devices, in-room CT (fan beam and cone beam), ultrasound, stereoscopic X-ray devices, or combinations thereof. These techniques, in order to be realistically applied require a thorough understanding of anatomy and physiology and cannot be implemented without proper preparation (preferably based on multimodality and 4D imaging techniques).

Extracranial stereotactic radiotherapy is a rapidly expanding treatment modality, being offered to an increasing number of patients for an increasing number of indications. In this book, the various techniques, including linac-based systems using the ELEKTA Body System®, Novalis®, CyberKnife®, and tomotherapy, will be described in detail. The radiobiological aspects of stereotactic radiotherapy and the use of new imaging modalities are discussed and the clinical results of extracranial stereotactic radiotherapy for various tumor sites, including liver, lung, prostate, spine, and head and neck are presented.

2

The ELEKTA Stereotactic Body Frame®

Jörn Wulf

Department of Radiotherapy, University of Würzburg, Würzburg, Germany

INTRODUCTION

The stereotactic body frame (SBF) 23has been created and developed by Ingmar Lax, Ph.D. and Henric Blomgren, M.D., Ph.D. at Karolinska Hospital, Stockholm, Sweden. It is the merit of these two authors having introduced the successful concept of stereotactic irradiation of cerebral lesions into treatment of extracranial targets at the beginning of the 1990s (1–4). While high precision of stereotactic irradiation of cerebral tumors is achieved by sharp fixation of the skull or tight mask systems, it is more difficult in extracranial tumors, e.g., in the lung or liver. Sharp fixation of the patient's body is impossible and the targets and organs at risk are potentially mobile due to breathing motions or changing organ fillings. Additionally, marks on the patient's body surface are less accurate than marks attached to a mask system due to subcutaneous fat tissue, different fillings (e.g., of the abdomen) or breathing motions of the body. Nevertheless, stereotactic irradiation according to the concept of Blomgren and Lax consists of precise application of very high fraction doses, e.g., 2×15 or 3×10 Gy prescribed to the PTV-enclosing 65%-isodose and normalized to 100% at the isocenter (1–4). Therefore, introduction of this concept into clinical practice requires a high-precision approach. For that purpose the SBF was developed and since the mid-1990s, marketed by ELEKTA Instruments (ELEKTA AB, Stockholm, Sweden). It has come into clinical use by groups all over the world (1–8).

ELEKTA Instruments, ELEKTA AB, Stockholm, Sweden.

SYSTEM DESCRIPTION

The technical concept of the SBF addresses three basic requirements for extracranial stereotactic radiotherapy, i.e., the need for:

1. patient fixation,
2. an external reference system for determination, localization, and alignment of the stereotactic coordinates, and
3. a mechanical tool for reduction of breathing mobility.

Patient Fixation

Patient fixation is achieved by a vacuum mattress, which is molded to the patient's individual body contour. Two sizes of 25 or 40 L are available to address different patient sizes. The mattress is fixed to a plastic shell by two screws. The shell–mattress unit is inserted into the body frame by a system of tongues and grooves. This allows a very easy and fast change of the shell–mattress unit for different patients without disconnecting the vacuum pillow.

Repositioning of the patient in the vacuum mattress for treatment is supported by an SBF-attached laser system at the trunk and the legs. After molding of the mattress, the patient's position is marked by small marks tattoos at the trunk (preferably the sternum) and both tuberositae tibiae. The position of the tattoos is indicated by a trunk laser attached to the stereotactic arc and a leg laser at a chosen position (Fig. 1, Nos. 6 and 7). For repositioning, the tattoos are aligned to the SBF-attached laser system at previously determined positions.

The body frame itself is open ventrally and at the head and foot ends (Fig. 1). It achieves rigidity by a honeycomb structured paper center embedded in a fiberglass surface. The wooden edges are rounded to avoid artefacts, e.g., at CT scans. The low-density material of the SBF sidewalls is aimed to reduce artefacts and to minimize absorption of irradiation. According to Lax et al. (3), the geometrical specifications of the SBF are within ±0.5 mm. The outer dimensions of the SBF are 111 cm in length, 50 cm in width, and 40 cm in height. The complete system including rulers, indicators, and a bottom plate for level control has a weight of about 9 kg.

The level control consists of a bottom plate loosely attached to the SBF left ground side and a rubber bladder, which is pushed between the bottom plate and ground side of the SBF. Inflating or deflating air into the bladder by a pump system (similar to a cuff for measuring blood pressure) allows precise alignment of the SBF in the anterior–posterior direction to the laser system of the CT or linac within a range of ±5 mm.

The Stereotactic Reference System

The SBF is not only used for patient fixation but also as external reference system for identification of the stereotactic isocenter. It consists of a

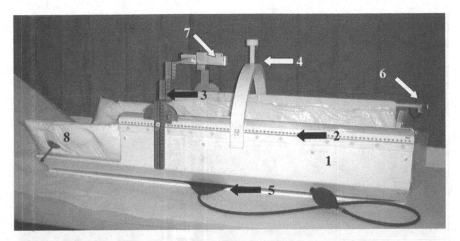

Figure 1 The ELEKTA stereotactic body frame (SBF). (1) Sidewall containing oblique and horizontal copper wires for CT-based measurement of longitudinal stereotactic coordinate. (2) Longitudinal stereotactic scale. (3) Stereotactic arc for lateral and AP coordinates. (4) Arc and scaled screw for diphragm control. (5) Level control. (6,7) SBF attached laser system (leg and trunk) for assistance at patient repositioning. (8) Vacuum pillow.

longitudinal scale in millimeters, which is bilaterally fixed to the outside of the frame sidewalls. The lateral and anterior–posterior position in millimeters can be read from a stereotactic arc, which is attached to both sidewalls of the SBF at a chosen longitudinal position. The stereotactic arc is also marked with a central notch (Fig. 2B), which allows precise alignment of the SBF at a defined coordinate to the laser systems of fluoroscopy, CT, or linear accelerator.

This outer system for adjusting the SBF to the isocenter at a certain stereotactic coordinate corresponds to an internal system, which allows deriving the stereotactic coordinate from each CT slice. This internal reference system consists of horizontal and oblique copper wires, which are embedded in a plexiglas shell attached to both sidewalls of the SBF (Fig. 2C). The same system is available with copper sulfate fill for use in MRI. The copper wires appear as fiducials in each CT slice (Fig. 2D). From these fiducials, the isocenter coordinates for each target can be calculated (Figs. 2D and 3).

Breathing Control

Breathing mobility of targets in the lung, liver, or abdomen can be reduced by a simple but effective mechanical tool: A pentagonal template is

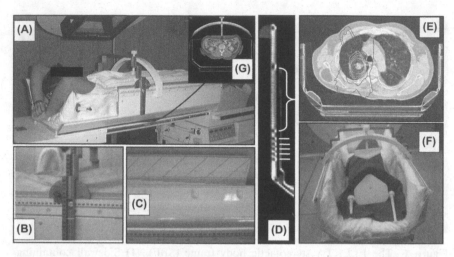

Figure 2 (A) Patient immobilized in the SBF with stereotactic arc and diaphragm control. (B) Isocenter alignment of the SBF. The stereotactic arc is attached to the frame at the planned longitudinal position, the AP and lateral coordinate can be read at the stereotactic arc. (C) The longitudinal position in the SBF can be seen in each CT slice due to a system of horizontal and oblique copper wires (D) e.g., five horizontal dots = 500, distance to the oblique wire =70 mm: longitudinal position = 570). (E) CT-slice of a patient immobilized in the SBF. (F) Two sizes of of templates and three sizes of screws are available. (G) Diaphragm control: A pentagonal template is pushed into the patient's epigastrium to increase abdominal pressure.

pushed into the patient's abdomen by moving a scaled screw fixed to an SBF-attached arc. With this procedure the abdominal pressure is increased, leading to decreased motions of the diaphragm muscle. Instead of large breathing motions up to 20 mm, the patient breathes with many smaller motions of about 5 mm. For adjustment of this "diaphragm control" to different patient sizes, a small and large template and three different lengths of screws are available. Theoretically, the amount of pressure can be reproduced just by pushing the screw to the same position as planned.

Dose Absorption of the SBF

For evaluation of dose absorption of the SBF, treatment plans including and excluding the SBF in the calculation model were compared. Two phantoms (Alderson phantom and thoracic phantom as described in the ICRU Report 42) were used. By means of ionization chambers and TLD measurements, the dose and dose distributions were compared with the results of the 3D-treatment planning system Helax TMS. While the difference between calculation and measurement was 5% at maximum if the SBF was

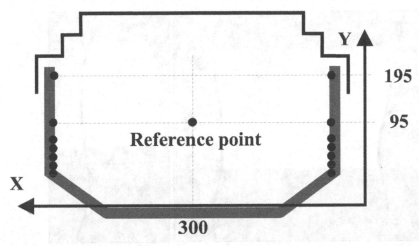

Figure 3 Schematic view of the SBF. The stereotactic coordinate can be derived and calculated from a system of oblique and horizontal copper wires in the SBF sidewalls. This internal system corresponds to marks in millimeters on the outer sidewall and the stereotactic arc, which allows precise alignment of the SBF to the isocenter of a CT or linac according to the calculated coordinates.

included into the calculation model, the difference increased by additional 10% if the SBF was excluded (9). Therefore, the SBF should be included into the calculation model. This approach additionally allows clinical estimation of the skin dose for targets close to the patient's surface, because the build-up effect is calculated more realistically.

ACCURACY OF PATIENT AND TARGET REPRODUCIBILITY IN THE SBF

The accuracy of target reproducibility for stereotactic irradiation of extracranial targets not only depends on the fixation device itself but also on the user's experience and the mobility of the targets chosen for treatment. Principally, external fixation by a vacuum pillow is more reliable in slim patients than in obese individuals. Nevertheless, an accuracy of about 2 mm can be achieved if the vacuum pillow is molded properly. Hence, a "double-S-shape" design of the vacuum pillow is desired (Fig. 4). It is achieved laterally by molding the pillow very tightly to the patient's waist, and longitudinally by molding the material to the patient's lordosis of the lumbar spine. The patient is asked to perform snake-like movements in the smooth vacuum pillow. To achieve vacuum, the pillow material is tightly pressed laterally to the patient's surface. A comfortable position for both arms has to be ensured while performing this.

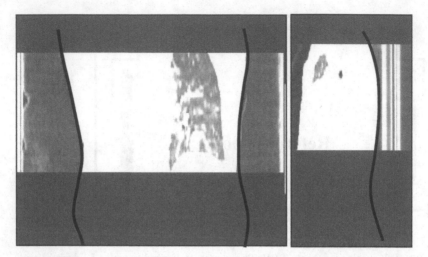

Figure 4 Accuracy of patient repositioning in the SBF is dependent on the quality of molding of the vacuum pillow. For a maximum of reproducibility, an "S"-shaped pillow is recommended. This is achieved by preparing a sufficient amount of pillow material at the anticipated waist and lordosis of the patient's back prior to positioning. By asking the patient to move "like a snake" with his/her back, the material is moved to the correct site molded to the patients anatomy and the pillow can be deflated.

Accuracy of treatment in the SBF can be evaluated at three different levels:

1. alignment of the SBF to the isocenter system of a CT or linac.
2. reproducibility of patient repositioning in the SBF especially in fractionated treatment.
3. reproducibility of the target.

The alignment of the SBF to the isocenter system, e.g., of the CT scanner, can be measured by comparing the aligned longitudinal coordinate to the measured coordinate in the corresponding CT slice. The results not only depend on the SBF but also on the accuracy of the laser system. Lax et al. (3) reported an accuracy of alignment of less than 1 mm derived from 10-mm CT slices. Our own evaluation revealed a standard deviation of 1.4 mm derived from a 5 mm slice thickness. Nevertheless, maximum deviations of up to 3.9 mm were observed, indicating that misalignment occasionally might occur and that correct alignment should be proved prior to proceeding with treatment planning or the treatment itself (10).

Accuracy of patient repositioning can be measured by comparing immobile patient structures such as bones to the external reference system of the SBF. Hence, for treatment planning the bony structures in the CT are compared to the position in a CT-verification at a defined coordinate.

The differences can be measured using the external reference system of the SBF. In our department, the first 32 targets were evaluated (10). The mean deviation of bony structures as derived from CT-verification was 2.9 mm (SD 2 mm) in longitudinal, 2.2 mm (SD 1.8 mm) in anterior–posterior, and 2 mm (SD 1.9 mm) in lateral directions. The mean 3D-vector was 4.7 mm (SD 2.6 mm). The reproducibility of bony structures can also be measured by comparison of digitally reconstructed radiographs (DRR) from the planning CT to portal films. In our analysis of 93–97 verification films for 32 targets, we found a mean deviation of 1.5 mm (SD 4.2 mm) in longitudinal, 0.1 mm (SD 2.3 mm) in anterior–posterior, and 0.1 mm (SD 2.5 mm) in lateral directions.

While repositioning accuracy in the SBF is about 2 mm, it is the concept of extracranial stereotactic radiotherapy, as introduced by Blomgren and Lax, to overcome isocenter verification relative to bony landmarks, a common practice in conventional radiotherapy. The only relevant structure to verify is the target relative to the stereotactic system and coordinates of the SBF. Lax reported the reproducibility of 30 tumors evaluated with 48 verification CTs treated in the current version of the SBF. The targets were located in the lung, liver, retroperitoneal space, and skeleton. The mean deviation of the target was 3.4 mm in the transverse and 5.5 mm in the longitudinal plane. In 98%, the transversal deviation was within 5 mm. The longitudinal deviation was at 95% within 8 mm and 100% within 10 mm (3). Additionally, according to Lax, it was generally possible to keep breathing mobility of mobile targets within 5 mm using the diaphragm control device. Based on these results, most groups use security margins for PTV-definition to address target deviation of 5 mm in transversal and 5–10 mm in longitudinal directions.

In our own analysis of 32 targets in the lung, liver, abdomen, pelvis, and bones, the SD of all targets was 3.4 mm in anterior–posterior (mean 1.1 mm), 3.3 mm in lateral (mean 0.7 mm), and 4.4 mm in longitudinal directions (mean 1.5 mm), which corresponded well to the results of Lax. Nevertheless, we occasionally found maximum deviations of up to 12 mm leading to a proportion of targets reproducible within 5 mm of 84% in anterior–posterior, 88% in lateral, and 91% in longitudinal directions. About 98% of targets deviated within 10 mm in anterior–posterior and lateral directions and 94% in the longitudinal direction. If a security margin for target variability of 5 mm in axial and 10 mm in longitudinal directions was used, these results indicate that about 12–16% of targets might be missed partially in anterior–posterior and lateral directions and 9% of targets in the longitudinal direction. Therefore, the conclusion was to recommend CT-verification prior to irradiation to detect those targets with decreased reproducibility.

Isocenter verification relative to bony landmarks seemed to be inappropriate, at least for mobile targets, because this approach implies that deviation of bony structures is representative for target deviation. To prove this hypothesis, the CT-verification data were analyzed and it was postulated that target deviation should be within 5 mm relative to bony landmarks. This was true in only 62.5% of all 32 targets. Differentiated to different types of targets as bony targets, soft tissue targets fixed to bony structures, and mobile soft tissue targets ± breathing control device, major difference were observed. While 100% of bony targets and 80% of fixed soft tissue targets deviated within 5 mm relative to bony reference structures, this was the case in only 37.5% of mobile soft tissue targets without breathing control and only 28.5% with breathing control (10). These results again indicate the importance of CT verification to eventually correct for major target deviation.

Nevertheless, the presented data are based on only one CT verification prior to treatment. Therefore, it seemed necessary to evaluate target reproducibility over a complete course of treatment, e.g., three fractions as first described by Blomgren and Lax. A study including three CT verifications in each of 22 lung tumors and 21 liver tumors was performed (11). The main goal of defining a planning target volume (PTV) is to ensure that the clinical target volume (CTV) will be covered by the prescribed reference dose despite target mobility. Therefore, the target reproducibility was evaluated by analyzing the CTV-dose by dose–volume histograms (DVH). For that purpose the CTVs derived from repeated CT-verifications were matched into the planning study using the fiducials of the SBF sidewalls as an independent, external matching system. Major target deviation exceeding the PTV-related reference isodose should result in decreased target dose to the CTV. Prior to this evaluation, the conformity of the stereotactic dose distribution to the PTV has been analyzed (12). For PTV definition, the commonly used security margins of 5 mm in axial and 5–10 mm in longitudinal directions were added to the CTV. The study revealed a decrease of target coverage to the CTV to less than 95% (5% of the CTV were not covered by the reference isodose) in 3 of 60 simulations for lung targets (5%) and 7 of 58 verifications for liver targets (12%). Related to targets in 2 of 22 lung tumors (9%) and in 4 of 21 liver tumors (19%), a decreased target coverage <95% was observed in at least one fraction. Two out of three major deviations in lung tumors were observed in a single patient after pneumonectomy and in liver targets six out of seven major deviations occurred in targets with a CTV >100 cm^3. These results again indicate the importance of CT verification to detect occasionally occurring major target deviation beyond the reference isodose. According to our study, patients with large liver tumors or mobile lung tumors, in whom breathing mobility cannot be sufficiently suppressed by the breathing control device (e.g., after pneumonectomy), are at higher risk for major target deviation (11). Theoretically an increase of security margins would be able to compensate for increased target mobility. Nevertheless, this seems not to be an appropriate approach, because the high-dose area should be kept as small as possible especially in a patient group not amenable to surgery due to impaired medical condition.

TREATMENT PLANNING AND DELIVERY

Patient Positioning in the SBF and CT-Planning Study

Treatment planning can be performed within 30 min and starts with premolding of the vacuum pillow. It can be performed at the fluoroscopy or CT unit. First, the patient is asked to use a hospital shirt ventrally open to avoid too much clothing between the patient and the pillow. The hospital shirt also allows easier and more accurate moving of the patient by pulling the shirt as necessary. If application of i.v. contrast media is planned (e.g., for targets in the liver), the informed consent and an i.v. needle should be placed prior to positioning the patient in the SBF. Depending on the patient's size, the 25 or 40 L mattress should be chosen. The pillow should be prepared with a slight vacuum to avoid dislocation of the pillow material under the patient during the positioning procedure. After premolding, the pillow is attached to the plastic shell, which is inserted into the SBF. The SBF is positioned on the end of CT-/fluoroscopy-couch and the patient is asked to first sit down and then lay back onto the pillow. The SBF containing the patient is slipped to the scanning position, a standardized support device is positioned under the knees, and the arms are comfortably moved behind the head. In this position, the prevacuum is deflated and the patient is asked to perform some snake-like movements to achieve an optimal embedment in the vacuum pillow. Now the mattress can be deflated maximally while pressing the material laterally to the patient and supporting the arm to maximize comfort. At this point, the comfort of the patient should be queried because a change of the mattress or patient position from this point is impossible without repeating the complete procedure. If there is doubt on the optimal embedment of the patient, an investigatory CT slice can be performed to assess the quality of the embedment: The patient should be well enclosed by the vacuum mattress with full contact of the patient's back to the base of lateral and dorsal surface to the pillow. When the vacuum pillow is optimal, little tattoos are pricked into the patient's skin at the trunk and tibiae to ease later repositioning for treatment. For this purpose the leg and trunk laser are attached to the SBF at the chosen position, preferably at the sternum and tuberositas tibiae. At the trunk, tattoos not only at the midline but also laterally are recommended to detect rotational errors at the time of repositioning.

If patient positioning is performed at the fluoroscope, breathing mobility of the target should be evaluated there and—if necessary—diaphragm control should be used. If patient positioning is performed at the CT unit, breathing mobility is evaluated later. In the CT situation, the SBF is aligned to the isocenter of the CT by the use of the stereotactic arc. Correct alignment is proved by comparing the aligned position to the measured position of the internal fiducials in the SBF sidewalls. The planning study should be performed, only if alignment is correct, otherwise irreproducible oblique slices would be achieved.

The CT study for treatment planning starts with obtaining a reference slice, usually at the initially aligned position. From that position the target must be found by moving the scanner directly to the estimated target position. This procedure can be performed without obtaining a scout scan. After locating the target, breathing mobility must be evaluated if not performed previously. While tumors in the lung are usually easy to locate, targets in the liver might be assessed relative to vessels or the diaphragmatic dome. CT evaluation of target mobility can be performed optimally by multiple slice technique in modern CTs (13). Otherwise it can be evaluated by slow CT scanning over some seconds (14) or by continuous dynamic scanning at the same table position over a chosen period of time, e.g., 6–15 sec (10,11). While axial mobility can easily be measured in each CT slice, cranio-caudal mobility must be assessed by comparison of the target shape in several CT slices.

If breathing mobility is assessed to be more than 5 mm, the breathing control device can be used. A pentagonal template (two sizes are available) is positioned on the patient's epigastrium. The flexible arc is positioned at the SBF and a scaled screw (three sizes are available) is attached. The screw is moved on the template until a sufficient and patient-tolerable pressure is achieved. Breathing mobility is evaluated again until an optimum is achieved. Of course other modalities to decrease breathing mobility can be used, such as oxygen-supplied shallow breathing or the use of an active breathing control device (active breathing coordinator™, ELEKTA AB, Stockholm, Sweden), and evaluated alternatively (15–17). After breathing control is achieved the patient is ready for the CT-planning study.

Depending on the size and location of the target, the CT for treatment planning can be performed in 3–5 mm slice thickness. For lung tumors, i.v. contrast is only necessary if the target has to be differentiated from normal tissue structures; i.v. contrast is always required for liver tumors. To achieve an optimum of contrast, the planning study should be performed under almost diagnostic conditions. Therefore, an arterial and a portal-venous phase should be achieved using a volume scan. Sometimes, an additional venous phase is helpful to differentiate the target volume from normal liver tissue. After the planning study is finished the patient is removed from the SBF after being photographed to document the setup, e.g., the exact position of the arms.

Target Definition and 3D-Treatment Planning

3D-treatment planning requires definition of a patient model, CTV, PTV, and organs at risk. As described previously (9), the SBF should be included into the patient model. This not only increases reliability of the dose calculation but also allows assessment of skin dose due to a more realistic calculation of the build-up effect. No consistent data have been published concerning target definition. While some authors report adding security margins for PTV definition of 5–10 mm to the GTV, others add it to the CTV. Nevertheless, the goal of stereotactic irradiation is to achieve local control. Therefore, local tumor—including microscopic disease—should receive the planned dose to avoid local failure. The security margins for PTV-definition are exclusively necessary to address potential target mobility and setup inaccuracy. Generally, the security margins should be added to the GTV or CTV using a digital tool to ensure a 3D PTV-model.

For 3D-treatment planning of dose distribution, again different doses, irradiation techniques, and normalization procedures are used. Generally, a reference isodose is created, which should encompass the PTV as conformal as possible. For that, 5–7 static beams individually modeled by multileaf collimators or rotational beams are created. Non-coplanar beams and/or wedges can be added, but it should be considered that these approaches might prolong treatment time. Especially in lung tumors, dose calculation should be performed by a collapsed cone (point-kernel) algorithm with low photon energy, because the widely used pencil beam algorithm neglects the secondary charged particle disequilibrium at the tumor–lung interface and therefore might overestimate the target dose considerably (18–21).

Target Verification and Irradiation

A treatment session usually lasts for 30–60 min depending on the target verification procedure and the irradiated dose. While patient setup and repositioning in the SBF can be performed within five minutes of target verification, the check of the correct isocenter coordinates relative to the target is more time consuming. As described above, CT verification is preferred compared to isocenter verification relative to bony landmarks.

Usually CT verification is performed at the CT scanner with subsequent transport of the patient in the SBF to the treatment room. This approach requires additional isocenter verification at the linac to detect patient dislocation due to transport and to document the correct isocenter coordinates. Because patient dislocation can be detected by comparing bony structures relative to the stereotactic coordinates, this procedure can be performed by comparison of digital reconstructed radiography (DRR) from the CT-verification study to portal images.

For CT verification the patient is repositioned in the SBF. The accuracy of repositioning is eased by matching the laser of the trunk and leg to the tattoos on the patient's skin at the determined positions. The diaphragm control device is also positioned and adjusted as determined at the CT for treatment planning. The SBF is aligned to the CT at the planned longitudinal stereotactic isocenter coordinate. Beginning from this position, one or multiple CT slices are generated to find the slice with the target shape that best matches the shape of the isocenter slice from treatment planning. For mobile tumors, sufficient suppression of breathing mobility by the diaphragm control device has to be controlled also. If breathing mobility is increased compared to the planning study the diaphragm control device must be adjusted by increasing pressure until a sufficient result is achieved. Under this condition it is usually necessary to repeat the procedure to reproduce the target shape at the planned isocenter slice. Finally, the stereotactic coordinates for irradiation of the current target position can be measured relative to the internal SBF reference system (Figs. 3 and 5). While the procedure determining the isocenter coordinates by CT verification is identical, performing this process directly on the treatment couch has obvious advantages: The patient will not dislocate due to transport, the immobilization time of the patient is shortened. Therefore potential changes, e.g., the abdominal pressure by the diaphragm control are less probable. An example of CT verification at the treatment couch using a mobile CT with gantry movement is shown in Figure 5.

After CT- and/or isocenter verification are performed, the patient is aligned to the isocenter of the linac at the current coordinates. Depending on the practice of each department, the correct field size, MLC positions, and plan parameters should be checked prior to irradiation. Ideally, this

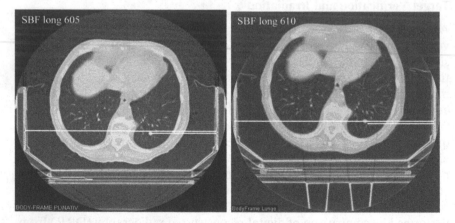

Figure 5 The CT verification of a small lung metastasis in the left lower lobe. The verification is performed directly on the treatment couch using a mobile CT (Philips Tomoscan M). The CT gantry moves over the patient positioned in the SBF as if for treatment. A carbon fiber couch allows scanning without artefacts in diagnostic quality. Compared to the planning study (*right*) according to CT-verification (*left*) the target is dislocated 5 mm cranial (SBF longitudinal position 610 vs. 605), 4 mm ventrally, and 4 mm medially of the isocenter position in the center of the tumor. Again, the effectiveness of the breathing control device can be evaluated on the treatment couch by using the dynamic scan procedure.

can be performed parallel to evaluation of the CT verification to shorten the overall immobilization time.

CONCLUSION

The SBF is an easy to handle and reliable stereotactic system. During 6 years of use with more than 150 patients, no unforeseen events occurred, e.g., leakage of the vacuum pillow or breakage of important parts. The patient can be immobilized sufficiently upto an hour, which might be occasionally necessary for patient repositioning, target verification, and irradiation. Nevertheless, initial procedures such as molding of the vacuum pillow, tattooing, and setup can be performed within 15 min due to the easy-to-handle system. Patient setup at the linac as well is possible within 10 min.

With a properly molded vacuum pillow, repositioning accuracy of about 2 mm can be achieved. Nevertheless, individual accuracy depends on the patient's condition and is more accurate in slim than in obese patients. Target reproducibility as influenced by breathing mobility can be sufficiently decreased to 5–8 mm using the mechanical breathing control device and again is dependent on individual factors. Therefore, target mobility and reproducibility should be individually evaluated and controlled using CT verification, if the commonly used security margins for PTV definition of 5 mm in axial and 5–10 mm in longitudinal direction are chosen.

REFERENCES

1. Blomgren H, Lax I, Göranson H, Kräpelien T, Nilsson B, Näslund I, Svanström R, Tilikidis A. Radiosurgery for tumors in the body: clinical experience using a new method. J Radiosurg 1998; 1(1):63–74.
2. Blomgren H, Lax I, Näslund I, Svanström R. Stereotactic high dose fractionation radiation therapy of extracranial tumors using an accelerator. Acta Oncol 1995; 34:861–870.
3. Lax I, Blomgren H, Larson D, Näslund D. Extracranial stereotactic radiosurgery of localized targets. J Radiosurg 1998; 1(2):135–148.
4. Lax I, Blomgren H, Näslund I, Svanström R. Stereotactic radiotherapy of malignancies in the abdomen. Methodological aspects. Acta Oncol 1994; 33: 677–683.
5. Wulf J, Haedinger U, Oppitz U, Thiele W, Ness-Dourdoumas R, Flentje M. Stereotactic radiotherapy of targets in the lung and liver. Strahlenther Onkol 2001; 177:645–655.
6. Nagata Y, Negoro Y, Aoki T, Mizowaki T, Takayama K, Kokubo M, Araki N, Mitsumori M, Sasai K, Shibamoto Y, Koga S, Yano S, Hiraoka M. Clinical outcomes of 3D conformal hypofractionated single high dose radiotherapy for one or two lung tumors using a stereotactic body frame. Int J Radiat Oncol Biol Phys 2002 Mar 15; 52(4):1041–1046.
7. Lee SW, Choi EK, Park HJ, Ahn SD, Kim JH, Kim KJ, Yoon SM, Kim YS, Yi BY. Stereotactic body frame based fractionated radiosurgery on consecutive

days for primary or metastatic tumors in the lung. Lung Cancer 2003 Jun; 40(3):309–315.

8. Timmerman RD, Papiez L, McGarry R. Extracranial stereotactic radioablation: results of a phase I study in medically inoperable stage I non-small cell lung cancer. Chest 2003; 125(5):1946–1955.

9. Richter J, Haedinger U, Bratengeier K, Flentje M, Wulf J. QA of stereotactic treatment techniques in the body region. Radiother Oncol 1998; 48(suppl l):733.

10. Wulf J, Haedinger U, Oppitz U, Olshausen B, Flentje M. Stereotactic radiotherapy of extracranial targets: CT-simulation and accuracy of treatment in the stereotactic body frame. Radiother Oncol 2000; 57:225–236.

11. Wulf J, Haedinger U, Oppitz U, Thiele W, Flentje M. Impact of target reproducibility on tumor dose in stereotactic radiotherapy of targets in the lung and liver. Radiother Oncol 2003; 66:141–150.

12. Haedinger U, Thiele W, Wulf J. Extracranial stereotactic radiotherapy: evaluation of PTV coverage and dose conformity. Z Med Phys 2002; 12:221–229.

13. Hof H, Herfarth KK, Muenter M. The use of the multislice CT for the determination of respiratory lung tumor movement in stereotactic single-dose irradiation. Strahlenther Onkol 2003: 179(8):542–547.

14. Lagerwaard FJ, Van Sornsen de Koste JR, Nijssen-Visser MR, Schuchhard-Schipper RH, Oei SS, Munne A, Senan S. Multiple "slow" CT-scans for incorporating lung tumor mobility in radiotherapy planning. Int J Radiat Oncol Biol Phys 2001 Nov 15; 51(4):932–937.

15. Wong JW, Sharpe MB, Jaffray DA, Kini VR, Robertson JM, Stromberg JS, Martinez AA. The use of active breathing control (ABC) to reduce margin for breathing motion. Int J Radiat Oncol Biol Phys 1999; 44(4):911–919.

16. Dawson LA, Brock KK, Kazanjian S, Fitch D, McGinn CJ, Lawrence TS, Ten Haken RK, Balter J. The reproducibility of organ position using active breathing control (ABC) during liver radiotherapy. Int J Radiat Oncol Biol Phys 2001 Dec 1; 51(5):1410–1421.

17. Onishi H, Kuriyama K, Komiyama T, Tanaka S, Ueki J, Sano N, Araki T, Ikenaga S, Tateda Y, Aikawa Y. CT evaluation of patient deep inspiration self-breath-holding: how precisely can patients reproduce the tumor position in the absence of respiratory monitoring devices? Med Phys 2003 Jun; 30(6):1183–1187.

18. Scholz C, Schulze C, Oelfke U, Bortfeld T. Development and clinical application of a fast superposition algorithm in radiation therapy. Radiother Oncol 2003; 69:79–90.

19. De Jaeger K, Hoogeman MS, Engelsman M, Seppenwoolde Y, Damen EM, Mijinheer BJ, Boersma LJ, Lebesque JV. Incorporating an improved dose-calculation algorithm in conformal radiotherapy of lung cancer: re-evaluation of dose in normal lung tissue. Radiother Oncol 2003 Oct; 69(1):1–10.

20. Haedinger U, Krieger T, Flentje M, Wulf J. Influence of the calculation model on dose distribution in stereotactic radiotherapy of pulmonary targets. Int J Radiat Oncol Biol Phys 2005 Jan 1; 61(1):239–249.

21. Wulf J, Haedinger U, Oppitz U, Thiele W, Mueller G, Flentje M. Stereotactic radiotherapy for primary lung cancer and pulmonary metastases: a noninvasive treatment approach in medically inoperable patients. Int J Radiat Oncol Biol Phys 2004 Sep 1; 60(1):186–196.

3

Novalis®

Paul Medin

Department of Radiation Oncology, UCLA Medical Center, Los Angeles, California, U.S.A.

Dirk Verellen

Department of Radiotherapy, Oncology Center, Academic Hospital, Vrije Universiteit Brussels (AZ–VUB), Brussels, Belgium

INTRODUCTION

The history of radiation therapy is one of continuous development of new skills and new approaches. Often many of the desirable concepts were understood years ago but it is only with recent developments in physics, engineering, and computing that the techniques have become practicable. The latest developments in radiotherapy have allowed surgically precise delivery of radiation dose distributions to cure the patient without damaging healthy tissue. Conformal radiation therapy (CRT) and intensity-modulated radiation therapy (IMRT) have been the subject of many research projects during the last decade and are becoming clinically available today. High resolution IMRT treatments will probably result in improved outcomes and definitely better quality of life for patients compared to treatments based on conventional planning and dose delivery. The dynamic delivery of intensity-modulated beams provides homogenous dose coverage of the lesion as well as a much steeper dose fall-off at the lesion's boundaries. Yet, the current positioning techniques do not match the accuracy needed to perform CRT/IMRT adequately. In fact, difficulties with accurate target localization have represented the most significant obstacles to full exploitation of the capabilities of CRT/IMRT treatments. The clinical

---

Novalis System, BrainLAB AG, Heimstetten, Germany.

implementation of CRT is only feasible when two important requirements are fulfilled simultaneously: the ability to generate conformal dose distributions and to ensure accurate target localization (clinical knowledge of the target region as well as ensuring positioning accuracy during treatment). The latter requires an appropriate safety margin around the clinical target that increases with increasing uncertainty of the actual position of the tumor during irradiation. Margins of typically 1 cm are needed to make sure that the tumor will be irradiated sufficiently. This is in contradiction to the millimeter precision that can be achieved with modern radiotherapy techniques. Only when both aspects are covered adequately can one truly use the term stereotactic body radiation surgery or stereotactic body radiation therapy (SBRT).

SYSTEM DESCRIPTION

The Novalis® system (BrainLAB AG, Heimstetten, Germany) provides the user with an integrated system featuring treatment planning (BrainSCAN), automated patient positioning, and image-guidance (ExacTrac/Novalis Body) and treatment delivery (Novalis) for non-invasive stereotactic radiosurgery (SRS) and SBRT. All aspects of the treatment chain are seamlessly integrated in the process, avoiding common problems related to communication between different systems and vendors. Target delineation (based on multimodality imaging), image-guided target positioning (referencing the treatment isocenter to external or internal localization markers), virtual treatment simulation, dose calculation, and treatment verification are all supported by the treatment planning system. All treatment parameters (including the desired patient position necessary for automated patient setup) can be transferred to the treatment machine. The latter (Novalis) is a 6 MV single photon energy dedicated linac with build-in mini-multileaf collimator capable of different treatment modalities, such as conformal beam, dynamic field shaping arc, and IMRT. The field size ranges from $3.0 \times 3.0 \, mm^2$ to $98.0 \times 100.0 \, mm^2$ at isocenter distance with inner leaves of 3.0 mm (the mini-MLC features two banks with 26 leaves each, with varying leaf width from 3.0 mm for the 14 central pairs, to 4.5 mm for the next three, and finaly 5.5 mm for the outer three leaf pairs). Each leaf can over travel by 50 mm, and a central straight edge allows the leaves to touch when closed, with full interdigitation possible. In addition, a set of conical collimators can be attached to the head of the machine for very small tumors and functional treatment. Image-guided radiation therapy (IGRT) is provided by the ExacTrac/Novalis Body system that automatically aligns the target volume with the treatment beam based on infrared tracking of external IR/CT bodymarkers and/or automated registration of bony structures and implanted radio-opaque markers (using stereoscopic X-ray imaging). The systems also offers dedicated tools for quality assurance (QA), which will be explained in later chapters.

A detailed summary of the different features of the Novalis system is provided.

PATIENT POSITIONING

Description

Introduction

The SBRT or CRT generally is clinically not feasible without the appropriate target localization and tools for patient setup that matches the accuracy needed, especially if one considers that, to increase the therapeutic range, smaller and smaller margins are used between the clinical target volume (CTV) and planning target volume (PTV) (1,2). Often these margins are reduced with the introduction of CRT and IMRT techniques, in spite of the fact that the applied margin should reflect the accuracy that can be realistically obtained in clinic. Moreover, with the introduction of highly sophisticated and computer-guided treatment modalities, patient positioning procedures should evolve and develop equally, and should, ideally, be integrated in the treatment planning process.

Geometric accuracy for the SBRT/CRT/IMRT procedure is basically image-guided, and several solutions have been proposed in the last decade. Electronic portal imaging devices (EPIDs) (3–5) have been embraced with the expectation of achieving the required accuracy. A comprehensive overview of existing EPID techniques was published recently by Herman et al. (4), which acknowledges that the initial expectation has not led to widespread clinical application of EPIDs. Most studies present developments by research centers (in collaboration with manufacturers) to cover their individual needs, and commercial systems are often (arguably) limited to replacements of portal film and do not allow automated correction of setup errors. The clinical application of EPIDs for patient setup verification can generally be classified into two approaches: on-line (or intra-fractional) (6–19) and off-line (inter-fractional) (20–24). The latter, also coined adaptive radiation therapy (ART), monitors the position of the patient during a limited number of fractions and adapts the safety margins and/or treatment plan accordingly. This approach does not allow for decreasing the treatment margins sufficiently for aggressive SBRT. The intra-fractional approach offers the possibility of reducing all treatment execution errors (both systematic and random), yet is considered to be time consuming, requiring automated control of the treatment couch and mostly limited to two-dimensional setup errors (7–9,15–18). While EPIDs suffer from the lack of soft tissue imaging, ultrasound (US) (25) and kilovoltage X-ray–based (26–29) image-guidance systems have been proposed as a promising alternative. Some kV X-ray–based solutions under investigation include:

1. computed tomography (CT), either in-line CT scanners installed inside the treatment room (30,31) or kV cone-beam CT (26),
2. stereoscopic X-ray imaging systems (27–29).

The ExacTrac 3.0/Novalis Body system resides in the latter classification as it combines visualization of internal structures based on stereoscopic X-ray imaging with real-time infrared (IR) tracking of the patient's surface. The system is designed to be a positioning tool ensuring accurate positioning a priori fulfilling the following basic requirements: (a) integrated in the treatment planning process, (b) perform as a fully automated positioning tool (not verification tool) allowing highly accurate positioning of the target volume based on treatment planning data, (c) does not increase the number of actions required for patient setup compared to conventional methodologies (believed to be one of the major reasons for the limited clinical use of EPIDs to date), and (d) perform this task within an acceptable time frame (i.e., a typical treatment including positioning should not exceed 15 min) (29,32,33). Some centers combine this technique with minimal patient fixation (32,33), while others prefer more elaborate fixation devices (see Chapter 11 on spinal tumors). This chapter will be restricted to a detailed description of the image-guided technology with a limited summary of immobilization tools that can be used in combination.

For the reader's interest the positioning hardware of the Novalis system can be classified as ExacTrac 1.0/Novalis Body (IR system only), ExacTrac 2.0/Novalis Body (IR and stereoscopic X-ray imaging, with only one amorphous silicon (AmSi) detector mounted to the treatment couch), and ExacTrac 3.0/Novalis Body (IR and stereoscopic X-ray imaging making use of two AmSi detectors mounted to the ceiling). Basically, the positioning algorithms used in the latter two systems are based on similar principles but adapted to the hardware differences. All versions allow for automated computer-guided movement of the treatment couch.

Real-Time IR Tracking System

Hardware: The real-time IR tracking device is a system developed for automated positioning of patients by detecting IR-reflective/CT markers placed on the patient's surface, comparison of marker location with stored reference information, and instructing the treatment machine to move the patient to a preplanned position by moving the treatment couch (ExacTrac 1.0). The markers are visible by two IR cameras and one video camera that are mounted to the ceiling of the treatment room (Fig. 1). The patient's movements can be monitored in 3D real time with the IR cameras in the room, and consequently the patient's position can be controlled on-line either using a hand-pendant or computer-assisted commands

Software and settings: The IR-reflective/CT markers are automatically localized in the treatment planning system (Fig. 2) and the planned isocenter is referenced to this marker configuration. The IR tracking system is able to match a variable number of IR-reflective markers, visible at the time of

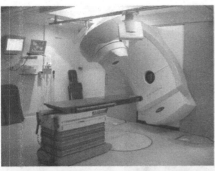
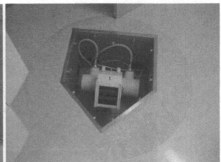
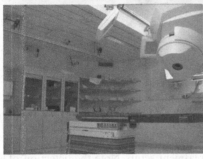

Figure 1 Room with Novalis system. Note the IR-cameras and AmSi detectors mounted to the ceiling and the X-ray tubes embedded in the floor. (ExacTrac 3.0/ Novalis Body courtesy of BrainLAB, AG.)

positioning, onto a set of markers (not necessarily of equal number) that were detected in the planning CT scan. As such the planned isocenter (based on the marker configuration detected during planning) can be localized with respect to the treatment isocenter of the linac (Fig. 3). The algorithm uses an unsorted

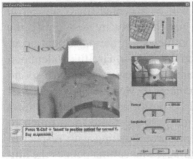
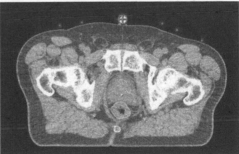

Figure 2 *Left*: Patient with IR reflective marker. (Note that the camera system has identified the markers indicated by the circles, and the coincidence with the planned position indicated by the small crosses.) *Right*: CT-image showing IR marker (localized by software), contours of CT, PTV, and rectum, and position of the treatment isocenter. (*See color insert.*)

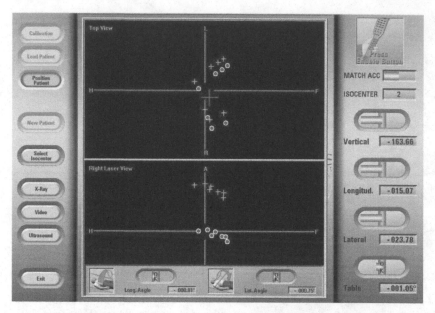

Figure 3 Illustration of the graphical interface of ExacTrac 3.0/Novalis Body with the patient on the treatment couch prior to treatment setup. Note the detection of transversal and rotational patient position at the right side and bottom of the image. The circles indicate the actual position and the crosses indicate the planned position where the patient will be moved. (*See color insert.*)

points match to solve the problem of matching the CT-localized marker with the corresponding visible IR-reflective markers. The markers are subjected to possible skin shift and do not represent a rigid body and, therefore, a number of assumptions and settings are needed. One of these settings is the maximum distortion of the marker configuration that will be accepted for a successful match. This setting reflects the search area for the software to identify the IR-reflective markers and has no noticeable influence on the positional accuracy of the isocenter. The latter is performed by least-square-fits, calculated by using different subsets of the markers. From the isocenters that correspond to the different subsets, the algorithm calculates a weighted average that becomes the isocenter where the patient will be positioned. The latter allows the system to recognize when one or more markers are shifted too much to be taken into consideration. Another, more important setting with respect to positional accuracy is the level of required accuracy. This setting defines the limits within which the isocenter position is considered acceptable, preventing infinite trials in reaching the exact isocenter position by computer-controlled couch movement. As mentioned earlier, the system allows for detection of patient movement as well as being used for computer-controlled couch movement to adjust the patient's position in real time.

Stereoscopic X-Ray Imaging Device

Hardware: The X-ray imaging system is fully integrated into the IR tracking device described above and consists of a generator, two X-ray tubes (MP 801 X-ray generator and comet X-ray tubes; K&S Röntgenwerk, Bochum, Germany) embedded in the floor, and two amorphous silicon (AmSi) detectors (PerkinElmer Optoelectronics GmbH, Wiesbaden, Germany) mounted to the ceiling (Fig. 1). The angle between both X-ray tube–detector pairs is approximately 90°, and approximately 42° tilted from the horizontal. In addition, a key board-controlled interface (using a particular key combination) has been developed allowing remote computer-assisted control of patient movement to predefined positions (final treatment position) from outside the treatment room. The X-ray system produces diagnostic photon beams ranging from 40 to 150 keV in exposure mode and from 40 to 125 keV in fluoroscopic mode, and projects a field size of approximately $20 \times 20\,cm^2$ on the AmSi-detector. The detectors have an active area of $22 \times 22\,cm^2$. A calibration is needed to define the spatial relationship between X-ray tubes and AmSi detectors on one hand, and the relationship with respect to the treatment machine's isocenter on the other. The spatial relationship with respect to the treatment isocenter is established by defining a relationship between the X-ray system and the IR tracking system with radio-opaque markers inside and IR-reflective markers outside a specially designed calibration phantom. Patient and treatment couch movements are controlled by real-time tracking of the IR-reflective markers. This system is referred to as the ExacTrac 3.0/Novalis Body system. The ExacTrac 2.0/Novalis Body refers to a previous setup with the X-ray tubes mounted to the ceiling and only one AmSi detector mounted on the treatment couch.

Software and positioning procedure: Once the patient is positioned on the treatment couch, two options are provided: (a) Using the predefined IR-reflective marker configuration that defines the planned isocenter based on CT data (see earlier). The advantage is that, once the patient is recognized by the system, the initial position does not need to be close to the actual treatment position. From that point on the entire positioning procedure is computer driven and performed from outside the treatment room. (b) A preliminary isocenter position is defined by the user that does not require a predefined IR-reflective marker configuration on the patient's skin and can even consist of IR-reflective markers rigidly fixed to the treatment couch. The latter has the advantage that breathing movements are eliminated and is therefore more stable. The disadvantage is that the system is no longer able to track patient movements during the positioning process and assumes that the patient is perfectly motionless. This option requires the entire positioning procedure to start from an a priori assumed correct treatment position (which will be corrected afterwards), after which the remaining procedure

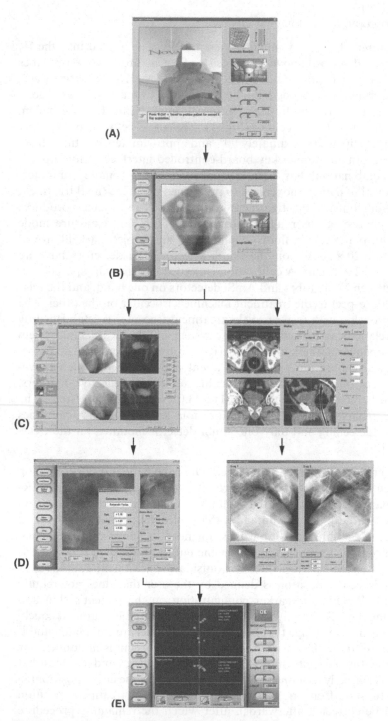

Figure 4   (*Caption on facing page*)

is again remote controlled and computer assisted. A video image can be provided during the automated setup procedure for patient's safety.

Once both X-ray images have been acquired, again two options are provided: (a) automated fusion of the actual X-ray images and DRRs representing the ideal patient position, and (b) matching implanted radio-opaque markers. The former procedure is considered an improvement in patient setup compared to conventional methods, although it is not able to cope with internal organ movements and therefore still requires a substantial internal target margin (ITV) (2). The implanted markers offer a more realistic assessment of the target volume's actual position and therefore enables reduction of treatment margins suitable for SBRT. A clinical example of appropriate treatment margins for treatment of the prostate follows, offering a detailed description of both procedures, with an illustration of the procedure given in the flowchart (Fig. 4).

Automated fusion of X-ray images and DRRs.   In this setup, a 2D/3D co-registration algorithm is applied to align a 3D CT patient data set with two X-ray images. Assuming that all components of the system are properly calibrated (i.e., the exact position of the X-ray tubes and detectors are known with respect to the machine's isocenter), it is possible to generate digitally reconstructed radiographs (DRRs) from the planning CT (representing the ideal patient position) and compare these with the acquired X-ray images. For accurate positioning both the location and orientation of the patient need to be assessed, taking into account all six degrees-of-freedom (6 DOF) for the image co-registration (translations as well as rotations). An automated fusion algorithm is used based on gradient correlation, which optimizes a similarity measure for each image pair (34). The similarity measure relies primarily on edges and gives a high response if strong edges are visible in the same place. In a first phase, the two pairs of corresponding X-rays and DRRs are fused and the amount of 2D translations necessary to register the image pairs can be used to compute a first course 3D correction vector (this is possible since the spatial relations and magnification factors between X-ray tubes and patient are known). This was the only option in the ExacTrac 2.0/Novalis Body system. This 2D/3D correction vector is then used as a starting value for the second phase, being the 6 DOF co-registration. The latter is obtained from an iterative optimization cycle to determine values for the rotation and the translation of the 3D CT data set to maximize the similarity measure

---

Figure 4   *(Facing page)* Flowchart illustrating the different steps in the positioning procedure using ExacTrac 3.0/Novalis Body. From top to bottom: **(A)** Patient on the treatment couch with IR reflective markers. **(B)** Acquisition of X-rays (only one shown). **(C–D)** Calculation of 3D correction vector based on either automated fusion of X-ray images with DRRs representing the ideal position *(left)* or matching of implanted radio-opaque markers *(right)*. **(E)** Automated patient positioning. *(See color insert.)*

between the corresponding DRRs (each time re-calculated from the previous values for rotations and translations) and the actual X-ray images. The latter requires an efficient algorithm for rendering DRRs (since some hundred DRRs will be used in the registration process), an efficient optimization, and automated fusion algorithm. If the automated fusion should fail, a backup procedure is offered to manually shift the DRR images until an acceptable registration is obtained; the user can define regions of interest in the images (eliminating regions of high contrast that are not related to the patient's anatomy such as patient immobilization devices that may influence the automated fusion), or limit the search area (avoiding that the system drifts-off to find an unrealistic solution).

Matching implanted markers. Again, assuming a calibrated X-ray system, implanted radio-opaque markers previously located in the planning CT volume set will be projected on the X-ray images (Fig. 4). When the initial patient setup is correct these projections will coincide with the images of the markers on the X-ray image. In case of a setup error, each marker projection can be clicked and dragged by mouse to coincide with the corresponding image of the actual position. The combined marker translations/rotations in each X-ray projection allow for calculation of a full 6 DOF correction assuming a rigid configuration. If the marker configuration deviates too much from the expected configuration (indicating possible marker migration), the system will fail to match the markers and the "migrated" marker will have to be eliminated in the software.

VERIFICATION AND CLINICAL VALIDATION

Phantom Measurements

Verification tests have been performed on anthropomorphic phantoms containing a humanoid skeleton to assess the precision and accuracy of the positioning system. A summary will be given of the results that have been published previously (29) on the system's performance for detection and correction of known translational setup errors with and without rotational errors in the pelvic region. In this study a segmented phantom (Alderson Rando Phantom for radiotherapy: Radiology Support Devices, CA) has been used consisting of 25-mm thick axial segments and allowing insertion of hidden targets to evaluate the entire procedure from CT scanning to treatment and verifying the alignment of treatment beam and target (assessment of the residual setup error). The phantom also allowed for insertion of radio-opaque markers to test the system's performance with matching of implanted markers. CT scans with 2-mm slice thickness and spacing between consecutive slices were acquired of the phantom together with the IR-reflective markers. The image data sets were transferred to a dedicated treatment planning system (BrainScan V 5.1: BrainLAB AG, Heimstetten, Germany) to define an appropriate treatment isocenter, after which these data, in turn were transferred to the positioning system on the treatment machine. Due to the segmented construction, inter-segment movements may have affected the obtained results and a rigid anthropomorphic phantom (a human skeleton embedded in resin with the shape of a human torso) had been introduced to validate the results obtained with the segmented phantom for the automated fusion of bony structures, and to investigate the possible influence of slice thickness in the acquisition of CT data (2 vs. 5-mm slice thickness and spacing).

Known setup errors have been applied to the phantoms and, after automated positioning based on either fusion of bony structures or matching implanted radio-opaque markers, the residual error was obtained with the hidden target test (HTT) known for quality assurance of stereotactic radiosurgery procedures (35,36). A lead bead of 2-mm diameter had been inserted in the segmented anthropomorphic phantom and defined as being the treatment isocenter. The phantom followed the entire procedure from CT scanning to treatment planning and automated positioning with the Novalis Body system. The treatment beam, collimated with a 10-mm circular collimator, had been used to generate portal films (X-OMATIC cassette with T-MAT L/RA film: Kodak, Rochester, NY) from 0° to 90° gantry angles. The center of the projected image of the lead bead had been measured with respect to the center of the circular field with a ruler (0.5 mm precision) on film with a magnification of 1.5 (focus–isocenter–distance = 100 cm; focus–film–distance = 150 cm). This procedure not only yielded an experimental estimate of the corrected setup error but also offered a comprehensive test of the entire treatment procedure, including, target localization on CT images (accuracy limited by voxel size) and mechanical uncertainties of treatment table and linear accelerator.

The following tests have been performed to assess the setup accuracy of the Novalis Body system using both the automated fusion of bony structures and matching of implanted radio-opaque markers:

1. automated positioning in the absence of shifts
2. automated positioning in the presence of shifts, each coordinate has been evaluated separately
3. automated positioning in the presence of combined shifts in the three principle directions
4. automated positioning in the absence of shifts with a rotation around one of the principle axes
5. automated positioning in the presence of combined shifts with a rotation around one of the principle axes
6. automated positioning in the presence of combined shifts and combined rotational setup errors

As mentioned before the automated fusion of bony structures is only applicable for SBRT of lesions that do not show much internal movement with respect to the bony structures used for positioning purposes. An investigation of the first version of the fusion algorithm (based on correcting three degrees-of-freedom only—omitting rotations—where the amount of 2D translations necessary to register the image pairs was used to compute a 3D correction vector for the patient) yielded an overall 3D accuracy (for combinations of both translational and rotational setup errors: up to 30 mm and 4° about all three axes) of 0.7 mm (SD: 0.8 mm) and 0.4 mm (SD: 0.9 mm) with the segmented and rigid phantom, respectively (Table 1). Reducing rotational setup errors below 0.5° prior to the positioning process increases this accuracy to 0.4 mm (SD: 0.5 mm) and 0.5 mm (SD: 0.7 mm). Breaking apart the measurements (rotations about a single axis in combination with translational setup errors) revealed an increased sensitivity with respect to rotations around the table axis (i.e., a 3D setup deviation vector of 2.0 (SD: 0.3 mm) versus 0.9 mm (SD: 0.4 mm) for rotations around the longitudinal and lateral axes). The largest residual error observed for combinations of induced translational and rotational setup errors was 2.7 mm, whereas the use of a 5 mm CT data set resulted in a 3D setup deviation vector of 2.0 mm (SD: 0.9 mm). Note that the DRRs were not re-sampled during the matching process and only a shift has been calculated rather than a full 6 DOF motion. The latest 6 DOF software version as described earlier has not yet been analyzed in detail but preliminary results look promising. The use of implanted radio-opaque markers increases the accuracy even more to 0.3 mm (SD: 0.4 mm) and 0.5 mm (SD: 0.3 mm) with and without rotational setup errors. The largest residual error observed for combinations of induced translational and rotational setup errors was 1.7 mm. Separate analyses of individual translations in combination with a particular rotation did not show any specific directional sensitivity. It must be recognized that although detected, the rotational setup errors have not been corrected for. The systems includes the detected rotational error in the calculation of the required translations to position the planned isocenter with respect to the treatment machine's isocenter. The phantom setup procedures have not been timed explicitly, but typically required less than 5 min and 3 min using the ExacTrac 2.0/Novalis Body or ExacTrac 3.0/Novalis Body system, respectively.

Patient Studies

A study has been performed in three steps to investigate the clinical performance of the ExacTrac/Novalis Body system for treatment of prostate cancer (see Chapter 10 on prostate and other pelvic tumors). The aim of the study was to reduce rectal toxicity while maintaining equal outcome for the patient. The latter can be realized only when the conventional PTV margins can be reduced without compromising the dose coverage of the CTV. As the PTV margin is introduced to cope with positional uncertainties (both internal organ movement—internal margin or IM—and uncertainties related to patient positioning and alignment of the treatment beam—setup margin or SM) (2) a reduction can be warranted only by increased knowledge of the patient's position and/or the actual position of the target volume. Once the positional uncertainty is quantified, an appropriate PTV margin can be realized by means of any appropriate CRT technique. Both dynamic field shaping arc and IMRT (37) have been adopted by the AZ-VUB for treatment of the prostate, and the reader is again referred to Chapter 10 on prostate and other pelvic tumors for more details on the treatment protocols. The different phases in this study were related to the introduction of more accurate methodologies of target positioning and defining the appropriate PTV margins for each technique:

Step 1: Patient positioning based on IR-skin markers using ExacTrac 1.0. This study included 19 patients (553 treatment fractions in total). All patients were treated for prostate cancer by dynamic field shaping arc with the mini-MLC of Novalis. Patients were treated in the supine position, stabilized by a vacuum cushion (12/19) or with conventional head and knee supports only (7/19). A comparison was made between conventional (using skin drawings and room lasers) and IR positioning (32).

Step 2: Patient positioning based on automated fusion of X-rays and DRRs using ExacTrac2.0/Novalis Body. Fifteen patients were followed with a total of 261 treatment sessions. All patients were treated in the supine position and stabilized with conventional head-and-knee support. A comparison was made between conventional IR positioning and the DRR-fusion (33).

Step 3: Patient positioning based on matching radio-opaque implanted markers using ExacTrac 3.0/Novalis Body. The study included 12 patients (122 treatment fractions analyzed), again treated in the supine position with conventional head-and-knee support. A comparison was made between conventional IR positioning, DRR-fusion, and implanted marker matching. An objective verification (residual error after automated positioning) of the patient positioning was performed on orthogonal megavoltage films taken at gantry 0° and 90°.

In the step 1 and 2 study the distances of the isocenter to the midline and to lines tangential to the superior and ventral border of the os pubis were measured on coronal and sagittal reconstructions of the planning CT data set (with an intrinsic voxel size of $1.0 \times 1.0 \times 3.0\,\text{mm}^3$) (Fig. 5). These measurements were repeated on the megavoltage film by a radiation oncologist using a standard ruler (1 mm scaling). For the step 3 study, the coordinates of the implanted markers with respect to the isocenter (both on the CT-data set and orthogonal megavoltage films) were used to define the residual setup error. In all cases the patient was assumed to remain in the initial treatment position during acquisition of the additional megavoltage films. Again, one

Table 1 Average Residual Setup Error (mm) and Standard Deviation (in Parentheses) With and Without Rotational Setup Errors After Automated Positioning Based on One of Both Calculation Algorithms (Fusion of DRR and X-Ray Image or Matching Implanted Markers)

	DRR fusion			Marker matching		
	No rotation	Rotation	All	No rotation	Rotation	All
Vertical	0.32	−0.39	0.05	0.15	−0.33	−0.20
	(0.65)	(1.12)	(0.92)	(0.65)	(0.41)	(0.52)
Longitudinal	−0.09	−1.05	−0.46	−0.16	−0.17	−0.17
	(0.56)	(1.38)	(0.06)	(0.33)	(0.40)	(0.38)
Lateral	−0.36	−1.68	−0.48	−0.38	−0.14	−0.21
	(0.62)	(0.99)	(0.80)	(0.77)	(0.45)	(0.55)

The residual error is obtained from hidden target data representing the remaining error measured with portal films at gantry angles 0° and 90° with a 10 mm circular beam of the isocenter represented by a 2 mm bead, after automated positioning based on the corrected shift.

must note that the DRR fusion used in these studies was not the full 6 DOF version.

In this chapter, for comparison purposes, the results from the three studies have been pooled into one data base and re-analyzed yielding an overall 3D residual error equal to 1.1 mm (SD: 11.7 mm), 1.4 mm (SD: 7.1 mm),

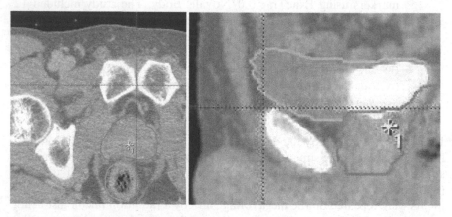

Figure 5 Illustration of the distances taken to define the position of the treatment isocenter with respect to bony structures for verification with portal film. The distance of the isocenter to the midline and to the lines tangential to the superior and ventral border of the os pubis are measured according to the dotted line. (*See color insert.*)

0.5 mm (SD: 4.6 mm), and 1.2 mm (SD: 3.8 mm) for positioning based on conventional methods, infrared, DRR fusion, or marker matching, respectively. For the first three results the comparison was based on bony references, whereas the last figure results from the actual marker coordinates and as such the only indication of the actual target positioning including organ movement. These results show a striking reduction in the spread of data going from conventional to marker matching method. To obtain an estimate of the distribution of systematic errors in setup for all patients, the standard deviation (SD) of the mean deviation of individual patients was calculated. The random component was determined by calculating the SD of the individual deviations (pooled data) after subtractions of their corresponding mean. These results are shown in Figure 6. Table 2 shows the percentage of moderately large (≥ 5 mm) and large errors (≥ 10 mm) for the pooled patient data. Only the third study allowed assessment of the difference between positioning based on bony structures and implanted markers, which can be interpreted as an indication of organ movement. Overall differences of 1.6 mm (latero-lateral), 2.8 mm (antero-posterior), and 2.3 mm (cranio-caudal) have been observed between both positioning methods in this patient data set. Based on these results the following rules for PTV margin have been proposed at the

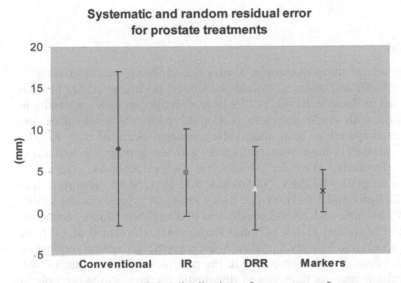

Figure 6 An estimate of the distribution of setup errors for prostate treatments resulting from positioning with (left to right) skin markers and room-laser alignment, IR tracking, automated fusion between DRR and actual X-ray images, and matching of implanted markers. The systematic error is calculated as the SD of the mean deviation of individual patients. The random error is defined as the SD of the individual deviations of all patients after subtraction of the corresponding mean.

Table 2 Percentage of Moderate (≥5 mm) and Large (≥10 mm) Errors for the Pooled Data Base Along One of the Principle Axes

	Moderately large errors (≤5 mm)	Large errors (≤10 mm)
Conventional	41	12
IR	21	2
DRR fusion	8	1
Marker matching	3	0

AZ-VUB: 6.0 mm latero-lateral, and 10.0 mm antero-posterior and cranio-caudal when DRR-fusion is used for positioning; 5.0 mm antero-posterior and cranio-caudal, and 3.0 mm latero-lateral when implanted markers are used for positioning. Clinical use of the ExacTrac 2.0/Novalis Body sytem required a total linac time (patient entering treatment room to patient leaving treatment room) of 14′51″ (SD: 4′18″). The X-ray-assisted patient positioning required 7′54″ (SD: 3′43″) (33). No specific time measurements have been performed since the introduction of the ExacTrac 3.0/Novalis Body system, but the total linac time never exceded 11′, the X-ray-assisted setup was below 4′.

Discussion

The approach of using diagnostic X-rays for verifying treatment setup is not new (38–40) and offers a twofold advantage: (a) image quality [a well-documented problem in EPIDs (4,17,19)] is no longer an issue, especially in combination with AmSi detectors (4,41); (b) patient dose becomes less important compared to daily megavoltage images acquired with EPIDs. Dose measurements have been performed with an appropriate ionization chamber (Dosimax, Welhöfer Dosimetrie, Schwarzenbruck, Germany) covering a range of 50–125 kV, 50–160 mA, and 50–1250 mS, yielding values between 22.9 µSv and 1.640 mSv per X-ray image. A typical clinical setting of 100 kV, 100 mA, and 100 mS resulted in 0.513 mSv per image. Based on the work of Motz and Danos (42) and Rogers (43), Herman et al. (4) have shown a strong link between signal-to-noise ratio (SNR), spatial resolution, and patient dose. For the same dose to the patient, the SNR is much lower at megavoltage energies than that at diagnostic energies. In the example of a 78 Gy prostate treatment, some simple mathematics show that (assuming 3 MU—or 30 mSv at depth of maximum dose—per EPI and requiring minimal two images for 3D information) patient doses of 2340 versus 40 mSv are delivered with electronic portal imaging and kilovoltage imaging, respectively, i.e., a ratio of 58. Moreover, the combination with real-time monitoring of patient positioning is not limited to patient observation, but also offers the possibility of controlling the treatment beam based on that information (28,29,44,45). The feasibility of implanted radio-opaque markers has been investigated in this and other studies (6,29,46–50) and shows promising results. It is evident, however, that a detailed clinical study must be performed to investigate the influence of migration and possible variations in target shape on setup accuracy.

The prostate studies shown in the previous discussion made use of immobilization devices only in the first study where a subset of patients were treated supine with a vacuum cushion and another subset with the conventional head-and-knee support. Although it was not the aim of that study (32), there was no evidence that the immobilization devices altered the positional accuracy, which is confirmed in other studies (51). The use of implanted radio-opaque markers not only proved to be more accurate it also allowed localization of the actual organ, and hence assessment of internal organ movement. Observations from the AZ-VUB study showed average deviations of 1.6 mm (latero-lateral), 2.8 mm (antero-posterior), and 2.3 mm (cranio-caudal) between bony landmarks and implanted markers. These results agree with observations made with consecutive CT measurements (52,53) and assessments of intra-fractional movement based on MRI (54). Ultrasound studies (55,56) show significantly larger (i.e., a factor 2) organ motions, which may be attributed to the technique more than actual internal organ movement (57,58). All studies show that organ movement is largest in the antero-posterior and cranio-caudal directions. So far no marker migration has been observed in the AZ-VUB studies (CT prior, during, and after termination of treatment). Yin et al. performed a similar study on the usefulness of the ExacTrac 2.0/Novalis Body system for radiosurgery for spinal tumors (59). This group did use the system in combination with a vacuum body-fixing device (combining a vacuum bag and a piece of special plastic wrap from Medical Intelligence) and an alpha cradle. A verification of positional accuracy obtained from comparison with orthogonal portal films and DRRs from the planning CT data set yielded a 3D isocenter deviation of less than 2 mm. The deviation was attributed by the authors to various sources such as CT slice thickness (2 mm), patient breathing, and positioning system accuracy. The system's performance for other extracranial sites such as liver metastases and lung tumors is currently under investigation. First results at the AZ-VUB show promising results, yet one limitation of the Novalis Body system can already be identified. Contrary to pelvic lesions where a suficient amount of bony landmarks is present, abdominal or thoracic lesions that are located laterally in the patient do not offer sufficient bony landmarks and failures of the automated fusion algorithm occur more often. Implanted radio-opaque markers become a necessity in these cases. Moreover, lesions where the vertebrae are the major bony landmarks the automated fusion algorithm might be off by one vertebra due to the cylindric symmetry.

TREATMENT PLANNING AND TREATMENT DELIVERY

Dynamic Arc

The accelerator is equipped with an integrated miniMLC consisting of two banks with 26 leaves each. The leaf width varies at isocenter distance from 0.30 cm for the 14 central pairs, 0.45 cm for the next three, and finally 0.55 cm for the outer three leaf pairs. A maximum field size of $9.80 \times 10.00\,cm^2$ can be generated, again at isocenter distance. Each leaf can overtravel by 5.00 cm. A central straight edge (the other two straight edges correspond to the field divergence at full extension and full retraction) allows the leaves to touch when closed and full inter-digitation is possible. A detailed description of the miniMLC is given by Cosgrove et al. (60) and Xia et al. (61).

The dynamic conformal arc technique is a merging of traditional "arcing" radiosurgery and conformal beam irradiation. Radiation is delivered while the linac gantry rotates around the patient and the field shape is modified dynamically by the Novalis multileaf collimator to conform to the target shape for each gantry angle (37). The dynamic conformal arc concept is illustrated in Figure 7, which shows eight consecutive "beam's eye views" (BEVs) from a 70° arc in 10° increments. The yellow line surrounding the target (green) indicates the conformal field shape created by the multileaf collimator. The spinal cord (magenta) is shown running vertically through each frame. Parameters such as arc length, dose, and the margin between the field edge and the tumor are specified by the user. Dose distributions may be customized

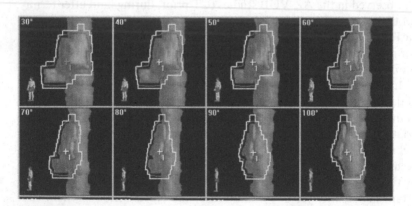

Figure 7 Beam's eye views of a dynamic arc (10° gantry steps). The yellow line surrounding the target (green) indicates the conformal field shape created by the multileaf collimator. The spinal cord (magenta) is shown running vertically through each frame. Parameters such as arc length, dose, and the margin between the field edge and the tumor are specified by the user. Dose distributions may be customized using software tools that allow for preferential sparing of organs at risk (OARs) and for graphical editing of field shapes in any BEV. (*See color insert.*)

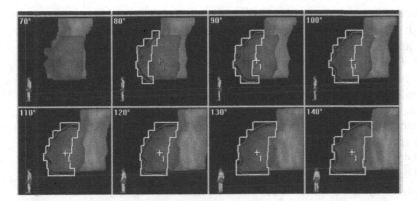

Figure 8 Beam's eye view of a dynamic arc with an "organ at risk" (OAR). The field shape (yellow) intentionally blocks part of the target (purple) in order to minimize the dose to the OAR behind it. (*See color insert.*)

using software tools that allow for preferential sparing of organs at risk (OARs) and for graphical editing of field shapes in any BEV. An arc that incorporates OAR sparing is shown in Figure 8. The field shape (yellow) intentionally blocks part of the target (purple) in order to minimize the dose to the OAR behind it. The dynamic conformal arc combines the most advantageous aspects of traditional radiosurgery and conformal beam irradiation by minimizing the dose to surrounding structures by use of a large number of beam angles and by effectively custom shielding healthy tissue in every beam. The dynamic conformal arc is the most expedient delivery method because the dose can be delivered to a large number of beam angles in one fluid motion. The $9.8 \times 10.0 \, cm^2$ maximum field size of the Novalis collimator obviates the need for multiple isocenters in the case of larger lesions.

The TPS (BrainSCAN V 5.1: BrainLAB AG, Heimstetten, Germany) comes with the shaped beam radiosurgery linac, which allows for both forward and inverse planning. The former is used to calculate the dose resulting from dynamic conformal arc treatments. The dose calculation is based on the pencil beam algorithm; two different calculation grids are used: (a) an adaptive grid (i.e., the grid size is locally reduced in high dose gradient areas) that can be refined with the zoom function for 2D display of isodoses, and (b) a fixed grid of $0.2 \times 0.2 \times 0.2 \, cm^3$ for calculation of the CDVH.

IMRS

The Novalis system is able to generate intensity-modulated treatment fields by means of SMLC and DMLC treatment delivery (again, a sliding window). The latter was created with the interpreter developed by Agazaryan et al.

(62), which corrects for transmission through MLC leaves by an iterative method. Leakage between opposing and neighboring leaves is also minimized and individual leaves are synchronized to reduce the tongue-and-groove (TaG) effect. The inter-digitation and 5.00 cm overtravel yield maximum IMRT field sizes of 9.80×10.00 cm^2. The resolution of the beam elements (pixel) in the direction of leaf travel can be specified arbitrarily and has been set to 0.20 cm for this study. The system guarantees that only bixels smaller or equal to the set value will be used. Perpendicular to the direction of leaf travel the resolution of the bixels is defined by the leaf width (i.e., 0.30, 0.45, and 0.55 cm).

The TPS (BrainSCAN V 5.1: BrainLAB AG, Heimstetten, Germany), used for the dynamic conformal arc in the previous section, yet in the inverse mode, was also used but with using the so-called treatment constraints. The optimization is based on the dynamically penalized likelihood method developed by Llacer (63), which is a variation of the maximum likelihood estimator known from inverse problems in positron emission tomography. A filtering term is included in the optimization loop that also penalizes solutions that yield bixel weights substantially different from their neighbors (64).

The Novalis approach to IMRS can be outlined as follows:

- Planning targets and organ(s) at risk are identified.
- An isocenter and beam angles are defined analogous to conformal beam planning.
- Various calculation parameters are prescribed.
- Clinical dose–volume constraints are specified.
- Multiple planning solutions are calculated with different priority relationships between treatment volumes and OARs.
- Planning solutions are compared and one is selected.
- The treatment plan is verified and delivered.

Only objects with PTV, OAR, or Boost status are considered during IMRS planning. All of these objects are contoured and defined on MR/CT images with Novalis software tools. The IMRS treatment planning process begins in the same way as conformal beam planning. An isocenter is defined and beam angles are selected. A maximum of 24 beams may be added to each isocenter but excellent dose distributions are usually achieved using 6 to 8. Unlike standard conformal SRS/SRT planning, the distribution of beams around the isocenter is not necessarily driven by OAR constraints. Often the best plans result when beams are non-coplanar with maximal geometric separation. One advantage of the Novalis system over others is that a wide range of angles is available over which to spread beams including the patient's posterior. In most cases, a full 360° of gantry angle is available for treatment in the axial plane and approximately 50° of anterior gantry angle is available for nonaxial planes.

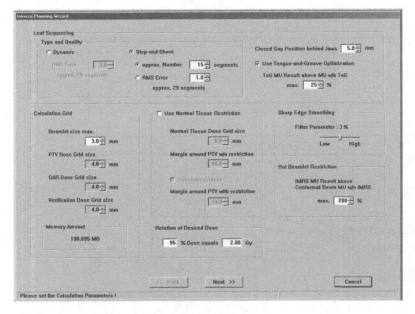

Figure 9 Novalis inverse planning wizard.

Once the physical beam directions have been set, inverse planning calculation parameters are specified using a *planning wizard* (Fig. 9). The five major parameter groups include: leaf sequencing, calculation grid, normal tissue restriction, sharp edge smoothing, and hot beamlet restriction.

A detailed description of all inverse planning parameters is beyond the scope of this chapter but the following example from UCLA is typical for prostate and spine treatments:

- step-and-shoot, approximate 15 segments
- closed gap position behind jaws = 5.0 mm
- tongue-and-groove (TaG) optimization = ON
- tag MU result above MU w/o TaG = 25%
- sharp edge smoothing filter parameter = 5%
- hot beamlet restriction maximum = 150–200%.

Dose–volume constraints are prescribed graphically for the PTV and each OAR by dragging adjustment points to shape the desired dose–volume histogram (DVH). The dose–volume constraint window for a prostate plan is shown in Figure 10. Dose–volume constraints for individual objects can be saved and recalled so that planning for a group of patients can be done under the same criteria. The relative importance of critical objects can be weighted for optimization using the "Guardian" slider.

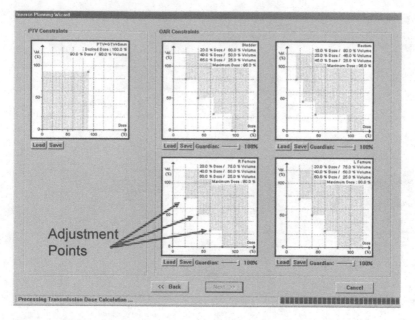

Figure 10 Clinical dose–volume constraints for a prostate plan.

Once constraints have been specified, Novalis software generates four treatment plans with optimization based on differing priorities for the OARs. The four results are called *PTV only, OAR low, OAR normal,* and *OAR high.* Dose distributions and DVHs from the four plans are displayed side by side for evaluation (Fig. 11). Forward calculations are processed for whichever plan is selected.

TREATMENT VERIFICATION

The AZ-VUB Approach

Introduction

Intensity-modulated radiation therapy is now accepted by the radiotherapy society as a feasible treatment technique and is gaining momentum in the clinical environment. Indeed, with the clinical implementation of IMRT the attention is shifting from feasibility studies toward patient-based studies and the investigation of treatment efficiency. However, off-the-shelf systems are still scarce and the clinical implementation of IMRT requires a substantial effort from the individual centers. The technology has not yet reached maturity and the step from phantom verification to patient treatment is, in many respects, a jump in the dark. The clinical implementation

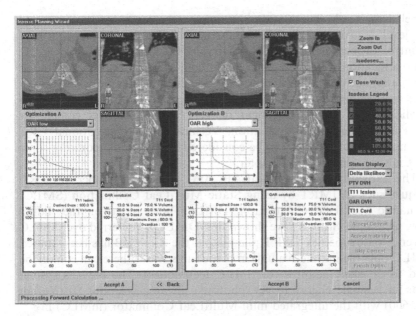

Figure 11 Plan optimization window. (*See color insert.*)

of IMRT requires the establishment of a complete chain of processes, starting with inverse planning and going right through to verification. Analysis of the QA needs to include careful delineation of the planning and delivery process, documenting where important decisions are made, how information is transferred, what kind of errors are likely or possible, and the sensitivity of various parts of the process to errors—in short "hazard analysis." It is important to understand what has not been verified with the applied QA procedure. The QA program can be divided into three classes: machine-related QA, pretreatment QA, and treatment QA. Only the latter two, in principle, involve patient-based issues. Unfortunately, the conventional methods are no longer valid and the intuition from conventional radiotherapy is lost. In vivo dosimetry becomes difficult and hand calculation is no longer feasible due to the complexity of the treatment. Moreover, target localization and target volume motion become major parameters in the delivered dose distribution, which is difficult to assess. There is no ideal solution and some of the options are either to perform individualized extensive verification tests prior to each treatment, or generalized verification of the so-called class solutions. The verification procedure in turn can be designed to analyze all variables of the treatment process in detail or to be comprehensive. The machine-related QA can be seen as a pyramid-shaped approach in that the upper level is build on the quality of the level underneath. The base level comprises basic QA of the linac and MLC; level 2 covers small field dosimetry, small amounts of MUs, and leaf-control properties; level 3, dosimetry of IM beams; and level 4, 3D IMRT verification. In this chapter, treatment verification will be limited to verification of dose delivery as target localization has been extensively covered in elsewhere in this book. Moreover, special emphasis will be given to verification of IMRT treatment delivery, which with its complexity requires a more extensive evaluation. Verification of conventional CRT and dynamic arc techniques can be considered special cases requiring some of the tools described in this chapter.

The Novalis system (BrainLAB AG) offers a number of CRT techniques such as IMRT by using Static MultiLeaf Collimation (SMLC) or Dynamic MultiLeaf Collimation (DMLC) both based on the sliding window technique. Studies have shown that DMLC is preferred over SMLC for several MLCs (65,66). IMRT planning at the AZ-VUB has been limited to DMLC only (again, the evaluation procedures shown here can equally be applied to or easily adapted for SMLC techniques). The Novalis system consists of a single energy (6 MV photons) linear accelerator (l) (Varian Clinac 600) with the integrated mini-MultiLeaf Collimator (mMLC) m_3^{TM} (BrainLAB AG), which is described in detail by Cosgrove et al. and Xia et al. (60,61), the Treatment Planning System (TPS) BrainSCAN (Brain-SCAN V 5.1, BrainLAB AG, Heimstetten, Germany), and the automated positioning tool Novalis Body as described in the previous chapter. The interface between the linac and the TPS is realized with the VARIS record and verify system (Varian, Medical Systems, Milpitas, CA). The inverse planning modality for IMRT has also been described earlier. After arranging the static beam configuration in the conformal beam and preplanning and defining the calculation parameters and constraints to be used, the inverse planning optimizes four plans with different priorities to OARs using a dynamically penalized likelihood algorithm (63). The calculated fluence maps are used in the forward calculation of the dose distribution using the pencil beam dose calculation algorithm (67–69). The user can chose one of the four calculated plans or change the calculation parameters and constraints to achieve the required dose distribution.

The use of the mMLC enables a higher degree of conformity of the dose distributions produced by the BrainSCAN IMRT planning system (37,70). With the increasing degree of complexity and sophistication of a treatment technique such as the IMRT technique, the clinical implementation requires a more comprehensive QA procedure than conventional radiation therapy. At the moment there is no general protocol established for the QA procedure of IMRT, therefore each clinical site is forced to create an individualized QA procedure to verify the correctness and accuracy of the TPS calculations and treatment delivery. This chapter summarizes the procedure followed at the AZ-VUB for the QA of IMRT with the mMLC.

The QA procedure for IMRT at the AZ-VUB is divided into the following major parts:

Non-patient-related QA:

- Evaluate the overall functionality of the system (similar to acceptance testing).
- Analyze class solutions for different treatment sites (similar to commissioning of the complete system).

Patient-related QA:

- Pretreatment tests of the confirmed plan for a patient prior to the first fraction.
- Prefraction tests designed to eliminate the risk of mistreatment.

To ensure that the system is operating within specifications, general non-patient-related tests are regularly performed as well as sample verifications of actual patient treatments (e.g., once a month). The patient sample verification consists of a comprehensive test that includes mapping of the treatment plan into a cubic or anthropomorphic phantom with absolute (TLD and ionization chamber measurements) and relative (EDR-2, gamma evaluation of dose distributions) dose verification. This procedure allows sufficient confidence in the system's performance and reducing the patient-specific QA. The latter consists of verification of fluence maps and independent calculation of monitor units (MU). The AZ-VUB policy is to perform a comprehensive QA procedure of class solutions for the different treatment sites and to limit the verification prior to each patient treatment.

Evaluation of Overall Functionality

In MLC-based IMRT, complex movement of the MLC leaves is used to deliver the desired nonuniform dose distribution in the treatment field. This complex leaf movement is controlled by the operating system of the linac (Varis, Varian Medical Systems, Milpitas, CA, U.S.A. for the Novalis system). Due to these complex leaf movements, the acceptance of the mMLC requires additional tests compared to conventional acceptance tests for the verification of the linac's accuracy and reliability to ensure the accuracy of the mMLC when delivering intensity-modulated treatment fields. The validation of the mMLC includes tests for: (a) leaf positioning accuracy, (b) speed stability, (c) beam on/off stability, (d) gravity influence, and (e) MLC reliability.

    a. The calibration of an MLC to be used for the delivery of intensity profiles needs special attention because the tolerances of the leaf positioning accuracy used for conventional treatments (1–2 mm) are no longer stringent enough for IMRT treatments. The leaf positioning is especially critical for the step-and-shoot technique.

If the shaping of every segment is not accurate, the dose of the total intensity map can be changed. The leaf position is checked by static light field projection on graph paper ruled in millimeters positioned at the couch top at isocenter distance, or with radiographic film positioned at isocenter distance horizontally between solid water phantom at the depth of maximum dose (d_{max}). The positional accuracy of the leaves of the mMLC is smaller than 0.50 mm, the acceptable accuracy for IMRT treatments.

b. The leaf speed stability is critical for the DMLC technique since this parameter defines the formation of the segments for the sliding window during the irradiation. The leaf speed test is conducted by moving the leaves over a defined distance during a specified time, or while irradiating a certain amount of monitor units (MU) at a certain dose rate. Use the test files provided by Varian Medical Systems for the "MLC dynamic treatment acceptance procedure" to perform this test. With the dynamic file viewer application available from Varian, an error histogram table is generated for the performed tests that allows one to readily evaluate the tests.

c. To deliver intensity-modulated beams (IMBs) with either step-and-shoot or dynamic multileaf collimation accurately, the beam hold-off (i.e., the period where there is no irradiation because the leaves are in motion) must be controlled correctly. The MLC dynamic treatment acceptance procedure from Varian also provides test files to verify if the periods of beam hold-off appear at the planned times.

d. To ensure that the mMLC operates accurately under variable influences of gravitation (variable gantry angles), a gravity test must be performed. This can be done by verifying the leaf speed with a maximum and minimum influence of gravitation. Therefore, the leaf speed test is conducted at three different gantry angles of 0°, 90°, and 270°.

e. The mMLC reliability or repositioning accuracy is verified by running an autocycle of a number of mMLC fields where the last field setup is the same as the initial one. After about 50 cycles, the leaf positions of the first field are compared with those of the last field. The reposition accuracy of the leaves of the mMLC is within 0.50 mm.

The accuracy must be verified on a regular (e.g., weekly) basis. Therefore it is desirable to have a test for routine QA that is simple and quick to give an overall assessment of the accuracy of all leaf pairs of the MLC simultaneously by visual inspection of the irradiated radiographic film.

During the installation of the BrainSCAN V5.1 software, an IMRT phantom was copied to the TPS. On this phantom some fluence distributions are predefined to test the performance of the MLC in both step-and-shoot IMRT and DMLC IMRT. The fluence distributions simulate a chessboard pattern and a garden fence pattern as shown in Figure 12. The procedure to deliver these fluence distributions is described in the "Acceptance Checklist for BrainSCAN IMRS" working instruction provided by BrainLAB.

When these fluence distributions are delivered to radiographic film, the resulting dose pattern will show whether or not there is a positional error for a particular leaf or leaf pair. For instance, in the garden fence test a positional error will result in either the location or the thickness of the dark line that will be different from the lines generated by the other leaf pairs. To be able to compare the performance of the mMLC in step-and-shoot IMRT with DMLC IMRT, the same dose must be delivered to the radiographic film in both delivery types to result in the same amount of blackening of the film.

Another QA pattern is created at the AZ-VUB based on patterns already in use by other medical departments. Figure 13 displays the daily QA pattern that is delivered with the collimator rotated to 90° so that the leaves move from left to right over the pattern. All profiles in the pattern give an idea about the positional accuracy of the leaves. The wedge profiles help to evaluate the leaf speed stability by measuring the relative doses of the different steps of the profiles. Relative doses can also be verified with the two black areas, the gray area, and the white circle that have a 100%, 50%, and 0% dose, respectively. The TaG underdosages will appear clearly in the gray area and allow one to judge the influence of the TaG effect.

When the leaf patterns are evaluated, it is more important to look at the resulting geometry than at absolute doses. Absolute doses are verified during the acceptance of the pencil beam calculation algorithm, of the TPS.

For the acceptance of the pencil beam calculation algorithm, the beam parameters of the Novalis linac are measured as prescribed in the "Beam Measurements for Pencil Beam" operating instruction provided by BrainLAB and

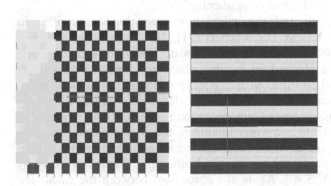

Figure 12 Chessboard and garden fence intensity map.

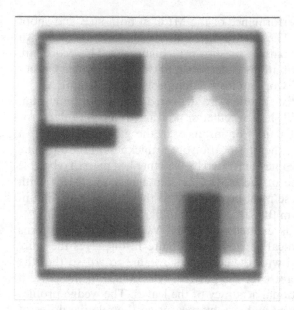

Figure 13 Daily QA pattern used at the AZ-VUB to check the mMLC performance.

defined in the BrainSCAN planning system. The beam data measurements require accurate small field dosimetry with a micro-ionization chamber or diamond detector to ensure that the TPS will accurately calculate the dose delivered by small segments often appearing in IMBs. At the AZ-VUB, the beam data measurements were performed with the NAC007 micro-ionization chamber (Wellhöfer Dosimetrie GmbH, Schwarzbruck, Germany), which is a waterproof chamber with a high spatial resolution due to its small active volume ($0.007 \, \text{cm}^3$) that can be used for both relative and absolute dosimetry. The small active volume makes the chamber particularly suitable for measurements of small fields and high-dose gradients.

The defined beam and the calculation algorithm are verified in accordance with the AAPM TG23 report (71). 2D dose profiles are measured with the NAC007 chamber in a cubic water phantom and compared with the distributions planned on a cubic phantom. Absolute doses were also verified at several positions with respect to depth and off-axis position. The agreement between the calculated and the delivered dose was within 2% or 2 mm in a water phantom, as recommended in the ICRU42 report (72). In addition to verification in a water phantom, the algorithm was also verified for calculations for different locations on an anthropomorphic phantom (Alderson Rando Phantom for Radiotherapy, Radiology Support Devices, California, U.S.A.). Again the agreement between the calculated and actual delivered dose was within 2% or 2 mm.

Analysis of Class Solutions

The verification of the quality of the resulting treatment plan can be performed in two ways. A first possibility is to work top–down with an absolute and relative verification of the complete plan (the comprehensive approach). verification is broken into separate parts of the calculation and delivery process if a discrepancy in the result of the comprehensive test has been observed. A second possibility is to work bottom–up, where all parts of the plan are verified separately to achieve complete plan verification. Analysis of the verification is straightforward with the latter approach but the procedure is time consuming. The first approach requires less time, yet the discrepancy analysis is much more complicated; it has been adopted by the AZ-VUB.

Phantoms: Two types of phantoms are used at the AZ-VUB for the verification of IMRT. The first is a homogeneous polystyrene cubic phantom with external dimensions of $16.50 \times 16.50 \times 17.80 \, cm^3$ containing 20 polystyrene spacers of $13.90 \times 12.70 \times 0.60 \, cm^3$ for inserting film sheets. The spacers can be oriented according the three orthogonal directions allowing transversal, coronal, and sagittal measurements of the relative dose distribution. In some of the spacers, holes with a $0.50 \, cm$ diameter and $0.08 \, cm$ depth are drilled, where TLDs can be placed in for absolute dosimetry. An adaptation of the phantom allows insertion of the NAC007 micro-ionization chamber. The second phantom is a humanoid phantom (Alderson Rando Phantom for Radiotherapy) and is used to verify clinically relevant treatment plans where tissue inhomogeneities can have a large influence on the resulting dose distribution. Film sheets can be inserted between the slabs of this phantom and, at specified locations in some of the slabs, holes are drilled to allow performance of absolute dosimetry with TLDs. Sequential CT images with $0.20 \, cm$ slice width and $0.20 \, cm$ slice spacing were generated with both phantoms. The obtained sets of images were imported in the TPS for the calculation of the verification plans. Target localization and phantom positioning for all verification measurements were performed by ExacTrac3.0/Novalis Body (BramLAB AG, Heimstetten, Germany) for both the homogeneous cubic phantom and the humanoid phantom.

Dosimeters and calibration: The dose distributions were examined relatively with radiographic film (X-OMAT V and EDR-2 ready pack; Kodak, Rochester, New York, U.S.A.) and absolute dosimetry performed with ThermoLuminescent Detectors (TLD) [LiF: 700 pellets (Vinten Instruments, Surrey, U.K.)] with $0.50 \, cm$ diameter and $0.08 \, cm$ thickness and the NAC007 micro-ionization chamber (Wellhöfer Dosimetrie GmbH, Schwartzbruck, Germany).

The prescribed dose of the verification plans was 0.50 or 2.00 Gy for the irradiation of the X-OMAT V film and the EDR-2 film, respectively, resulting in a net optical density within the approximate linear range of the response of the radiographic film. The original radiographic film was cut into smaller sheets that fit into the phantom. To create a sensitometric curve allowing the conversion of the optical densities into absorbed dose distributions, a calibration procedure was developed and validated in our department yielding an accuracy of 3% (1 SD). The film sheets used to calculate the sensitometric curve were calibrated with $5.00 \times 5.00 \, cm^2$ fields against ionization chamber measurements. The calibration film sheet was developed (Kodak X-Omat 3000RA processor: Kodak, Rochester, New York, U.S.A.) simultaneously with the measurement film sheets. The films were digitized using the WP102 film scanner with an aperture of 0.08 cm and the WP700V3.51 software (Wellhöfer Dosimetrie, Schwarzenbruck, Germany), and compared to calculated dose distributions using an in-house developed version of the gamma-method (4% dose difference/4 mm distance-to-agreement tolerances) (73), dose difference maps, and cumulative dose histograms in a MATLAB environment (MATLAB® V5 Student Edition: The MathWorks Inc., Littlefield, Texas, U.S.A.).

For the absolute dosimetry with TLD, the prescribed dose was set to 1.00 or 2.00 Gy, the dose to which the TLDs were calibrated. The detectors were individually calibrated with the 6 MV photon beam of the Novalis linac, yielding a reproducibility of 3% (1 SD). The TLDs were positioned in the transversal plane. Alternatively, the plan could be mapped into the cubic phantom allowing insertion of the NAC007 micro-ionization chamber.

Verification plans: Verification plans have been evaluated for different treatment sites such as prostate, head and neck, and brain lesions, and once a month a sample plan is run, selected from the patients under treatment. These cases have been simulated on the anthropomorphic phantom and/or mapped to the cubic phantom. The latter is a useful evaluation feature of the TPS where the complete set of treatment parameters is superimposed on another image set, e.g., an anthropomorphic or a geometrical phantom. In this case the isocenter of the patient's plan is placed into an appropriate place in the phantom to ensure a relevant verification measurement of the treatment. The treatment plan (geometrical settings, beam arrangement, leaf settings, MUs are used from the patient's plan) is then recalculated using the contours and densities of the phantom, allowing relative and absolute dosimetry of the patient's plan. Special care needs to be given to the choice of the phantom; when important variations in tissue density are present at the treatment site, the homogeneous phantom may not be appropriate and offer a false sense of confidence as seen in Figure 14. The "dose export" tools of the BrainSCAN TPS allow the comparison of the calculated with the measured doses and dose distributions. The dose distributions of the overall plan as well as the fluence distributions of every treatment beam used in the plan can be exported from the TPS. The correspondence between the planned and the measured doses and dose

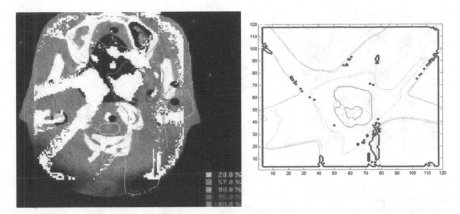

Figure 14 The importance of the choice of an appropriate phantom when mapping treatment parameters from a patient treatment to a phantom for verification of dose distribution is illustrated here. The left-hand pane shows the result from mapping into an anthropomorphic phantom; the white "erased" pixels indicate regions where the gamma tolerance (4% DD, 4 mm DTA) is not met between measured and calculated dose distributions. The right-hand pane shows the same treatment mapped into a homogeneous cubic phantom; the "bold" pixels indicate regions where the gamma tolerance is not met. The homogeneous mapping does not show possible errors due to tissue heterogeneities and might give a false sense of confidence. (*See color insert.*)

distributions has then been analyzed using the gamma-method, dose difference maps, and cumulative dose histograms (Fig. 15).

Pretreatment Verification

Once an acceptable confidence level with respect to the overall performance of the entire system is achieved and maintained (test-pattern tests, class solution verification, and regular sample tests), the individual patient QA is reduced to verification of fluence patterns and absolute dose calculation.

The absolute dose check is performed prior to every patient treatment by mapping the patient's plan to a homogeneous polystyrene cubic phantom (identical to the one used for commissioning) that is modified so that the NAC007 micro-ionization chamber fits in the phantom. The patient's plan is recalculated and delivered to the phantom and the calculated dose to the chamber is compared with the actual delivered dose measured by the chamber. Care should be taken while positioning the dose distribution, allowing an absolute dose measurement in a low-dose gradient region of the dose distribution.

A second patient-specific test is an independent MU verification. A simple spreadsheet-based program has been developed that uses as few as possible parameters from the plan to re-calculate the dose given in the

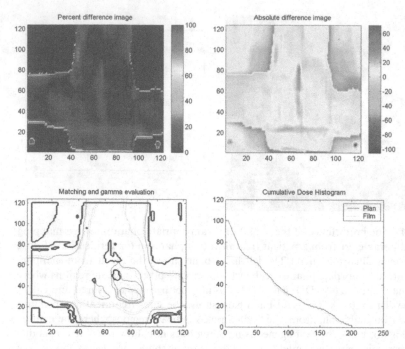

Figure 15 Illustration of in-house developed tool for verification of dose distribution (measured and calculated) at the AZ-VUB showing percent difference, absolute difference, and gamma map overlayed with both dose distributions and a cumulative dose histogram. (*See color insert.*)

normalization point by the IMBs used in the treatment plan (65). The parameters imported in the program from the treatment plan are the MU per IMB, shapes and relative weights for each segment (written in the beam shape file that can be exported with the "Export Beam Data" tool from the TPS), and the equivalent depth to the normalization point. The parameters used in the program that are not imported from the treatment plan are the tissue maximum ratio (TMR) data, the output factors (OF), and the off axis ratios (OR). These parameters are taken from the original measured beam data.

First, the contribution of each segment of the IMB to the dose in the normalization point is determined. Therefore the relative weight of that segment (w_i) is defined by subtracting the indices from the successive segments in the exported beam shape file. For each segment the contribution of the segment (con_i) to the normalization point dose is defined by determining if it covers the normalization point fully or partially (e.g., if the normalization point is located in the penumbra of the segment). For the segments that block out the normalization point, the leakage contribution is calculated. By multiplying the relative weight and the contribution with the total amount of MU of the IMB, the amount of MU of the IMB is divided over the contributing segments.

$$MU_i = MU_{IMB} \times w_i \times con_i \tag{1}$$

where MU_{IMB} is the total MU for IMB; MU_i, MU for segment i; w_i, relative weight of segment i; and con_i, contribution of segment i.

The dose that every segment delivers to the normalization point is calculated with this formula:

$$D_i = \frac{MU_i \times TMR_i \times OF_i \times OR_i}{D_{ref} \times CF_{SAD}} \tag{2}$$

where D_i is the dose of segment i; MU_i, MU for segment i; TMR_i, tissue maximum ratio for segment i; OF_i, output factor for segment i; OR_i, off axis ratio for segment i; D_{ref}, total dose in the normalization point; and CF_{SAD}, conversion factor for isocentric treatments.

$$CF_{SAD} = ((SSD_{norm} + d_{norm})/SID)^2. \tag{3}$$

The OF of every segment is defined according the equivalent square field that corresponds with the surface of every segment. The equivalent square field of the segment and the equivalent depth are used for looking up the TMR. To find the OR for every segment, the coordinates of the gravity point of the segment are calculated with respect to the coordinates of the normalization point. The OR for the segment is found in function of the equivalent depth and the distance to the normalization point.

To define the dose delivered by that IMB in the normalization point, the doses of all segments of the IMB are summed together.

This approach of recalculating the dose of an IMB in the normalization point eliminates the use of some parameters calculated by the TPS, such as the leaf sequencing factor (LSF), which is a parameter that is hard to verify, and any inaccuracy introduced by the recalculation of TMR data to PDD data done by the TPS.

The verification of the fluence patterns of the IMBs used in a treatment plan is the third part of the patient specific QA. With the use of the Varis MLC Shaper application, every IMB can be delivered with the adjusted amount of MU to result in a dose appropriate for the detector. The fluence patterns are verified with radiographic film positioned horizontally between solid water phantom at a depth of at least 5.0 cm. This depth is necessary since the beam profile of the Novalis at depth of maximum dose (≈ 1.6 cm) shows a dip in the center of the field of about 5%, which can greatly influence the measured fluence pattern. The measured pattern is compared with the pattern exported from the TPS. This exported fluence pattern is calculated at an entered equivalent depth (the depth used for the measurement) with a resolution of 0.5 mm and saved in a file that is spreadsheet compatible.

Figure 16 shows an example of one of the fluence maps of a prostate treatment. Figure 16A displays the exported fluence pattern; Figure 16B, the fluence pattern obtained with film measurement. Based on a visual comparison of both patterns, one can determine that the correct pattern is deliverd by that specific treatment beam.

Prefraction Verification

The prefraction verification is performed by the radiation technologists by comparing, during the creation of the chart, the shape of the first segment of each treatment beam to the printout of the plan. The DMLC scheme of that treatment beam is simulated with the Varis MLC shaper application to ensure that there are no initial problems in the scheme. Another technologist reviews all chart components to discover possible errors. Prior to the first fraction, a dry-run of the complete treatment is carried out to ensure that there is no equipment collision during the treatment. After the first positioning of the patient (either with the Target Positioner Box for brain or with ExacTrac 3.0/Novalis Body for extracranial treatments), the lasers are defined on the patient's mask or skin to create a visual reference for positioning of the patient during all following fractions of the patient's treatment.

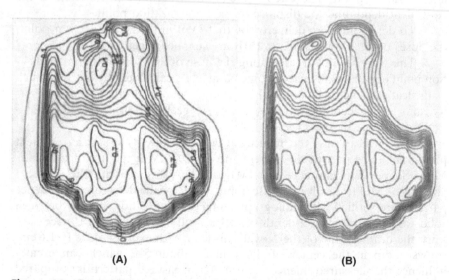

(A)   **(B)**

Figure 16 Comparison of fluence maps for a prostate treatment. (**A**) Fluence pattern exported from treatment planning system. (**B**) Measured fluence pattern.

The UCLA Approach

Rigorous QA measurements are performed to verify the accuracy of dose calculations and radiation delivery of every IMRS computer plan. The Novalis IMRS QA protocol at UCLA has been discussed in detail by Agazaryan et al. (62). A combination of film and ionization chamber measurements is performed to evaluate the absolute dose delivered at isocenter, the composite dose distribution, and the fluence maps of individual fields. Absolute dose and composite dose distributions are measured in one of two phantoms. The Benchmark IMRT Phantom™ (MED-TEC Inc., Orange City, Iowa, U.S.A.) is used for targets that are surrounded by largely homogeneous tissue and the Thorax IMRT Phantom (CIRS Inc., Norfolk, Virginia, U.S.A.) is used for targets that require irradiation through lung. Both phantoms are constructed with multiple axial planes for film measurements and multiple inserts for ionization chambers. After a treatment plan has been completed, Novalis software is used to map all planning parameters from the patient plan to a CT scan of the appropriate phantom. The treatment plan in Figure 17 is shown mapped to the MED-TEC and CIRS phantoms in Figures 18 and 19, respectively. The dose distributions in Figures 17 to 19 differ in appearance because identical treatments are delivered to each object; therefore, the resulting distributions are factors of the object's size, shape, and density. In-phantom dose distributions are exported to a file for digital qualitative comparison with film measurements. The dose to phantom isocenter is a standard printed plan parameter. Composite dose distributions are measured in the axial plane at isocenter using EDR2 film (Eastman Kodak Corp., Rochester, New York, U.S.A.). Exposed films are digitized and compared to the calculated dose distributions with the aid of software developed for this task. The measured and calculated dose distributions

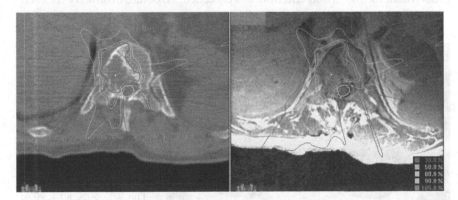

Figure 17   Eight-field IMRS dose distribution for T11 metastasis on fused CT/MR. The 30%, 50%, 80%, 90%, and 105% isodose lines are displayed. The maximum dose is 105%. (*See color insert.*)

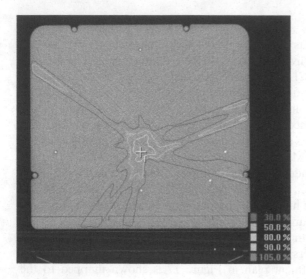

Figure 18 An eight-field IMRT plan mapped to a MED-TEC benchmark phantom. The 30%, 50%, 80%, and 90% isodose lines are displayed. (*See color insert.*)

are superimposed and positioned graphically using shift, rotate, and mirror tools, or by specifying isocenter coordinates and using fiducial marks. Dose difference, distance-to-agreement, and the gamma index (73) (minimum scaled multidimensional distance between a measurement and a calculation point determined in combined dose and physical distance space) are calculated along a specified isodose line. At UCLA, 3% dose difference and 3 mm distance is used as a scaling acceptability criterion. The results of an IMRT dose distribution analysis using the gamma index are shown in Figure 20. The solid black lines represent the calculated 20%, 50%, and 80% isodose lines while colorwash indicates the corresponding isodose lines from film. Dark green spots indicate areas where the 3%/3 mm criterion was exceeded. Absolute dosimetry for each

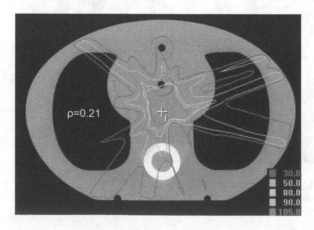

Figure 19 An eight-field IMRT plan mapped to a CIRS thorax phantom. The 30%, 50%, 80%, 90%, and 105% isodose lines are displayed. (*See color insert.*)

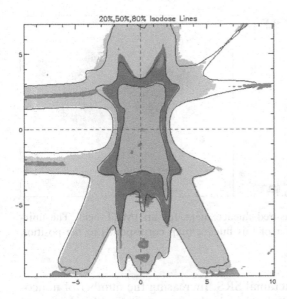

Figure 20 Comparison of a film measurement to calculation using gamma-index analysis for an IMRT dose distribution. Solid black lines are the calculated isodose lines; colorwash is the corresponding isodose lines from film. Dark green are the area where the dose criterian was exceeded. (*See color insert.*)

composite plan is performed using a $0.015\,cm^3$ ionization chamber inserted in the appropriate phantom. Fluence maps of individual fields may be analyzed either qualitatively or quantitatively.

Quantitative film dosimetry analysis was performed for the first 100 IMRT patients at UCLA using the same method described for composite distributions but this was replaced by qualitative visual analysis. It was decided that the information gained by quantitative analysis was not sufficient to justify the significant additional expense in time and film. Currently, individual fields are delivered to a sheet of XV2 film (Eastman Kodak Corp., Rochester, New York, U.S.A.) perpendicular to the beam for visual comparison with Novalis calculated fluence maps as shown in Figure 21.

Dynamic arc or static conformal fields are preferable for more regularly shaped tumors that do not wrap around the cord. Both treatment options are more expedient to deliver, require fewer MU, and require a lesser degree of QA than IMRS. IMRS delivery times are essentially twice as long as dynamic arc and conformal fields because the number of MU is approximately doubled and the beam is switched off between field segments. An increase in delivery time also increases the risk that a patient may move or become too uncomfortable to finish treatment. Additional monitor units result in a proportionally higher whole-body leakage dose to the patient that is considered undesirable. Patient-specific QA measurements are not generally performed for dynamic arc and static field therapy. Commissioning data along with daily, monthly, and annual QA (American Association of Physicists in Medicine, Task Group-40) (74) are considered adequate. The treatment planning principles followed when using dynamic arcs or conformal

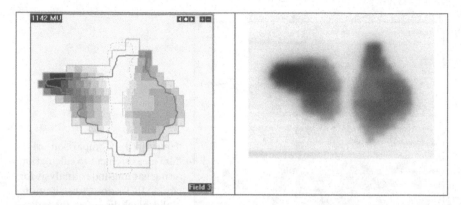

Figure 21 Calculated and measured fluence maps for an IMRT field. The unir-radiated canal through the center of this fluence map corresponds to the position of the spinal cord.

fields are the same as in intracranial SRS. Increasing the number of noncoplanar arc degrees or fixed fields spreads the dose over healthy tissue and provides tighter dose conformation to the target. Dynamic arc plans with three arcs and a 13-field conformal beam plan are shown in Figures 22 and 23, respectively.

Once a treatment plan is finished and approved, it is transferred to the ExacTrac computer in the linac control area. Practical information, such as the height of the isocenter above the treatment table and the distance to

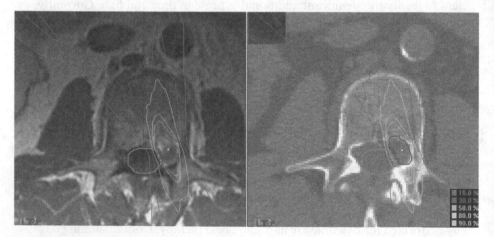

Figure 22 Dynamic arc dose distribution for L2 schwannoma on fused MR/CT. The 10%, 30%, 50%, 80%, and 90% isodose lines are displayed. The maximum dose is 100%. (*See color insert.*)

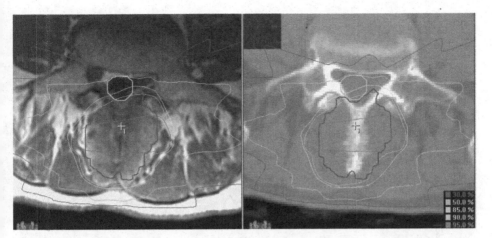

Figure 23 Conformal field dose distribution for L5 metastasis on fused MR/CT. The 30%, 50%, 85%, 90%, and 95%, isodose lines are displayed. The maximum dose is 100%. (*See color insert.*)

ExacTrac reflectors, is recorded as an additional means of patient positioning verification.

TREATMENT OF MOVING TARGETS

The characteristics of a novel, IR-based stereophotogrammetry system for patient positioning (ExacTrac, BrainLAB AG, Heimstetten, Germany) have been described previously (75). Subsequent investigations have been conducted at UCLA to evaluate the capabilities of the Novalis ExacTrac systems for tracking motion in real time (76). For these studies, patients were placed in a supine position and four to seven IR-reflecting markers were attached at various locations on the anterior chest, abdomen, and pelvis. Prior studies have shown that the ExacTrac system is capable of reproducing the position of a point to within 0.2 mm when the markers are attached to a rigid object (75). On a nonrigid object, system accuracy is clearly degraded. However, Wang et al. demonstrated that using an over-determined set of markers (greater than 3) could improve localization accuracy (75). Subjects were monitored for approximately 20 min during which time the three spatial coordinates of each marker were sampled at a rate of 5 Hz. Figure 24 shows the displacement in the vertical direction of three markers affixed to a single volunteer as a function of time. For clarity only the first 60 sec are shown, though the sinusoidal pattern corresponding to respiratory motion, with a frequency of approximately 0.2–0.3 Hz, can be observed for the entire 20-minute study duration.

Additional studies were performed to investigate patient motion characteristics in 3D. In this case, the individual coordinates of the IR

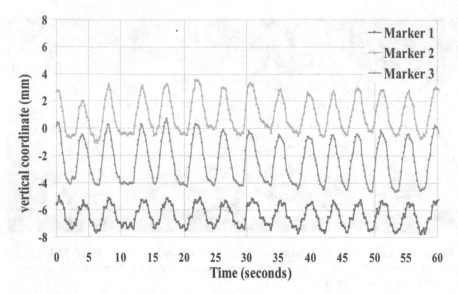

Figure 24 Vertical isocenter displacement as a function of time for three markers attached to the anterior surface of one patient. Though data are shown only for the first 60 sec, the pattern repeats over the entire 20 min. (*See color insert.*)

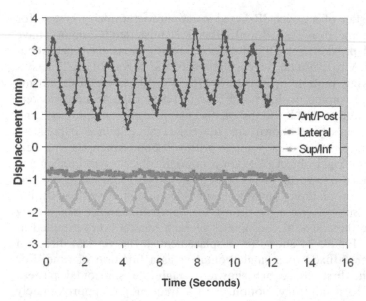

Figure 25 Marker displacement as a function of time for a single marker attached to the anterior surface of one patient. The steresophotogrammetry system is capable of reporting marker coordinates at a frequency of up to 10 Hz. (*See color insert.*)

marker locations were recorded, again at a frequency of 5.0 Hz. Not surprisingly, the greatest motion was observed in the anterior–posterior (A/P) and superior–inferior (S/I) directions; motion in the lateral direction was essentially non-existent. Figure 25 shows an example of the real time, 3D motion characteristics of one patient. Subsequent observations in many patients indicated significant variation of the amplitudes of the A/P motion relative to the S/I motion; that is, different patients breathe in different ways. Based on this observation, the 3D motion function (Eq. 4) described by Baroni et al. (77) was adopted for many subsequent interventions (including gating studies).

$$F = \left\{ \sum_j^N \left[Z_j((x - x_j)^2 + (y - y_j)^2 + (z - z_j)^2)^{\frac{1}{2}} \right]^2 \right\}^{\frac{1}{2}} \quad (4)$$

To facilitate gated delivery using the Novalis, a software module designed at UCLA was added to the ExacTrac control system (78). The module displays

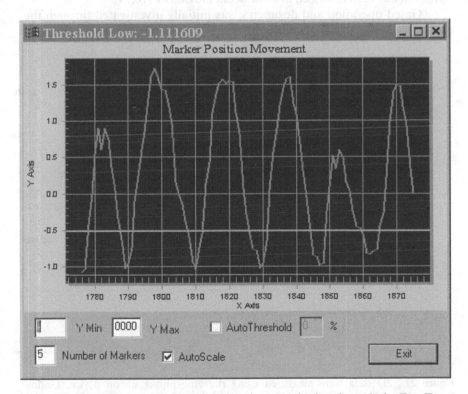

Figure 26 The gating control software monitors respiration through the ExacTrac, calculates and displays ths Baroni F-function, establishes gating windows or thresholds, and triggers the Novalis via the MHOLDOFF/status bit. (*See color insert.*)

the 1D or 3D position of any marker or combinations thereof as well as the
Baroni *F*-function calculated from the marker positions. Gating is facilitated
through the selection of an amplitude-based gating window measured in absolute units of mm, as in percentage of respiratory amplitude, or as a percentage
of duty cycle (Fig. 26). The modified ExacTrac system was used to control the
gated operation through a commercial respiratory gating interface installed on
the Novalis. The gating interface consists of a 25-pin connector inserted between
the dynamic MLC (dMLC) cable and the console backplane. A 3-pin connector
provides access for a 12 V DC signal to the MHOLDOFF/status bit on the console backplane. A beam inhibit is triggered whenever this bit is low. Gating is
controlled through a switching device connected between pins 1 and 2 of the
3-pin connector. An open switch generates an initial position (IPSN) interlock
on the accelerator controller. For dynamic treatments, the absence of an IPSN
interlock ensures that neither the dose nor the collimator position varies more
than 0.2 MU and 0.2 cm, respectively. Thus this interlock halts both radiation
and leaf motion and is cleared immediately upon closure of the switch. System
operation has been described in some detail previously (76,79).

   Gated operation and dosimetry was initially investigated through the
use of a simple signal generator. For open fields, FWHM, flatness and

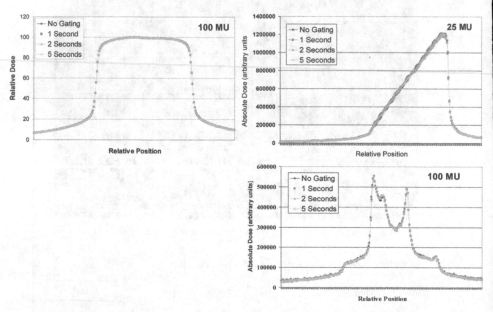

Figure 27 2D data were measured using the amorphous silicon device. Gating
frequencies of 0.2, 0.5, and 1.0 Hz were used in addition to non-gated conditions.
Profiles are shown for an open $10 \times 10 \, \text{cm}^2$ square field (*top left*), a dynamic wedge
(*top right*), and arbitrary intensity map (*bottom right*). (*See color insert.*)

symmetry as well as absolute dose were evaluated as a function of gating frequency (76,79). Images were obtained using film and using an amorphous-silicon (a-Si:H) imaging system (Scanditronix Medical/Wellhöfer Dosimetrie, Uppsala, Sweden). The a-Si:H system consists of a 256×256 flat panel array coupled to a personal computer. The size of individual detector elements is 0.8 mm per pixel. Each image was corrected for pixel sensitivity and the dark signal was removed appropriately based on the number of acquired frames. Dosimetric properties of this device have been described previously (80). Measurements were repeated for MU ranging from 25 to 200 with no gating and at the gating frequencies between 0.2 and 1.0 Hz. At each MU and gating frequency level, non-gated images were subtracted from gated to facilitate analysis. Frames were acquired every 80 msec and integrated to obtain an absolute dose map. Dynamic wedge and IMRT delivery were evaluated in a similar manner. Profiles for an open $10 \times 10 \text{ cm}^2$ field, a dynamic wedge, and an arbitrary IMRT intensity profiles are shown in Figure 27.

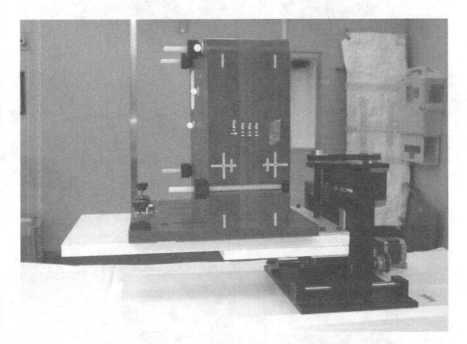

Figure 28 The gating stage was constructed to verify proper operation of the gating system and to evaluate imaging and dosimetry characteristics. The stage accommodates a variety of phantoms; note the infrared makers attached to the MedTec phantom. The stage can be programmed to move in a periodic manner or can accommodate patient-specific motion acquired with the ExacTrac system.

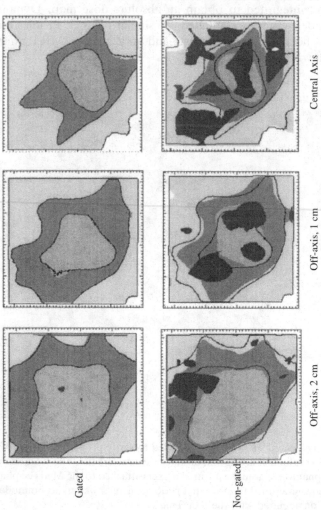

Figure 29 Composite film dosimetry results for a 5-field IMRT liver plan. The dosimetry phantom is moving according to the liver function described by Lujan et al. (81,82). The Novalis is operated in either normal (non-gated) or gated mode. Measurement in colorwash is overlaid on calculations (*solid lines* with the 80%, 50%, and 20% levels displayed). Dark areas indicate poor agreement between measurement and calculation as quantified using the γ index. *Source:* From Ref. 78.

Central Axis

Off-axis, 1 cm

Off-axis, 2 cm

Gated

Non-gated

Using the modified ExacTrac system interfaced to the Novalis, Hugo et al. have subsequently studied gated IMRT dosimetry in a series of extracranial sites (78). For this work, a gating stage (Fig. 28) was constructed to provide respiratory motion to phantoms of various designs. Investigations were performed using several motion patterns including a 1D liver function described by Lujan et al. (81,82) and a 2D lung function. Several treatment locations were considered, including IMRT delivery for a liver target. Figure 29 shows one example of the resulting dosimetric characteristics of gated delivery. This strongly supports the assertion that gated delivery can significantly reduce the dosimetric errors associated with extracranial radiosurgery and IMRT in anatomical sites that may be influenced by respiratory motion. However, as pointed out subsequently by Hugo et al., equal consideration must be given to imaging studies (e.g., gated CT acquisition) if treatment planning is to be performed properly (83).

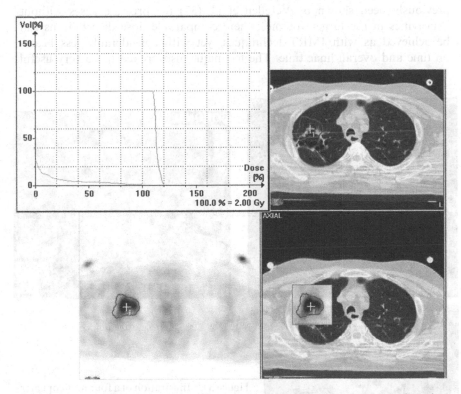

Figure 30 Example of target localization for a lung lesion using co-registration information from PET and CT imaging, with cumulative dose–volume histogram resulting from a coplanar dynamic conformal arc treatment. (*See color insert.*)

CAPABILITIES AND LIMITATIONS OF THE TECHNIQUE

By far the largest limitation of the Novalis system with respect to SBRT is its limited field size of $9.8 \times 10.0 \, \text{cm}^2$. Although arguments can be found to dismiss tumors exceeding these dimensions for aggressive stereotactic radiotherapy or radiosurgery, a work-around has been presented by Linthout et al. (84). This study showed that using partially overlapping intensity-modulated beams assigned to different isocenters to enlarge the treatment region was indeed feasible, and introduced smaller dose inhomogeneities in the resultant dose distribution than in the case of abutting treatment fields. The resultant dose distribution proved to be less sensitive to positioning errors of the used treatment isocenters. Based on film and TLD measurements, the magnitude of the maximum dose inhomogeneities varied by -8% per mm (for shifts ranging from -3 to $+3$ mm).

An interesting feature of the Novalis system is the dynamic conformal arc technique, which is extremely efficient both in treatment planning (see the section on "Treatment Planning and Treatment Delivery"). The latter has previously been shown by Verellen et al. (37) for prostate cases without concavities in the target volume, where comparable dose distributions can be achieved as with IMRT techniques, yet with considerably less beam-on time and overall linac time. The technique also proved to be very useful

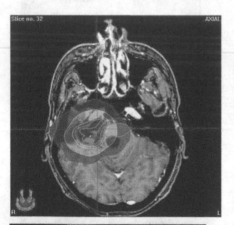
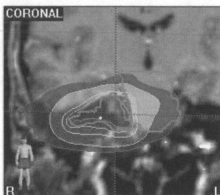
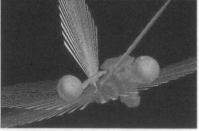

Figure 31 Illustration of a four non-coplanar dynamic conformal arc technique for a meningioma. The 30%, 50%, 90%, 98%, and 100% isodose lines are shown. (*See color insert.*)

for hypofractionated treatment of lung (Fig. 30) and liver metastasis in combination with the high positional accuracy that can be obtained with the ExacTrac 3.0/Novalis Body system. Due to possible collisions with non-zero table angles, the dynamic conformal arc technique for abdominal and pelvic regions is limited to coplanar arcs only. Therefore, the technique is limited in its performance for target volumes that present large concavities. However, for head-and-neck and cranial treatments the dynamic conformal arc technique is capable of competing with most IMRT proposals. Figure 31 illustrates a treatment of a meningioma using four non-coplanar beams, yielding high conformality without compromising dose homogeneity.

ACKNOWLEDGMENTS

The authors wish to express their gratitude to the nurses (for daily setup of the patients) and the members of the respective physics teams for support. In particular Drs. Nadine Linthout, Koen Tournel, and Swana Van Acker who largely collaborated in the work presented here. Dr. Guy Soete is greatly acknowledged for setting up the prostate studies at the AZ-VUB, gathering the raw data (input of some thousands of figures), and making the data available for the author for the pooled analysis. We also thank S. Froehlich and A. Wäckerle and their teams from the BrainLAB company for a very dynamic and interesting collaboration on the Novalis Body project.

REFERENCES

1. International Commission on Radiation Units and Measurements: Prescribing, Recording and Reporting Photon Beam Therapy. ICRU Report 50. Maryland: Bethesda, 1993.
2. International Commission on Radiation Units and Measurements: Prescribing, Recording and Reporting Photon Beam Therapy. ICRU Report 62. Maryland: Bethesda, 1999.
3. Boyer AL, Antonuk L, Fenster A, et al. A review of electronic portal imaging devices (EPIDs) Med Phys 1992; 19(1):1–16.
4. Herman MG, Balter JM, Jaffray DA, et al. Clinical use of electronic portal imaging: Report of AAPM radiation therapy committee task group 58. Med Phys 2001; 28(5):712–737.
5. Munro P. Portal imaging technology: past, present, and future. Semin Radiat Oncol 1995; 5(2):115–133.
6. Alasti H, Petric MP, Catton CN, et al. Portal imaging for evaluation of daily on-line setup errors and off-line organ motion during conformal irradiation of carcinoma of the prostate. Int J Radiat Oncol Biol Phys 2001; 49(3): 869–884.
7. Bel A, Petrascu O, Van de Vondel I, et al. A computerized remote table control for fast online patient repositioning: implementation and clinical feasibility. Med Phys 2000; 27(2):354–358.

8. De Neve W, Van den Heuvel F, Coghe M, et al. Interactive use of on-line portal imaging in pelvic radiation. Int J Radiat Oncol Biol Phys 1993; 25:517–524.

9. De Neve W, Van den Heuvel F, De Beukeleer M, et al. Routine clinical on-line portal imaging followed by immediate field adjustment using a tele-controlled couch. Radiother Oncol 1992; 24:45–54.

10. Ezz A, Munro P, Porter AT, et al. Daily monitoring and correction of radiation field placement using a video-based portal imaging system: a pilot study. Int J Radiat Oncol Biol Phys 1992; 22(1):159–165.

11. Gildersleve J, Dearnaley DP, Evans PM, et al. A randomised trial of patient repositioning during radiotherapy using a megavoltage imaging system. Radiother Oncol 1994; 31(2):161–168.

12. Herman MG, Abrams RA, Mayer RR. Clinical use of on-line portal imaging for daily patient treatment verification. Int J Radiat Oncol Biol Phys 1994; 28(4):1017–1023.

13. Petrascu O, Bel A, Linthout N, et al. Automatic on-line electronic portal image analysis with a Wavelet-based edge detector. Med Phys 2000; 27(2): 321–329.

14. Van de Steene J, Van den Heuvel F, Bel A, et al. Electronic portal imaging with on-line Correction of setup error in thoracic irradiation: clinical evaluation. Int J Radiat Oncol Biol Phys 1998; 40(4):967–976.

15. Van de Vondel I, Coppens L, Verellen D, et al. Microprocessor controlled limitation system for a stand-alone freely movable treatment couch. Med Phys 1998; 25(6):897–899.

16. Van de Vondel I, Coppens L, Verellen D, et al. Remote control for a stand-alone freely movable treatment couch with limitation system. Med Phys 2001; 28(12):2518–2521.

17. Van den Heuvel F, De Neve W, Coghe M, et al. Relations of image quality in on-line portal Images and patient individual parameters for pelvic field radiotherapy. Eur Radiol 1992; 2:433–438.

18. Van den Heuvel F, De Neve W, Verellen D, et al. Clinical implementation of an objective computer-aided protocol for intervention in intra-treatment correction using electronic portal imaging. Radiother Oncol 1995; 35:232–239.

19. Verellen D, De Neve W, Van den Heuvel F, et al. On-line portal imaging: image quality defining parameters for pelvic fields - A clinical evaluation. Int J Radiat Oncol Biol Phys 1993; 27:945–952.

20. Bel A, van Herk M, Lebesque JV. Target margins for random geometrical treatment uncertainties in conformal radiotherapy. Med Phys 1996; 23:1537–1545.

21. Bel A, Vos PH, Rodrigus PT, et al. High-precision prostate cancer irradiation by clinical application on an offline patient setup verification procedure, using portal imaging. Int J Radiat Biol Phys 1996; 35:321–332.

22. van Herk M, Bruce A, Kroes AP, et al. Quantification of organ motion during conformal radiotherapy of the prostate by three dimensional image registration. Int J Radiat Oncol Biol Phys 1995; 33:1311–1320.

23. Yan D, Wong JW, Gustafson G, et al. A new model for "accept or reject strategies" in off-line and on-line megavoltage treatment evaluation. Int J Radiat Oncol Biol Phys 1995; 31:943–952.

24. Yan D, Wong J, Vicini F, et al. Adaptive modification of treatment planning to minimize the deleterious effects of treatment setup errors. Int J Radiat Oncol Biol Phys 1997; 38:197–206.
25. Holupka EJ, Kaplan ID, Burdette EC, et al. Ultrasound image fusion for external beam radiotherapy for prostate cancer. Int J Radiat Oncol Biol Phys 1996; 35(5):975–984.
26. Jaffray DA, Siewerdsen JH, Wong JW, et al. Flat-panel cone-beam computed tomography for image-guided radiation therapy. Int J Radiat Oncol Biol Phys 2002; 53(5):1337–1349.
27. Shirato H, Shimizu S, Shimizu T, et al. Real-time tumor-tracking radiotherapy. Lancet 1999; 353:1331–1332.
28. Shirato H, Shimizu S, Kitamura K, et al. Four-dimensional treatment planning and fluoroscopic real-time tumor tracking radiotherapy for moving tumor. Int J Radiat Oncol Biol Phys 2000; 48(2):435–442.
29. Verellen D, Soete G, Linthout N, et al. Quality assurance of a system for improved target localization and patient set-up that combines real-time infrared tracking and stereoscopic X-ray imaging. Radiother Oncol 2003; 67:129–141.
30. Aoki Y, Akanuma A, Karasawa K, et al. An integrated radiotherapy treatment system and its clinical application. Radiat Med 1987; 5(4):131–141.
31. Takeuchi H, Yoshida M, Kubota T, et al. Frameless stereotactic radiosurgery with mobile CT, mask immobilization and micro-multileaf collimators. Minim Invasive Neurosurg 2003; 46(2):82–85.
32. Soete G, Van de Steene J, Verellen D, et al. Initial clinical experience with infrared reflecting skin markers in the positioning of patients treated by conformal radiotherapy for prostate cancer. Int J Radiat Oncol Biol Phys 2002; 52(3): 694–698.
33. Soete G, Verellen D, Michielsen D, et al. Clinical use of stereoscopic X-ray positioning of patients treated with conformal radiotherapy for prostate cancer. Int J Radiat Oncol Biol Phys 2002; 54(3):948–952.
34. Penney GP, Weese J, Little JA, et al. A comparison of similarity measures for use in 2D–3D medical image registration. IEEE Trans Med Img 1998; 17(4): 586–595.
35. Schell MC, Bova FJ, Larson DA, et al. AAPM Report No. 54, Stereotactic Radiosurgery: Report of AAPM Task Group 42, 1995.
36. Verellen D, Linthout N, Bel A, et al. Assessment of the uncertainties in dose delivery of a commercial system for linac-based stereotactic radiosurgery. Int J Radiat Oncol Biol Phys 1999; 44(2):421–433.
37. Verellen D, Linthout N, Soete G, et al. Considerations on treatment efficiency of different conformal radiation therapy techniques for prostate cancer. Radiother Oncol 2002; 63:27–36.
38. Biggs PJ, Goitein M, Russell MD. A diagnostic X-ray field verification device for a 10 MV linear accelerator. Int J Radiat Oncol Biol Phys 1985; 11: 635–643.
39. Schewe J, Lam K, Balter J, et al. Development of a room-based diagnostic imaging system for use in radiotherapy. Med Phys 1995; 22:939–940.

40. Shiu AS, Hogstrom KR, Janjan NA. Technique for verifying treatment fields using portal images with diagnostic quality. Int J Radiat Oncol Biol Phys 1987; 13:1589–1594.
41. Munro P, Bouius DC. X-ray quantum limited portal imaging using amorphous silicon flat-panel arrays. Med Phys 1998; 25(5):689–702.
42. Motz JW, Danos M. Image information content and patient exposure. Med Phys 1978; 5(1):8–22.
43. Rogers DW. Fluence to dose equivalent conversion factors calculated with EGS3 forelectrons from 100 keV to 20 GeV and photons from 11 keV to 20 GeV. Health Phys 1984; 46(4):891–914.
44. Adler JR, Chang SD, Murphy MJ, et al. The cyberknife: a frameless robotic system for radiosurgery. Stereotact Funct Neurosurg 1997; 69:124–128.
45. Murphy MJ. An automatic six-degree-of-freedom image registration algorithm for image-guided frameless stereotaxic radiosurgery. Med Phys 1997; 24(6): 857–866.
46. Balter JM, Lam KL, Sandler HM, et al. Automated localization of the prostate at the time of treatment using implanted radiopaque markers: technical feasibility. Int J Radiat Oncol Biol Phys 1995; 33(5):1281–1286.
47. Balter JM, Sandler HM, Lam K, et al. Measurement of prostate movement over the course of routine radiotherapy using implanted markers. Int J Radiat Oncol Biol Phys 1995; 31(1):113–118.
48. Gall KP, Verhey LJ. Computer-assisted positioning of radiotherapy patients using implanted radiopaque fiducials. Med Phys 1993; 20(4):1153–1159.
49. Lam KL, Ten Haken RK, McShan DL, et al. Automated determination of patient setup errors in radiation therapy using spherical radio-opaque markers. Med Phys 1993; 20(4):1145–1152.
50. Vigneault E, Pouliot J, Laverdiere J, et al. Electronic portal imaging device detection of radiopaque markers for the evaluation of prostate position during megavoltage irradiation: a clinical study. Int J Radiat Oncol Biol Phys 1997; 37(1):205–212.
51. Song PJ, Washington M, Vaida F, et al. A comparison of four patient immobilization devices in the treatment of prostate cancer patients with three dimensional conformal radiotherapy. Int J Radiat Oncol Biol Phys 1996; 34:213–219.
52. Stroom JC, Koper PC, Korevaar GA, et al. Internal organ motion in prostate cancer patients treated in prone and supine treatment position. Radiother Oncol 1999; 51(3):237–248.
53. Zelefsky MJ, Crean D, Mageras GS, et al. Quantification and predictors of prostate position variability in 50 patients evaluated with multiple CT scans during conformal radiotherapy. Radiother Oncol 1999; 50(2):225–234.
54. Mah D, Freedman G, Milestone B, et al. Measurement of intrafractional prostate motion using magnetic resonance imaging. Iht J Radiat Oncol Biol Phys 2002; 54(2):568–575.
55. Chandra A, Dong L, Huang E, et al. Experience of ultrasound-based daily prostate localization. Int J Radiat Oncol Biol Phys 2003; 56(2):436–447.
56. Little DJ, Dong L, Levy LB, et al. Use of portal images and BAT ultrasonography to measure setup error and organ motion for prostate IMRT: implications for treatment margins. Int J Radiat Oncol Biol Phys 2003; 56(5):1218–1224.

57. Langen KM, Pouliot J, Anezinos C, et al. Evaluation of ultrasound-based prostate localization for image-guided radiotherapy. Int J Radiat Oncol Biol Phys 2003; 57(3):635–644.

58. Van den Heuvel F, Powell T, Seppi E, et al. Independent verification of ultrasound based image-guided radiation treatment; using electronic portal imaging and implanted gold markers. Med Phys 2003; 30(11):2878–2887.

59. Yin FF, Ryu S, Ajlouni M, et al. A technique of intensity-modulated radiosurgery (IMRS) for spinal tumors. Med Phys 2002; 29(2):2815–2822.

60. Cosgrove VP, Jahn U, Phaender M, Bauer S, Budach V, Wurm RE. Commissioning of a micro multi-leaf collimator and planning system for stereotactic radiosurgery. Radiother Oncol 1999; 50:325–336.

61. Xia P, Geis P, Xing L, Ma C, Findley D, Rorster K, Boyer A. Physical characteristics of a miniature multileaf collimator. Med Phys 1996; 26(1):65–70.

62. Agazaryan N, Solberg TD, DeMarco JJ. Patient specific quality assurance for the delivery of intensity modulated radiotherapy. J Appl Clin Med Phys 2003; 4(l):40–50.

63. Llacer J. Inverse radiation treatment planning using the dynamically penalized likelihood method. Med Phys 1997; 24(11):1751–1764.

64. Llacer J, Solberg T, Promberger C. Comparative behaviour of the dynamically penalized likelihood algorithm in inverse radiation therapy planning. Med Phys Biol 2001; 46:2637–2663.

65. Linthout N, Verellen D, Van Acker S, Van de Vondel I, Coppens L, Storme G. Assessment of the acceptability of the Elekta multileaf collimator (MLC) within the Corvus planning system for static and dynamic delivery of intensity modulated beams (IMBs). Radiother Oncol 2002; 63(1):121–124.

66. Low DA, Sohn JW, Klein EE, Markman J, Mutic S, Dempsey JF. Characterization of a commercial multileaf collimator used for intensity modulated radiation therapy. Med Phys 2001; 28(5):752–756.

67. Mohan R, Chui C, Lidofsky L. Differential pencil beam dose computation model for photons. Med Phys 1986; 13(1):64–73.

68. Mohan R, Chui C, Lidofsky L. Energy and angular distributions of photons from medical linear accelerators. Med Phys 1985; 12:592–597.

69. Mohan R, Chui C. Use of fast fourier transforms in calculating dose distributions for irregularly shaped fields for three-dimensional treament planning. Med Phys 1987; 14:70–77.

70. Bortfeld R, Oelfke U, Nill S. What is the optimum leaf width of a multileaf collimator? Med Phys 2000; 27(11):2494–2502.

71. American Association of Physicists in Medicine (AAPM). Radiation treatment planning dosimerty verification. AAPM Report 55 of Task Group 23 of the Radiation Therapy Committee. Woodbury, NY: American Institute of Physics, 1995.

72. International Commission on Radiation Units and Measurements (ICRU). Use of Computers in External Beam Radiotherapy Procedures with High-Energy Photons and Electrons. ICRU Report 42. Baltimore, MD: ICRU, 1987.

73. Low DA, Harms WB, Mutic S, Purdy JA. A technique for the quantitative evaluation of dose distributions. Med Phys 1998; 25(5):656–661.

74. Kutcher GJ, Coia L, Gillin M, Hanson WF, Leibel S, Morton RJ, et al. Comprehensive QA for radiation oncology: report of AAPM radiation therapy committee task group 40. Med Phys 1994; 21(4):581–618.
75. Wang LT, Solberg TD, Medin PM, Boone RA. Infrared patient positioning for stereotactic radiosurgery of extracranial tumors. Comput Biol Med 2001; 31: 101–111.
76. Solberg TD, Paul TJ, Boone RA, Agazaryan NN, Urmanita T, Arellano AR, Llacer J, Fogg R, DeMarco JJ, Smathers JB. Feasibility of Gated IMRT. Proceedings of the World Congress on Medical Physics and Biomedical Engineering, Chicago, IL, July 23–28, 2000.
77. Baroni G, Ferrigno G, Orecchia R, Pedotti A. Real-time three dimensional motion analysis for patient positioning verification. Radiother Oncol 2000; 54:21–27.
78. Hugo GD, Agazaryan N, Solberg TD. An evaluation of gating window size, delivery method, and composite field dosimetry of respiratory-gated MRT. Med Phys 2002; 29:2517–2525.
79. Solberg TD, Paul TJ, Agazaryan NN, Urmanita T, Arellano AR, Llacer J, Boone RA, Fogg R, DeMarco JJ, Chetty I, Smathers JB. Dosimetry of Gated Intensity Modulated Radiotherapy. In: Schlegel W, Bortfeld T, eds. The Use of Computers in Radiation Therapy. Berlin: Springer-Verlag, 2000:286–288.
80. Paul TJ, Solberg TD, Leu MY, Rosemark PJ, Smathers JB. Independent real-time verification of dynamically shaped intensity modulated radiotherapy (IMRT) using an amorphous silicon (a-Si:H) detector array. Med Phys 1999; 26:1065.
81. Lujan AE, Baiter JM, Ten Haken RK. Determination of rotations in three dimensions using two-dimensional portal image registration. Med Phys 1998; 25(5):703–708.
82. Lujan AE, Larsen EW, Baiter JM, Ten Haken RK. A method for incorporating organ motion due to breathing into 3D dose calculations. Med Phys 1999; 26:715–720.
83. Hugo GD, Agazaryan N, Solberg TD. The effects of tumor motion on planning and delivery of respiratory-gated MRT. Med Phys 2003; 30:1052–1066.
84. Linthout N, Verellen D, Van Acker S, et al. Dosimetric evaluation of partially overlapping intensity modulated beams using dynamic mini-multileaf collimation. Med Phys 2003; 30(5):847–855.

4

Whole-Body Radiosurgery with the CyberKnife®

Achim Schweikard

Luebeck University, Luebeck, Germany

Hiroya Shiomi

Osaka University Hospital, Osaka, Japan

Minaro Uchida and John R. Adler

Stanford University Medical Center, Stanford, California, U.S.A.

INTRODUCTION

In the 1950s, Professor Lars Leksell of the Karolinska Institute in Sweden coined the term "radiosurgery" to define a neurosurgical procedure that combined precision targeting with a large number of cross-fired beams of ionizing radiation. By directing a very large dose of highly collimated radiation at a discrete location in the brain, the objective of Leksell's operation was to make a lesion (ablate brain tissue) without "cutting," arguably thereby achieving the ultimate in minimally invasive surgery. At the time (1950s and 1960s) the clinical motivation for such a procedure was a class of operations broadly referred to as functional neurosurgery, which includes thalamotomy for the tremor of Parkinson's disease and anterior capsulotomy for treating obsessive–compulsive disorder.

Leksell investigated multiple irradiation technologies for fulfilling his vision, including linear accelerator and heavy particle based concepts, before focusing his development efforts on the radioactive cobalt-based

CyberKnife®, Accuray, Sunnyvale, California, U.S.A.

GammaKnife®, (ELEKTA AB, Stockholm, Sweden). The eventual design of this instrument was such that it could only be applied to the brain. The first GammaKnife was built in the late 1970s, and has since undergone a series of changes to accommodate a gradual evolution in usage. Leksell always envisioned that his system would be used for non-invasive functional neurosurgery. However, in the 1970s, computed tomography (CT) scanning arrived and, with it, the opportunity to visualize mass lesions in the brain, especially tumors. Quickly the role of the GammaKnife and the principles of radiosurgery were redirected to facilitate the treatment of brain tumors and vascular malformations. By incorporating the effectiveness and minimally invasive nature of radiosurgery into the neurosurgical armamentarium, the past 20 years have witnessed a revolution in the management of many neurosurgical procedures. Over this period new radiosurgical technologies evolved, including more spatially accurate linear accelerator-based methods (compared to Leksell's earliest experience) and heavy particle beams. Furthermore, the influence of radiosurgery on neurosurgery continues to expand as indications and treatment parameters are refined.

Technological Limitations

The near ubiquity of radiosurgery within modern neurosurgical practices, there are inherent shortcomings to present-day technology that limit potential new applications. In particular, the GammaKnife and other related linac-based technologies all require stereotactic frames for accurate beam targeting. Such skeletal fixation causes enough pain to preclude flexible treatment fractionation. Since the principle of administering a dose of radiation over more than one session is an essential element of all modern radiation oncology, this limitation is not trivial; basic radiobiology and clinical experience have demonstrated the superiority of using fractionation to treat most malignant tumors and/or lesions involving critical yet sensitive anatomic structures, such as the optic apparatus. Furthermore, current radiosurgical instruments are isocentric-based, constraining all beams to converge on a common point. This design restricts some types of more flexible and conformal treatment planning. While these limitations by themselves might not serve as an impetus for designing a new concept in radiosurgery, an even greater rationale is provided by the opportunities to perform radiosurgery outside the brain.

At its core, radiosurgery involves two elemental principles: (a) precision targeting and (b) the application of ablative doses of radiation using limited if any fractionation. From a biologic and therapeutic perspective such principles could be of generic interest to all surgeons. Therefore, to address the above limitations and meet the needs of potential new extracranial therapies, a system for image-guided robotic radiosurgery was implemented.

Why Image-Guided Robotic Radiosurgery?

In developing a system for extracranial targeting and treatment, it was critical to begin by defining the specific clinical rationale for such a technology. Not surprisingly it was decided that the specifications for an extracranial radiosurgical system should be consistent with Leksell's original definition for "radiosurgery." In particular, such an instrument should enable the highest possible targeting accuracy (essentially near millimeter RMS errors) and enable ablative doses of radiation to be administered with a maximal use of solid angle. It is important to emphasize that the intent was to administer ablative doses of radiation and thereby enable surgeons to replace open surgical resection or invasive tissue destruction with a non-invasive procedure. This radiosurgical objective is to be distinguished from precision radiation therapy and intensity-modulated therapy (IMRT), where accuracy is less important, and the principles of conventional fractionation play a more important role in clinical outcome. An instrument utilizing image-guided robotics seemed uniquely able to achieve these objectives.

By extrapolating from the huge prior experience with brain radiosurgery, various surgical specialists are finally in a position to develop new extracranial radiosurgical applications for the CyberKnife (Accuray, Sunnyvale, California, U.S.A.). However, similar to other forms of surgery, the limits of human operative capability are not defined by tools alone. The imagination and diligence with which these instruments are directed towards relieving human suffering remain critical aspects of improving patient outcome.

This chapter gives a brief overview of the CyberKnife technology, and then presents two of the most innovative technical components of the CyberKnife: the planning sub-system and the motion tracking system for respiration compensation.

Related Work

Although radiosurgery is rapidly changing the scope of surgery, the vast majority of therapeutic irradiation is administered as part of a regimen of conventionally fractionated external beam radiotherapy. Medical linear accelerators (linac systems), which use a gantry construction for moving the linear accelerator, are the standard technology for delivering conventional radiotherapy. However, this mechanical construction was designed more than 40 years ago to deliver radiation from a limited number of directions during a single treatment. Meanwhile, its ability to compensate for target motion during treatment is inherently very limited. Several additional factors limit the accuracy of gantry-based systems, most notably mechanical flex and lack of fully computerized position/motion control.

Conventional linac-systems have six motion axes, which are sufficient to target any point within a given workspace from any angle. However, four of the six axes of the linac-gantry are built into the patient table. Compensating for respiratory motion is difficult with this construction. Motions of the patient table (especially lateral table tilting) are likely to cause involuntary counter-motion of the patient. Such involuntary motions lead to muscle contraction, changes in breathing patterns, and may cause substantial additional inaccuracy. Given the kinematic and size limitations of such systems, most researchers have investigated methods for motion detection rather than active motion tracking.

Respiratory gating is a technique that attempts to address the problem of breathing motion with conventional linac-based radiation therapy. Gating techniques do not directly compensate for breathing motion; that is, the therapeutic beam is not moved during activation. Instead the beam is switched off whenever the target is outside a predefined window. One of the disadvantages of gating techniques is the increase in treatment time. A second problem is the inherent inaccuracy of such an approach. One must ensure that the beam activation cycles are long enough to obtain a stable therapeutic beam.

Kubo and Hill (1) compared various external sensors (breath temperature sensor, strain gauge, and spirometer) with respect to their suitability for respiratory gating. By measuring breath temperature, it is possible to determine whether the patient is inhaling or exhaling. Kubo and Hill verified that frequent activation/deactivation of the linear accelerator does not substantially affect the resulting dose distribution. However, the application of such a technique still requires a substantial safety margin for the following reason: the sensor method only yields relative displacements during treatment, but does not report and update the exact absolute position of the target during treatment.

Tada et al. (2) report on the use an external laser range sensor in connection with a linac-based system for respiratory gating. This device is used to switch the beam off whenever the sensor reports that the respiratory cycle is close to maximal inhalation or maximal exhalation. However, typical variations in the respiratory motion patterns of 1–2 cm for the same patient (in pediatrics), and in the duration of a single respiratory cycle of 2–5 sec are reported in Ref. 3.

As noted above, respiratory motion is difficult to track with conventional linac-based systems, and the accuracy of such an approach would inherently be very limited. In contrast, modem robotic manufacturing relies on highly accurate motion control and high unit numbers. In the CyberKnife system, the radiation source (6 MV linear accelerator) is mounted on a robotic arm that can move with six degrees-of-freedom.

Recent research has extended CyberKnife brain and spine radiosurgery in such a way that respiratory motion can be compensated for by active motion of the robot. The basic advantage of this approach is that it is now possible for the robotic arm to track the motion of a lesion, and is therefore not necessary to gate the treatment beam.

To enable dynamic respiratory tracking, the stereo X-ray imaging system of the CyberKnife is combined with infrared tracking. X-ray imaging senses internal anatomy, while infrared tracking provides information on the motion of the patient surface. While X-ray imaging gives very accurate information about the internal location of a target, it is very difficult to obtain real-time motion information from X-ray imaging alone. In contrast, the motion of the patient surface can be tracked in real-time with commercial infrared position sensors. The central idea of our approach is to use a series of images from both sensors (infrared and X-ray), synchronizing one with the other. Thus, both X-ray image pairs and infrared data have time stamps. From a series of sensor readings and corresponding time-stamps, we can determine a motion pattern. This pattern correlates external to internal motion, and is both patient and site specific. A series of preclinical and clinical trials has since verified that we can accurately infer the placement of an internal target from a precalculated (and continuously updated) motion pattern.

SYSTEM OVERVIEW

Figure 1 shows the components of the CyberKnife. A robot arm moves a linear accelerator generating a 6 MV radiation beam. An X-ray camera system (two X-ray cameras with nearly orthogonal visual axes) records the position of natural or artificial markers (i.e., bony landmarks or implanted gold fiducials). An infrared tracking system records the external motion of the patient's abdomen.

For treatments of brain or spinal lesions, no respiration compensation is needed. In this case, infrared tracking is not active and the position of the target is computed from the stereo X-ray images alone. Two nearly orthogonal X-ray images show the position of the patient's skull within a carefully calibrated imaging space. Meanwhile, the position of the target is known with respect to the skull from the tomographic images. To compute the exact intratreatment position of the target, a registration step is necessary. This step spatially correlates the intratreatment (live) X-ray images to the pretreatment three-dimensional (3D) tomographic images. To this end, synthetic X-ray images are computed from the CT scans, for a series of positions and angles. Live X-ray images are then compared to synthetic images, to find the best matching pair of synthetic images. Because each synthetic image pair has one and only one position and angle associated with it, we can infer angular or positional displacement of the patient's skull, and hence perform the registration.

INVERSE PLANNING

During treatment the linear accelerator is moved in as step-and-shoot fashion to a series of fixed points in space. At each such point (also called node), the beam is activated for a certain duration. This duration determines the weight of each beam. Notice that we assume each node to represent a fixed

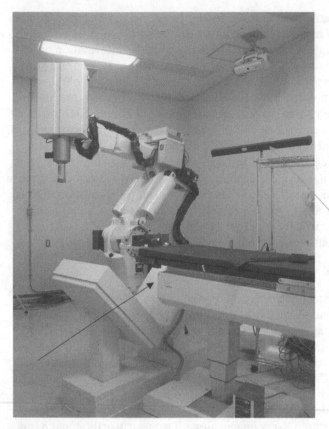

Figure 1 CyberKnife® system overview. (The arrows are pointing at the infrared tracking system camera bar and the left X-ray camera detector). Infrared tracking is used to record external motion of the patient's abdominal and chest surface. Stereo X-ray imaging is used to record the 3D position of internal markers (gold fiducials) at fixed time intervals during treatment. A robotic arm moves the beam source to actively compensate for respiratory motion.

position in space. However, this position may be adjusted during the respiration tracking process. Thus, at each node, the robotic arm performs very small corrective motions to compensate for respiratory motion when this compensatory system is activated.

To make full use of the kinematic flexibility of the six degree-of-freedom robotic arm, an inverse planning system has been designed. The planning process consists of two steps:

1. select nodes (beam configurations, positions, and orientations of the beam source),
2. adjust beam weights (i.e., activation durations of the beam).

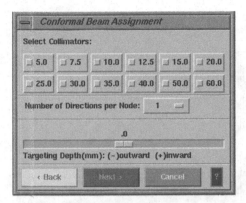

Figure 2   Collimator selection menu.

Phase 1: Node Selection

In phase 1, it is assumed that the tumor has been delineated previously in the tomographic image series. This results in a series of polygonal contours, where one contour corresponds to each tomographic slice. Furthermore, a collimator size is selected. The beam is cylindrical with collimator sizes ranging from 5 to 60 mm (Fig. 2). After delineation of the tumor, the process of beam selection is fully automatic. Up to 1200 beams are selected; greater numbers of beams are used for more complex, non-convex tumor shapes, or tumors near critical healthy structures. The rationale for the method underlying beam selection for targets of arbitrary shape is a mathematical extension of the (ideal) process that would be used if the tumor were strictly spherical. After beam selection, the user can interactively modify selected beam directions. For the principles underlying the automatic beam selection, the reader is referred to Ref. 4.

Phase 2: Beam Weighting

In phase 2, it is assumed the beam selection process has been completed. As noted above, this process is fully automatic once the tumor has been delineated in the tomographic images. To compute the optimal weights of the individual beams, it is necessary to delineate critical structures in the vicinity of the tumor. Furthermore, it is necessary to specify dose constraints. To this end, upper and lower threshold values for the target region are entered. Furthermore, threshold values are also entered for the critical regions, and for individual beams. After specifying the constraints, the process of computing weights is fully automatic and based on linear programming. Linear programming is a technique that has been proposed by several authors (5) in the context of radiation therapy planning due to the completeness properties of this method. "Completeness" in this context means that the

(A)

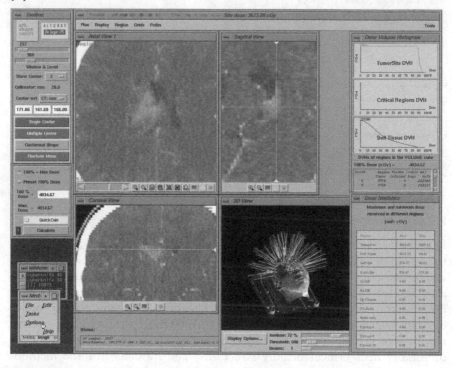

Figure 3A–C Inverse planning for robotic radiosurgery. (**A**) (*See color insert.*) Manual delineation of the target. Beam directions for optimized treatment of specific tumor shape (up to 1200, *lower left corner*) are computed automatically by the inverse planning system. (*Continued*)

algorithm is guaranteed to find appropriate weight distributions exactly fulfilling the given constraints, if such a distribution exists. Extensions of this method are described in Refs. 4 and 6.

An example for the planning process is given in Figure 3A–C.

RESPIRATION TRACKING

Tumors in the chest and the abdomen move during respiration. The ability of conventional radiation therapy systems to compensate for respiratory motion by moving the radiation source is inherently limited. Because safety margins currently used in radiation therapy increase the radiation dose by a very large amount, an accurate tracking method for following the motion of the tumor is of utmost clinical relevance. To track respiratory motion, the following basic method is used (7). Prior to treatment, small gold markers visible in X-ray images

(B)

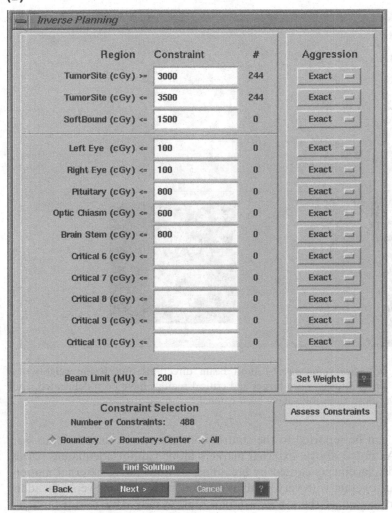

Figure 3 **(B)** Computing beam weights with linear programming. Dose threshold selection menu. (*Continued*)

aɪe anchored in proximity to the target organ. Stereo X-ray imaging is used during treatment to determine the precise spatial location of the implanted gold markers via automated image analysis. Using stereo X-ray imaging, precise marker positions can be established once every 10 sec. This time interval is too long to accurately follow respiratory motion.

In contrast, external markers (placed on the patient's skin) can be tracked automatically with optical methods at very high speed. Updated

(C)

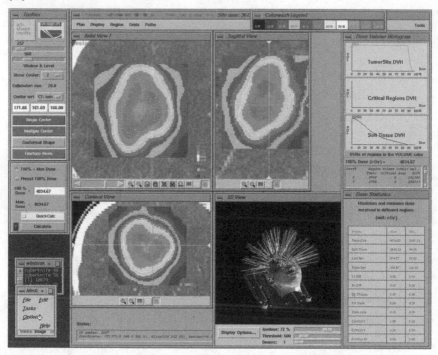

Figure 3 (C) (*See color insert.*) Both beam directions and beam weights are computed automatically, once target and critical regions have been delineated, and upper/lower dose thresholds have been entered.

positions can be reported to the control computer more than 60 times per second. As noted above, external markers alone cannot adequately reflect internal displacements caused by breathing motion. Large external motion may occur together with very small internal motion, and vice versa. In addition the direction of the visible external motion may deviate substantially from the direction of the target motion (Fig. 4).

Because neither internal nor external markers alone are sufficient for accurate tracking of lesions near the diaphragm, X-ray imaging is synchronized with optical tracking of external markers. The external markers are small active infrared emitters (IGT Flashpoint 5000, Boulder, Colorado, U.S.A.) attached to a vest. Notice that the individual markers are allowed to change their relative placement. The first step during treatment is to compute the exact relationship between internal and external motion, using a series of time-stamped snapshots showing external and internal markers simultaneously.

Although infrared tracking is combined with X-ray imaging, it is not necessary to detect the position of the infrared emitters in an X-ray image. Time

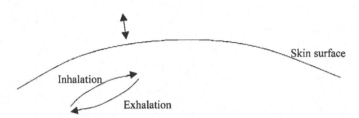

External Motion

Skin surface

Inhalation

Exhalation

Figure 4 Tracking of external markers/motion curves corresponding to inhalation and exhalation. While external motion is in an anterior/posterior direction, the internal motion of the target may be in a left/right direction.

stamps permit the positions of both marker types to be established simultaneously, and can therefore be used to determine the pattern of respiratory motion. Such patterns are patient specific and can be updated during treatment.

During the initialization stage of the procedure, a deformation model is computed, which describes the correlation between internal and external motion. To obtain the deformation model, we proceed as follows. A series of (stereo) X-ray image pairs of the target region are taken while the patient is breathing. When activating the X-ray sources, we record the point in time

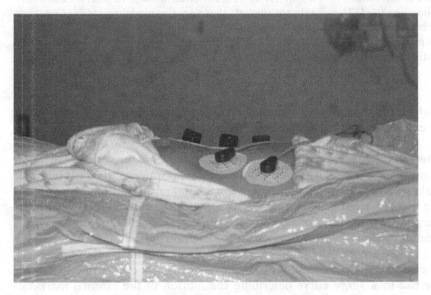

Figure 5 Infrared emitters attached to the patient's chest.

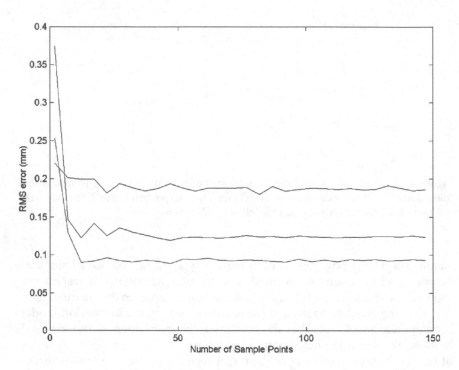

Figure 6 Dependency between number of model points in a correlation model and tracking accuracy. Test data were taken with an infrared tracking system alone, where a correlation model correlating external chest motion to external abdomen motion was used. The experiment suggests that very few model points are necessary to obtain an accurate model. The figure shows data for three different infrared emitters placed on a test person's chest, while inferring chest position from abdominal position alone via correlation.

at which the sources were activated. We also record the current position of the external sensors at the time of X-ray image acquisition.

Assume five X-ray image pairs have been taken in this way. These images have a sequence order, namely the sequence in which they were taken. In each image, we compute the absolute position of the gold internal markers. Note that we obtain their exact spatial position, as the X-ray imaging reports stereo images. Consider the first of the gold markers. By linear interpolation, the positions of this marker determine a curve in space. We compute such an interpolation curve for each of the gold markers.

There are six external markers and we compute the center of mass for these markers. During a motion, the series of center points thus obtained give rise to a single curve describing the motion of the external markers. As the treatment proceeds the curves for internal and external markers are used in the following way. A new pair of X-ray images is acquired every 10 sec. Let there be a time point at which no X-ray image is taken. We must then determine a predicted target placement based on the given deformation model. At the given time point, we read the external sensor positions. After computing the center of mass for the external markers, we can locate the closest point on the curve for the external motion in our deformation model. By linear interpolation this point determines corresponding points on the curves for the internal markers.

Linear interpolation extends directly to the case, where one or both curves are not line segments. In this case, points are connected by line segments, and we determine the lengths of the line segments in each curve. The parameter interval for each curve is then partitioned according to these lengths and the interpolation proceeds as above. This interpolation is sufficiently fast to update the given deformation model as the treatment proceeds. Specifically, as new X-ray images and matching sensor readings become available, the curves for the internal markers are updated. The updating scheme will be described in more detail in subsequent sections.

A difficulty arising in this context is to distinguish between voluntary patient movement and breathing motion. Clearly, the two types of motion must be processed in different ways. Patient movement can occur, e.g., as a result of muscle relaxation, sneezing, or voluntary movement. A patient shift must cause a shift of the deformation model, i.e., each curve must be shifted. In contrast, normal breathing should not shift these curves.

At first glance, distinguishing the two types of motion may seem difficult. However, the internal markers represent a "ground truth." Thus, our deformation model gives a predicted position for the internal markers, based on the position of the external markers. The location of internal markers can be predicted not only for time points in between X-ray imaging, but also for the times at which images are taken. Any deviation (exceeding a fixed threshold value δ) between predicted and actual placement is thus regarded as displacement caused by patient motion. Thus, the above linear interpolation scheme yields a predicted placement for each internal marker This predicted placement is a point in space. We compute the distance from the actual placement of this point. If this distance is larger than δ, the beam is switched off. A new deformation model is computed after respiration has stabilized.

Small values for δ give better accuracy but enforce frequent re-computations of the deformation model. Given differences in patterns of breathing between patients, it is reasonable to determine an appropriate value for during initialization, when the patient is asked to breathe regularly. The deviations observed during this interval of regular breathing (here for the external sensors alone) are used to determine δ.

A practical improvement of this technique for detecting patient motion allows for updating the deformation model without interrupting the treatment. Assume the deformation model consists of five X-ray image pairs together with matching infrared position data. Because we take a new pair of X-ray images at fixed time intervals during treatment (i.e., every 10 sec), the deformation model can be updated continuously in the following way. A table of position data with five entries is maintained. Each entry has a time stamp. In this table, we remove the earliest entry whenever a new set of position data (image pair with matching infrared positions) becomes available. The computation of the deformation model via linear interpolation can be carried out in real time after each update of the table data. This method can compensate both for systematic drift of the patient position and for small changes in the pattern of respiration during treatment.

CLINICAL TRIALS

Figure 7 shows representative results for respiration tracking in a clinical case. The figure shows the total correlation error. Thus, based on the

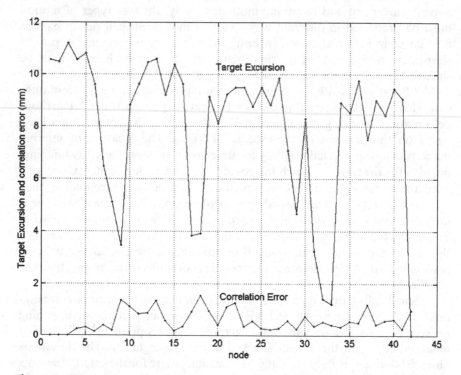

Figure 7 Total target excursion (*top curve*), and correlation error (*bottom curve*) in millimeters for a clinical case. The x axis gives the treatment beam direction number (X-ray live shot number); the y axis gives the error in millimeters.

(A)   **(B)**

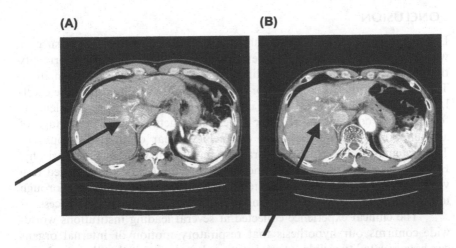

Figure 8 Treatment of a hepatocellular carcinoma (HCC) with fiducial-based respiration compensation as described in the text. (**A**) Before treatment; (**B**) 3 months after treatment. Total treatment time was 40 min per fraction for three fractions with 80 beam directions and 39 Gy.

correlation model, we compute the current position of the target based on the external infrared sensor signal alone. At this same time point, we also acquire a pair of X-ray images. We then plot the distance in millimeters from the placement inferred by the correlation model and the actual placement determined from the implanted fiducial markers in the image. The top curve in this figure shows the corresponding target excursion.

(A)   **(B)**

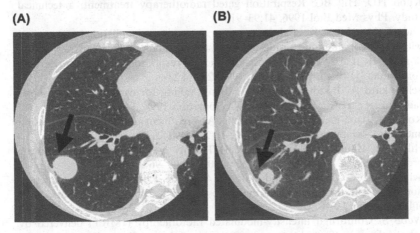

Figure 9 Treatment of an adenocarcinoma with fiducial-based respiration tracking (Osaka University Hospital), three fractions at 39 Gy.

CONCLUSION

Experience reported in the literature (8) suggests that robotic radiosurgery with cylinder collimators can achieve distributions with higher conformality than conventional multileaf collimators or micro multileaf collimators. There are two practical reasons for this: (a) Cylinder collimators have excellent penumbra characteristics. In contrast, penumbra remains problematic for multileaf collimators. (b) For spherical targets (a large percentage of all tumors), cylinder collimators can achieve near optimal distributions. The system selects beam configurations and beam weights automatically. However, beam configurations and input thresholds may be adjusted in a variety of ways. Selecting adequate parameters requires skill and thorough understanding of the principles underlying the inverse planning process.

The clinical experience collected at several leading institutions worldwide confirms our hypothesis that respiratory motion of internal organs can be correlated to visible external motion. It is necessary that the correlation model be updated automatically during treatment. To update the correlation model we use intratreatment stereo X-ray images. The clinical experience further suggests that any dose margin placed around a tumor to compensate for respiratory motion can be reduced by a very substantial amount. Because dose is directly proportional to volume, this could allow for higher doses in the tumor, and much lower doses in surrounding healthy tissue. For a variety of cancers with grim prognoses, this robotic technique could thus lead to far-reaching improvements in clinical outcome.

REFERENCES

1. Kubo HD, Hill BC. Respiration gated radiotherapy treatment: a technical study. Phys Med Biol 1996; 41:93–91.
2. Tada T, Minakuchi K, et al. Lung cancer: intermittent irradiation synchronized with respiratory motion—results of a pilot study. Radiology 1998; 207(3):779–783.
3. Sontag MR, Lai ZW, et al. Characterization of respiratory motion for pedriatic conformal 3D therapy. Med Phys 1996; 23:1082.
4. Schweikard A, Bodduluri M, Adler JR. Planning for camera-guided robotic radiosurgery. IEEE Trans Robotics Automation 1998; 14(6):951–962.
5. Rosen II, Lane RG, Morrill SM, Belli JA. Treatment plan optimization using linear programming. Med Phys 1991; 18(2):141–152.
6. Hilbig M, Hanne R, Schweikard A. IMRT-Inverse planning based on linear programming. Z Medizinische Physik 2002; 12:89–96.
7. Schweikard A, Glosser G, Bodduluri M, Adler JR. Robotic motion compensation for respiratory motion during radiosurgery. J Comput-Aided Surg 2000; 5(4):263–277.
8. Webb S. Conformal intensity-modulated radiotherapy (IMRT) delivered by robotic linac-conformality versus efficiency of dose delivery. Phys Med Biol 2000; 45:1715–1730.

9. Bzostek A, Inoesco G, Carrat L, Barbe C, Chavanon O, Troccaz J. Isolating moving anatomy in ultrasound without anatomical knowledge: application to computer-assisted pericardical punctures. Medical image-computation and computer-assisted intervention—MICCAI 98, Lecture Notes in Computer Science 1998; 1496:1041–1048.

10. Carol MP, Targovnik H 3D planning and delivery system for optimized conformal therapy. Int J Radiat Oncol Biol Phys 1992; 24:885–887.

11. Hofstetter R, Slomoczykowski M, Sati M, Nolte LP. Flouroscopy as an imaging means for computer-assisted surgical navigation. Comput-Aided Surg 1999; 4:65–76.

12. Lujan AE, Larsen EW, Balter JM, Haken RKT. A method for incorporating organ motion due to breathing into 3D dose calculations. Med Phys 1999; 26(5):715–720.

13. Morrill SM, Langer M, Lane RG. Real-time couch compensation for intra-treatment organ motion: theoretical advantages. Med Phys 1996; 23:1083.

14. Winston KR, Lutz W. Linear accelerator as a neurosurgical tool for stereotactic radiosurgery. Neurosurgery 1988; 22(3):454–464.

5

Serial Tomotherapeutic Approaches to Stereotactic Body Radiation Therapy

Bill Salter

Department of Radiation Oncology, The University of Texas Health Science Center, and Cancer Therapy and Research Center, San Antonio, Texas, U.S.A.

Martin Fuss

Department of Radiation Oncology, The University of Texas Health Science Center, San Antonio, Texas, U.S.A.

SYSTEM DESCRIPTION AND OPERATION

Serial tomotherapy represents an unusual delivery technique relative to the more traditional approaches typically employed in radiation therapy. As a result, the specifics of this approach are less familiar to many in our field. Most notably, the system is unusual in that it uses a *combination* of a moving gantry and intensity modulation. While many static-gantry systems are capable of delivering intensity modulated treatments, tomotherapy takes advantage of both the semi-infinite number of angles of approach afforded by an arcing method of delivery, and the ability to create convex-shaped distributions of dose, which comes from modulation of intensity. The Peacock system delivers its intensity modulated pencil beams through a binary collimator called the MIMiC (NOMOS Corp., Crannberry Township, Pennsylvania, U.S.A.) (Fig. 1A). The collimator is binary, i.e., each vane of the collimator can assume one of only two states, either opened or closed. Unlike so-called sliding leaf collimators, which can also be used to deliver

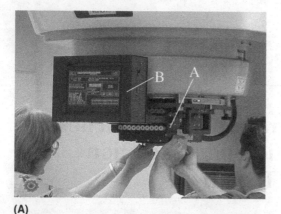

(A)

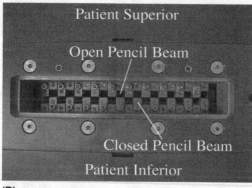

(B)

Figure 1   (A) Image depicting MIMiC (*A* in figure) and controller computer (*B* in figure). (B) Image looking into mouth or opening of MIMiC. Vanes are arranged in a checkerboard (opened and closed) pattern.

intensity modulated treatments, the MIMiC's leaves are pneumatically driven in very rapid fashion between these open and closed states, with typical open/close times of less than 100 ms. Figure 1B depicts a view of the collimator looking into the mouth or opening from which radiation emerges. The collimator consists of two rows of 20 tungsten vanes (40 total vanes) which are 8 cm in thickness. The leaves are stair-stepped in design, creating an interdigitation of adjacent vanes that allows for very low interleaf leakage values. Leaf/pencil-beam widths are constant at 10 mm and the pencil beam length can be varied among three user-selected dimensions (4, 8.5, and 17 mm) by varying the physical or effective length of retraction of the vane (1). During the treatment planning phase, pencil beam dimensions are chosen appropriate to the treated lesion's size and irregularity of shape. Modulation of intensity is accomplished by varying the amount of time that each pencil beam is open from a given gantry angle, and the fluence map for all pencil beams may be updated as frequently as every 5° of gantry rotation. Each of the 40 pencil beams are controlled independently from the others, thus allowing each arc of the gantry to deliver two completely different and separate fluence maps, corresponding to each of the two rows of vanes, each of which can be tailored to the unique shape of the target on that particular treatment slice. For the 340° arcs (net 320°) of radiation delivery typically used at our center, this allows for 128 different pencil beams for each delivered gantry arc, or 64 per treated slice of the target. This can be contrasted with typical values for static gantry approaches of 5–7, equivalent to the number of static gantry ports utilized. Because serial tomotherapy employs an arcing rotation of the slit-like MIMiC collimator, each rotation of the gantry treats a "slice" of the patient, much like axial computed tomography (CT) images a slice of the patient. Because of this similarity, serial tomotherapy has often been likened to CT image acquisition. A key difference between the two approaches is that for CT acquisition the input beam fluence is uniform, for the purpose of measuring the exiting non-uniformity as an indication of the tissue density encountered by the beam, whereas for intensity modulated radiation therapy (IMRT) the input beam fluence is intentionally non-uniform, for the alternate purpose of producing a uniform and conformal buildup of dose within the target. Because each rotation of the gantry typically treats a subsection of the target of thickness equal to $2 \times 4\,mm = 8\,mm$, $2 \times 8.5\,mm = 17\,mm$, or $2 \times 17\,mm = 34\,mm$, depending on the selected pencil beam size, the treatment table/patient must be sequentially, or serially, incremented following each delivered arc. Such increments must be performed very precisely to ensure an accurate abutment of each adjacent treatment slice to avoid the creation of hot or cold strips between the delivered slices. Gantry rotations are performed and the table is subsequently incremented until the entire target has been treated. Because current linear-accelerator-inherent couch positioning systems are not typically capable of positioning the patient to the precision required for serial tomotherapy (required accuracy $\leq 0.1\,mm$), the vendor supplies a system referred to as either the Crane® or AutoCrane® (NOMOS Corp., Crannberry Township, Pennsylvania, U.S.A.) (2) for performing this function (Fig. 2). The device performs the precise indexing of the patient necessary for serial tomotherapy, and is available in an automated version that can be controlled at the treatment console, obviating the need to return to the treatment vault for between-arc incrementing of the patient. The serial tomotherapeutic delivery approach has been shown to be capable of producing very conformal dose distributions (1–4).

PATIENT IMMOBILIZATION AND ALIGNMENT

A prerequisite to the utilization of conformal distributions of dose is the use of accurate patient fixation and alignment methods. The challenges of patient fixation and alignment that are unique to extracranial applications

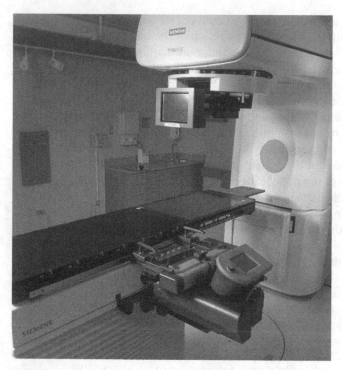

Figure 2 AutoCrane® mounted on linear accelerator table. The AutoCrane performs remote incrementing of the treatment couch and the patient.

have been discussed in previous chapters. The methods employed at our particular institution for serial tomotherapeutic delivery of extracranial stereotactic treatments will now be described.

Patient alignment and immobilization is facilitated through the use of a stereotactic, whole-body, double-vacuum-assisted immobilization system (BodyFIX, Medical intelligence, Schwabmünchen, Germany). Comprehensive characterizations of the repositioning accuracy of the system have been previously published (4,5).

In general, the system consists of a composite material base plate (variably sized), sealed vacuum cushions, a clear plastic foil covering the patient's torso and lower extremities, and a vacuum pump (Fig. 3). Depending on the need for stereotactic localization and targeting, an arch-like attachment can be affixed to the base plate, providing CT, magnetic resonance (MR), and positron emission tomography (PET) visible fiducials, as well as an integrated targeting system for stereotactic alignments in the treatment vault.

For immobilization device implementation, in preparation for treatment simulation, the patient is placed supine onto a vacuum cushion which is registered to the base plate by machined, clear-plastic registration bars that

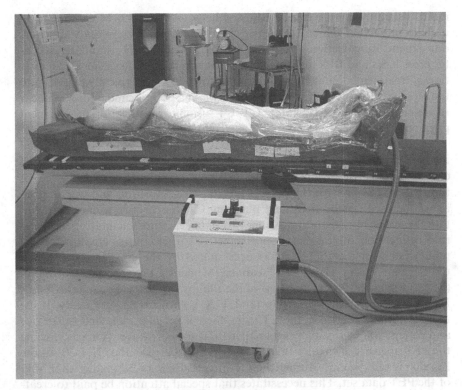

Figure 3 BodyFIX® immobilization system with vacuum pump.

insert onto protruding pins. The vacuum cushion, which is filled with small styrofoam BBs and has a valve attachment, allows for evacuation of the enclosed air space through a vacuum pump. A clear plastic cover sheet is attached by a sticky rubber strip to the left, right, and bottom/inferior sides of the vacuum cushion, covering the patient's lower body like a blanket up to the abdomen or thorax. The air between the clear plastic sheet, the patient, and the base vacuum cushion is evacuated, while the base cushion retains its enclosed air, causing the soft cushion to mold to the patient's posterior surface, providing a negative mold. Once the vacuum cushion is molded to the patient's back and sides, the enclosed air is evacuated from the cushion, creating a rigid, semi-permanent body cast. The vacuum cushions are available in various sizes, typically ranging in dimension from 180×65 to $220 \times 80\,\text{cm}$, with a constant Styrofoam-BB to air ratio maintained for all cushion sizes. Cushions are selected according to the patient's dimensions, thus enabling immobilization of both slender and relatively large patients in the same system. Once the full-body cast of the patient has been created, evacuation of the air between the clear plastic sheet, the patient, and the full-body cast creates a significant and valuable immobilization of the patient in the mold. Vacuum pressure can be adjusted between 0 and 120 Mbar to accommodate individual patient tolerance, and values most commonly used for our patients range between 60 and 100 Mbar. In addition to standard isocenter cross hairs and BBs that might be placed on the mold system for facilitation of treatment alignment, several other small BBs are typically placed onto the mold system, on each side of the patient, at a cranio-caudal location near the level of the tumor to facilitate CT/CT fusion for verification of treatment position, as will be discussed in a later section on Treatment Verification.

At our institution, the patient's BodyFIX mold system is often formed in the PET imaging suite prior to acquisition of a PET image study which can be utilized for fusion with the treatment-planning CT. Acquisition of the PET image set with the patient in the precise position and orientation, as will be used for the treatment planning CT, has proven to greatly facilitate the accurate registration of the two data sets, thus facilitating an accurate delineation of the metabolically active target. Initial creation of the mold system in the PET suite is necessitated by the smaller bore size of the Siemens ECAT-HR+ PET scanner (Siemens Corp., Berlin, Germany) (64 cm) versus the 70-cm aperture of the Philips PQ5000 CT scanner (Philips Medical Systems, Andover, Maryland, U.S.A.) utilized at our facility. If the mold is initially created in the CT suite, there is no guarantee that the device and patient will fit through the smaller PET aperture later. Ironically, while the PET aperture is smaller than the 70 cm CT aperture, the CT FOV of the PQ5000 is only 48 cm, causing the CT-imaged FOV to be smaller than that of the PET data set. This necessitates that special attention be paid to creating locations on the BodyFIX system for the placement of alignment and registration markers that will be visible on the 48 cm FOV CT image set.

TREATMENT PLANNING

The widely recognized ability of intensity-modulating delivery approaches to achieve conformality in even convex-shaped targets is achieved through an exploitation of the increased degrees of freedom afforded by such delivery schemes. Inherent to the increase in degrees of freedom is an enormous increase in solution space and, thus, complexity. Fortunately, the computational power of modern computing platforms has evolved to be capable of sufficiently addressing such complex solutions. Most, if not all, vendors of intensity-modulation-capable planning systems now employ so-called inverse planning approaches. The NOMOS Peacock serial tomotherapy approach used at our institution is supported by the Corvus Inverse Treatment Planning System (ITPS) Version 5.0 (NOMOS Corp., Crannberry Township, Pennsylvania, U.S.A.). The planning system employs a dose volume histogram (DVH)-based objective function and offers a choice between fast simulated annealing (FSA) and gradient descent optimization approaches. Because the more computationally intense FSA approach still progresses very quickly on modern hardware (as quickly as

5–6 min) and because FSA affords an optimization approach that can avoid becoming trapped in the local minima normally associated with DVH-based objective functions, we use the FSA approach for all clinical treatment plans.

Typical to all ITPSs, the Corvus objective function requires the entry of optimization parameters that characterize the nature of the problem to be solved by optimization. The Corvus system requires that the following parameters be entered for the target: (a) goal dose (the desired prescription dose to the target), (b) % volume below (the percentage volume of target tissue that can be below the goal value), (c) minimum dose (the minimum dose to the target that can be tolerated), and (d) maximum dose (the maximum target dose that can be tolerated). In addition to the previously listed parameters, the system also requires that a "target type" be selected. Inherent to the DVH-based objective function employed by the software are weighting arguments that assign importance to the previously listed user-supplied parameters. The importance of the maximum target dose, for instance, would be greater for a fractionated case (for which large hot spots are not acceptable), than for a radiosurgical application (for which hot spots inside the target might even be seen as advantageous). The selection of target type allows for a customized weighting of the importance arguments to the particular clinical application at hand. Interestingly, the implementation of such customized target types into the Corvus software evolved from our recognition in 1998 that in order to achieve clinically acceptable intracranial IMRS plans, such a customized approach would need to be implemented.

In addition to the target optimization parameters listed previously, the Corvus ITPS also requires that parameters be entered for all critical structures. As a minimum, the system always requires parameters to be entered for "healthy tissue," which represents, as a critical structure, all non-specific healthy tissue types. If other critical structures, which need to be individually controlled below specific dose levels, are present, parameters must be entered for them as well. These parameters include: (a) limit (the dose limit that the structure should be held below), (b) % volume above (the percentage of the structure that can be allowed to rise above the structure dose limit), (c) minimum (the structure dose below which there is limited value to further decrease of dose), and (d) maximum (the maximum tolerable structure dose). As for the target, each critical structure must be assigned a structure type, and multiple structure types are available, with each defining customized importance arguments unique to various clinical applications.

For the serial tomotherapeutic treatment of extracranial lesions at our institution, the following values for the previously described optimization parameters are "typically" used:

Target goal = 36–60 Gy in three fractions
Target % volume below = 3%
Target minimum dose = 95–97% of target goal

Target maximum = 200% of target goal and target type ⇒ IMRS
Tissue limit = Target goal
Tissue volume above = 0%
Tissue minimum = 0%
Tissue maximum = Target goal and tissue type ⇒ IMRS

These values generally correspond to the vendor's recommendation for the IMRS target and tissue types, and may be set up one time in the software as a user-named template that can be easily recalled by a click of the mouse. Because conformality and homogeneity are known to be competing factors, our utilization of the IMRS target and tissue types allows for the creation of extremely conformal distributions of dose, with an associated acceptance of increased hot spots inside the target. Interestingly, the large number of angles of approach afforded by the tomotherapy approach leads to what would still be considered by many to be relatively low-valued hot spots for such conformal plans. Hot spots, defined as the highest dose to any single dose voxel, are almost always less than 30% and are, most often, on the order of 10–15% of the prescribed dose value.

Other relevant TPS parameters typically used include:

Heterogeneity correction = ON during optimization and dose
                                            calculation
Number of couch angles = 1 (up to 3 for upper lung lobe tumors)
Couch angle = 180° (Varian)
Gantry angles = 350–10° (Varian)
Pencil beam size = 1 cm
Leaf transmission = 0–100% in 10% steps
Gantry step (for fluence map update) = 5°
Cost function = DVH
Optimizer = Continuous annealer
Iterations = More
Efficiency = 0
Benchmarks (i.e., relocation of isocenter) ⇒ As necessary to achieve
   target coverage from all gantry angles.

PTV margins are patient specific and evaluated based on full inhale and exhale CT evaluation, as discussed in the section on Treatment of Moving Targets. Typical values are 5 mm anterior, posterior, left, and right, with 10–15 mm inferior and superior.

For purposes of illustration an example case will now be presented.

Case Report

A 66-year-old female with diagnosis of stage 1 (T1N0M0) non-small-cell lung cancer (NSCLS), histopathologically confirmed in fine-needle aspiration. The patient was referred for SBRT due to medical inoperability second to severe chronic obstructive pulmonary disease (COPD).

The patient was immobilized using the BodyFIX double-vacuum whole body immobilization system for both CT simulation and FDG-PET imaging. For treatment planning, target volume delineation, anatomical tumor information derived from CT data, and metabolic tumor information derived from PET imaging were co-registered using a mutual information image-fusion software inherent to the AcQSim (Philips Medical Systems, Andover, Maryland, U.S.A.) virtual simulation software. Following target delineation, the CT data and the associated target volume were exported to the Corvus inverse planning platform by DICOM RT data transfer.

Inverse treatment planning parameters utilized were as follows:

Target goal dose = 60 Gy (3 × 20 Gy)
Target volume below = 3%
Target minimum dose = 96% of target goal (or 57.5 Gy)
Target maximum = 200% of target goal

The target volume type was specified as "IMRS target," emphasizing dose conformality over in-target dose homogeneity. The target volume was grown into a PTV by adding margins of 5 mm transversally and 10 cranio-caudally. Parameters for organs-at-risk (OAR) were set as follows:

Tissue limit = Target goal (60 Gy)
Tissue volume above = 0%
Tissue minimum = 0%
Tissue maximum = Target goal (60 Gy)
Tissue type ⇒ IMRS

Figure 4 depicts the Corvus prescription page with relevant critical structure parameters.

The pencil beam dimension chosen was 8.5 × 10 mm (1-cm mode) and the range of gantry rotation was 350–10°, with pencil beams delivered from 340° to 20°. While the presented treatment was delivered over a single, straight couch angle (Varian 180°), upper lobe lesions are sometimes treated using three couch angles (180°, 150°, and 210°, respectively).

The treatment plan was optimized utilizing typical ITPS parameters described previously, with a benchmark move equal to −40 mm (i.e., patient lowered from isocenter mark by 4 cm to allow laterally delivered pencil beams to have access to target). Figure 5 depicts the resulting dose distribution, with 100%, 90%, 70%, and 50% isodose lines displayed, and Figures 6 and 7 present the achieved/delivered structure statistics and DVHs. The dose distribution was normalized so that 95% of the PTV received 100% of the prescription dose. Thus, the GTV received no less than 61.4 Gy, with mean and maximum doses of 68.8 and 76.9 Gy, respectively.

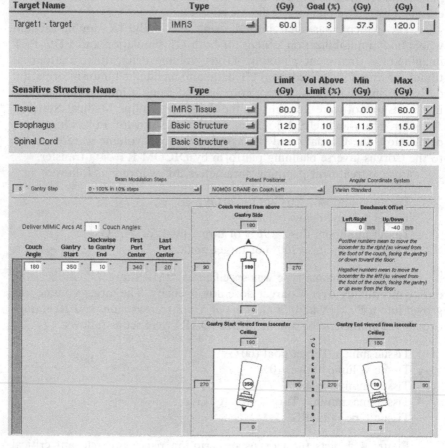

Figure 4 Corvus prescription page for the case report example containing ITPS input parameters.

OARs, namely the esophagus and the spinal cord, were predicted by the TPS to receive average doses of 6.9 and 4.2 Gy, with maximum doses of 13.9 and 4.2 Gy, respectively.

Following repeat control CT scanning in the immobilization system immediately prior to treatment to confirm accuracy of patient and target setup (as described in the following section of Treatment Verification), the treatment was delivered in three fractions separated by 48 hr using a 6 MV linear accelerator with 600 MU/min delivery capability. The number of couch indices, or treatment slices, was four. Figure 8 depicts the pencil beams and associated intensity levels utilized from a subset of five of the 64 actual arcing segments used for treatment. Note that for table indices 1, 2, and 3 (numbered

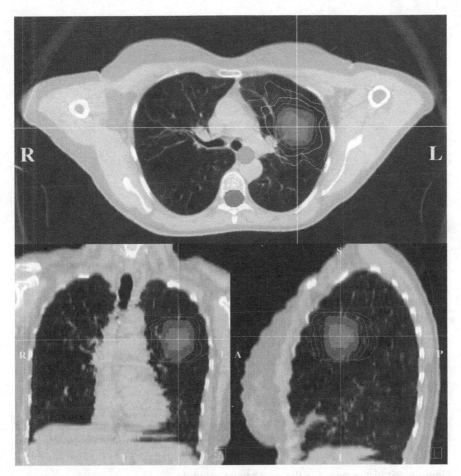

Figure 5 Isodose distribution for the case report example. Shown are the CTV (bright red), PTV (darker red), esophagus protection region (green), spinal cord protection region (blue), and isodose lines: 100% (dark blue) 90% (red), 70% (yellow), and 50% (green). (*See color insert.*)

at the left of Fig. 8 in white), both banks of pencil beams are delivering radiation and are modulated independently. At table index 4, only the cranially oriented bank of pencil beams "sees" the target, and accordingly only these pencil beams are utilized by the inverse planning system. As mentioned, the five arc-segments depicted are a subset of a total of 64 segments delivered for each gantry arc (each segment delivered over 5° gantry rotation). The central portion of Figure 8 also displays all utilized pencil beams over the entire gantry rotation, with each white dot on the patient surface representing an actual pencil beam delivered with non-zero intensity.

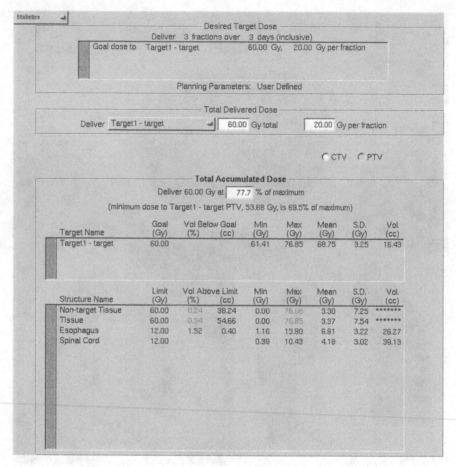

Figure 6 Statistics page for the case report example.

Total monitor units delivered were 43,037 for a net radiation delivery time of approximately 72 min. Including patient setup, control CT/image analysis, and treatment delivery, each fraction was completed in less than 100 min.

TREATMENT VERIFICATION

As mentioned previously, the effective and safe delivery of radioablative doses to extracranial targets requires a precise placement of the delivered high-dose region. While exhaustive efforts are undertaken at our institution to assure an adequate alignment and immobilization of the patient, as described previously, extensive experience gained from the greater than 200 SBRT treatments delivered at our facility (as of March 2004) have

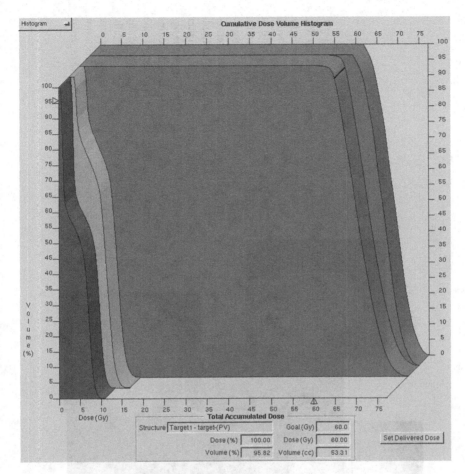

Figure 7 Cumulative dose volume histogram for the case report example. Shown (from back to front) are the CTV, PTV, esophagus, and cord. (*See color insert.*)

convinced us that such efforts must include a detailed verification of patient treatment position immediately prior to administration of treatment. While our previously published evaluation of the accuracy and reproducibility of the BodyFIX immobilization system used here for such treatments demonstrated mean target translations of 2.9, 2.3, and 3.2 mm in the x, y, and z directions, respectively, the occasional observance of larger values, which are capable of compromising adequate coverage by the previously stated PTV margins, is evidence of the need for pretreatment verification (4).

At our institution we have adopted a pretreatment verification approach which utilizes a three-dimensional (3D) data set provided by a repeat CT of the patient. Immediately prior to each day's treatment, the

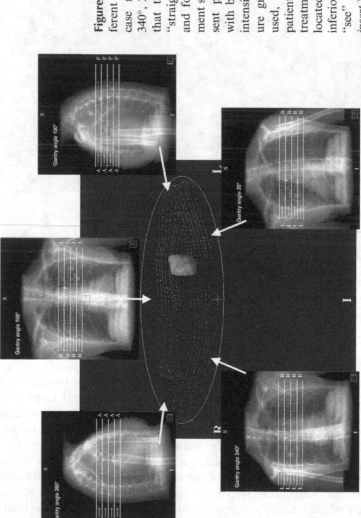

Figure 8 Depicting five of the 64 different intensity patterns used for the case report example (gantry angles 340°, 260°, 180°, 100°, and 20°). Note that the patient was treated with a "straight" couch (i.e., 180° Varian), and four couch increments (or treatment slices). The shaded squares represent pencil beam intensities utilized, with brighter shades indicating higher intensities. The central region of the figure graphically depicts pencil beams used, as dots on the surface of the patient. Note that the final arc of the treatment uses only the cranially located row of MIMiC vanes because inferior row of pencil beams does not "see" the target volume. (*See color insert.*)

patient is returned to the CT simulation suite, placed into the BodyFIX whole-body immobilization system, and re-imaged in the treatment position. The resulting CT data set, referred to as the Control CT, is transferred to the Corvus ITPS for fusion with the original treatment planning CT data set. The fiducial point matching fusion algorithm inherent to the Corvus ITPS is utilized to produce a registration of the two data sets relative to the BodyFIX whole-body cast. For such an approach to be valid, we must assume the BodyFIX cast to represent a rigid-body, which does not change shape during the course of a typical three-fraction treatment course, and the experience gained from 200+ such fusions has supported the validity of this assumption within reasonable limits (4). The registration of images is performed using the small BBs that were attached to the mold system during the treatment planning simulation, as described in a previous section. Fusion of the two CT data sets, based on the BodyFIX cast system, results in a near-perfect registration of the BodyFIX cast system between the two image sets, with any variation of patient position between the two imaging sessions apparent as movement of the patient anatomy observed when toggling between data sets. The Corvus ITPS allows for an overlay of the planned isodose distribution to be displayed on the Control CT dataset for that particular day's imaging session. Assessment of the pretreatment alignment quality is a straightforward matter of evaluating the coverage of the relevant isodose lines relative to the target and any other critical structures of interest. Based on such analysis, x, y, and z direction shifts required to correctly re-center the target in the high-dose region may be determined using the measurement tool inherent to the Corvus software. In our previously published report on the accuracy of the BodyFIX system, we observed that PTV margins of 5 mm transversally and 10 mm cranio-caudally would have provided adequate (i.e., target covered by at least the 90% isodose line) uncorrected target coverage in 87.1% of the 109 control CT data sets evaluated (4). Following determination of the 3D shifts necessary to return the target to the correct location within the delivered isodose distribution, all patients are shifted accordingly in the treatment room.

The utilization of a pretreatment control CT has the advantage of providing a high-resolution, high-contrast, 3D image set for precise evaluation of target location relative to treatment isocenter. The method allows for visualization of treatment isodose lines overlaid on the patient/target position for that particular day's CT control, thus providing reassurance of a proper 3D target position prior to treatment. The method has as a disadvantage the assumption of the validity of the CT control as a surrogate for the patient position on the treatment table. This assumption is valid only if one believes that the patient does not move within the BodyFIX cast between the time of imaging and treatment delivery. Because we currently do not have the ability to acquire a 3D image set in the treatment room, the CT control must be performed in the virtual simulation CT suite, which is located down a long hall from the treatment vault. Following CT control image acquisition, the patient is transferred to a transport-gurney by sliding the BodyFIX treatment board assembly from the CT table onto the gurney. The patient can then be wheeled down the hallway to the treatment vault where a similar procedure can be used to transfer the patient from the gurney to the linear accelerator treatment table. Ideally, the schedules of the CT suite and treatment vault are coordinated such that the patient may be transferred directly to the treatment vault. In reality this is often, but not always, the case. In such instances the patient may need to wait in a patient holding area, adjacent to a nurses station, for as much as 10–15 min, thus further testing the assumption of the CT control position as an acceptable representation of patient position at treatment time. As a coarse evaluation of this assumption, we also perform an assessment of patient position on the treatment table by comparison of pretreatment port films and CT-simulation-generated digitally reconstructed radiographs (DRRs). Any significant patient movement within the BodyFIX mold between the time of CT control and placement of the patient onto the treatment table is believed to be visible on such images. Ideally, of course, we would acquire the 3D CT data set in the treatment room, on the treatment table, and linear accelerator-based cone beam imaging and CT-on-rails approaches may hold promise for such applications, as will be discussed in a later section entitled Future Directions.

TREATMENT OF MOVING TARGETS

As discussed in previous chapters, the treatment of thoracic and upper abdominal targets must necessarily address the problem of respiration related motion, and numerous reports have characterized the nature and magnitude of target motion due to respiration (5–8). Current approaches aimed at addressing the treatment delivery aspects of such motion are seen to center around three general philosophies. The first is that of attempting to stop, or control, the motion to some degree by the application of breathing control approaches. Such approaches may be as aggressive as physically limiting when, and to what degree, the patient may breath; as moderate as reducing respiratory amplitude through the use of abdominal pressure applied via belts, plates or cushions; or as passive as coaching the patient to minimize the depth and frequency of respiration. In any case, investigators have reported an ability to effectively reduce the degree of target motion to acceptable limits. Such motion controlling approaches have the advantage of ensuring that the target remains in an acceptable treatment location, thus maximizing the amount of time spent delivering dose to the target, and minimizing dose delivered to healthy surrounding tissue. These approaches suffer from the disadvantage that the majority of patients undergoing treatment for thoracic lesions are compromised, to some degree, in their breathing efficiency. Many such patients are incapable of tolerating such limitations to their breathing cycle.

A second approach to addressing respiration related target motion is that of pulsing, or gating, the treatment beam. Such approaches may monitor the respiratory cycle of the patient through the use of various respiration sensors (e.g., belts, spirometers, and chest markers) and then quickly turn the treatment beam off when the target has moved beyond tolerable limits. Target position can also be ascertained through real-time tracking of implanted markers. Such approaches have the advantage of gating the treatment such that dose is not delivered when the target is out of position, but suffer from the disadvantage of increased treatment time due to time spent waiting for the target to return to an acceptable treatment position. Additionally, methods which rely on the rise and fall of the chest wall as an indication of target position must assume that the chest wall is a valid indicator of target position, and this assumption may be challenged by such factors as phase and amplitude differences between target and chest wall motion. The third general approach to dealing with target motion is, arguably, the least sophisticated. This approach addresses the problem of target motion by simply increasing the PTV margin to sufficiently accommodate the motion of the target. Numerous methods exist for defining the magnitude and nature of PTV increase, from sophisticated time, motion, and probability-related definitions, to methods which define the PTV as the physical intersection of the full inhale and full exhale PTV volumes, to even simpler methods that measure the maximum extent of motion in the three principle directions on the full inhale and exhale CTs. A so-called slow CT scan is often performed to generate a treatment-planning CT data set which represents the target as a larger "blurred" volume due to the slow scan-time, relative to target motion frequency. Because we currently lack technology necessary to support more sophisticated approaches, we are employing a combination of the latter of the previously described PTV-growth methodologies with abdominal pressure applied via the BodyFIX immobilization system. PTV margins are designed, on a patient specific basis, by the evaluation of full normal inhale and exhale maximum extent of target motion while immobilized in the BodyFIX system, and treatment planning CT data sets are acquired using slow CT scanning techniques. Moderate abdominal pressure, applied by the vacuum cushions inherent to the BodyFIX system, has been observed to provide a measure of respiratory amplitude reduction. While such an approach has proven clinically effective, it is, admittedly, less than ideal, and we are currently budgeted for and exploring the options for implementation of gating-related approaches. Such approaches appear to be capable of allowing for reductions in PTV margin and, therefore, subsequent reductions in volume of healthy tissue treated to prescription dose levels.

LOGISTICS OF THE METHOD

The method described here for stereotactic treatment of extracranial targets by use of a serial tomotherapeutic approach has been successfully employed at our institution since August of 2001 for the treatment of 82 patients by 260 delivered fractions. The tomotherapy approach utilized is, in all relevant regards, identical to the treatment approach utilized for the 50+ conventionally fractionated IMRT patients we treat each day. As such, it represents a proven delivery method which has been shown to present no significant technological challenges. The use of an arc-based delivery approach does require that consideration be given to linear accelerator/treatment-couch clearance issues, and we currently utilize a Varian ETR-Exact couch combination that has not posed any significant challenges to such clearance for treatment of lesions of the torso. The use of an intensity-modulating approach allows for the creation of extremely conformal distributions of dose, with the anticipated loss of treatment efficiency associated with such approaches. Monitor units (MU) required for delivery of any intensity modulated treatment may be increased by a factor of four to six times over standard, unmodulated delivery schemes, due to dose wasted to modulation. Serial tomotherapy's slicewise delivery approach further increases inefficiency by an additional factor approximately equal to the number of separate treatment arcs, due to its separate treatment of each slice of target. As a result, delivered monitor units for a 12-Gy fraction typically range from 15,000 to 25,000 MU, and beam-on times from 25 to 45 min on the 600 MU/min Varian 600CD accelerator used for such treatments at our facility. The average time from procedure start, defined as patient placed in the BodyFIX mold for CT control, to procedure finished, defined as all dose delivered, is on the order of 1 hr and 45 min. As such, the beam on time represents roughly 24–43% of the entire procedure time. Any reduction of the treatment procedure time is, of course, valuable in that it can allow for a reduction in the probability of patient movement, and for greater patient comfort. We are mindful, however, that a 25% reduction in beam-on time will still represent only a 6–11 min, or a 6–10%, reduction in procedure time. We are currently exploring methods for reducing beam-on time, as will be discussed in the Future Directions section, but such efforts must be weighed against improvements in conformality which are achieved through the use of such sophisticated, yet inefficient, delivery methods. Perhaps a more effective method for a significant reduction of procedure time would entail elimination of the need to perform two patient setups, with associated transport and wait time, subsequent to performing the control CT in a separate suite. Acquisition of the 3D positional data set on the treatment table could, theoretically, reduce the procedure time by 20–30 min, and such an approach is of significant interest to us, as will be discussed in the following section.

FUTURE DIRECTIONS

The Patient Immobilization and Alignment section alluded to logistical challenges associated with limited aperture and FOV issues that necessitated the creation of the BodyFIX mold in the smaller bore of the PET suite. In the near future it is envisioned that our acquisition of a large bore and extended FOV CT-PET combined unit will render such simulation arrangements unnecessary, allowing for a single imaging session and patient position for both the PET and CT planning data sets. For patients who do not require a fused PET data set, acquisition of a large-bore CT unit with 80+ cm aperture and 65+ cm FOV is envisioned to eliminate current FOV concerns, again, in the near future.

The section on Treatment Planning discussed the trade off between improvements in conformality associated with intensity-modulating approaches, such as Peacock approved, and the subsequent increases in treatment and procedure times due to reduced efficiency and increased required MU of such treatments. The Corvus ITPS possesses inherent capabilities which allow for user selection of the "complexity" desired in the resulting intensity-modulated treatment plan. The software accepts user input through the positioning of a slider bar, which ultimately affects the modulation frequency of the developed plan. Greater complexity equates to greater variation in the fluences of the delivered pencil beams used for treatment and, therefore, to larger numbers of "wasted" monitor units. We are currently systematically exploring the trade-offs between plan quality and increased efficiency. As mentioned in the previous section, improvements in efficiency can equate to reduced treatment time, which can subsequently result in reduced potential for patient movement and discomfort. However, such improvements must not come at the expense of clinically significant reductions in conformity.

The need for ascertaining the correct and accurate position of the patient was discussed in the section on Treatment Verification. In this section we presented our method for verifying pre-treatment patient position through the use of a Control CT. The reliance of this approach on an assumed validity of the CT Control as an acceptable surrogate for the position of the patient on the treatment table, at treatment time, was described. In the near future we anticipate the elimination of the need for such assumptions through the installation of a linear accelerator with in-room CT and/or on-board cone beam capabilities. Such in-room, three-dimensional imaging capability holds the promise of allowing us to explore the potential of these exciting new image guidance approaches, and to provide nearly real-time verification of patient treatment position, with associated reduction of total procedure time. Lastly, the section on Treatment of Moving Targets characterized our currently less-than-sophisticated approaches to addressing respiratory related target motion. We are currently budgeted for, and anticipate the installation of, respiratory-gated technology in the very near future. Such technology is believed to be capable of allowing for a clinically significant reduction in PTV margin and, therefore, dose to healthy tissue. The obstacles to implementation of gated technology in a tomotherapeutic environment are anticipated, and alternative scenarios are currently being explored.

REFERENCES

1. Salter BJ. NOMOS Peacock IMRT utilizing the Beak post collimation device. Med Dosim 2002; 26(1):37–45.
2. Salter BJ, Hevezi JM, Sadeghi A, Fuss M, Herman TS. An oblique arc capable patient positioning system for sequential tomotherapy. Med Phys 2001; 28(12): 2475–2488.
3. Fuss M, Salter BJ, Sadeghi A, Bogaev CA, Hevezi JM, Herman TS. Fractionated stereotactic Intensity-modulated radiotherapy (FS-IMRT) for small intracranial target volumes at the example of acoustic neuromas. Med Dosim 2002; 27(2):147–154.
4. Fuss M, Salter BJ, Rassiah P, Cheek D, Cavanaugh SX, Herman TS. Repositioning accuracy of a commercially available double vacuum whole-body immobilization system. Technol Cancer Res Treat 2004; 3(2):161–170.
5. Nevinny-Stickel M, Sweeney RA, Bale RJ, Posch A, Auberger T, Lukas P. Reproducibility of patient positioning for fractionated extracranial stereotactic radiotherapy using a double-vacuum technique. Strahlenther Onkol 2004; 180(2):117–122.
6. Balter JM, Lam KL, McGinn CJ, et al. Improvement of CT-based treatment-planning models of abdominal targets using static exhale imaging. Int J Radiat Oncol Biol Phys 1998; 41:939–943.
7. Balter JM, Ten Haken RK, Lawrence TS, et al. Uncertainties in CT-based radiation therapy treatment planning associated with patient breathing. Int J Radiat Oncol Biol Phys 1996; 36:167–174.
8. Davies SC, Hill AL, Holmes RB, et al. Ultrasound quantitation of respiratory organ motion in the upper abdomen. Br J Radial 1994; 67:1096–1102.
9. Kubo HD, Hill BC. Respiration gated radiotherapy treatment: a technical study. Phys Med Biol 1996; 41:83–91.

6

Anatomical and Biological Imaging

Frank J. Lagerwaard and Suresh Senan

Department of Radiation Oncology, VU University Medical Center,
Amsterdam, The Netherlands

INTRODUCTION

The growing clinical interest in extracranial stereotactic radiotherapy (ECSRT) is a logical consequence of the high control rates observed with hypofractionated intracranial stereotactic radiotherapy (SRT). In principle, similar SRT fractionation schedules can also be applied to extracranial sites, provided that treatment volumes are small and critical normal structures are avoided. Knowledge of patient-setup errors and (residual) mobility of both tumor and normal structures is essential in order to determine the smallest possible treatment planning margins without losing adequate tumor coverage. However, organ motion remains a major problem for extracranial sites, and methods to address this problem require considerable resources and are the subject of ongoing research.

It will be evident that the consequences of errors in the definition of target volumes and adjacent critical normal tissues will be far greater for hypofractionated stereotactic treatments than for conventionally fractionated treatments, and the characteristic steep dose-gradients obtained with stereotactic irradiation will increase even further the clinical impact of such geographical errors. In order to minimize the probability of such errors, two important issues that are specific to implementing ECSRT have to be solved: (1) the accuracy and reproducibility of patient positioning and (2) the internal mobility of tumors and normal tissues.

109

Optimal imaging techniques that precisely localize both the target volume and adjacent critical structures are a prerequisite for ECSRT. Although some form of image-based information has always been used to guide the radiotherapy treatment process, the availability and improved quality of digital data and the computerized 3D reconstruction of the patient's anatomy have permitted current "image-guided radiotherapy." Image guidance can be performed not only for diagnosis and treatment planning, but also for visualization during treatment delivery using either external reference systems that are attached to the patient (frame-based ECSRT) or using images that are registered relative to the patients anatomy (frameless ECSRT).

The implementation of image-guided approaches has expanded from using anatomical imaging techniques, such as computed tomography (CT), magnetic resonance imaging (MRI), and ultrasound, to include several biological imaging techniques, e.g., positron-emission tomography (PET) or magnetic resonance spectroscopy (MRS). However, the exact role of biological imaging in ECSRT planning is currently investigational, but co-registration of images from different anatomical and/or biological techniques can provide additional information in the determination of target volumes and critical structures.

This review will address current and ongoing developments in the role of image guidance in the phases of pretreatment selection, treatment planning, treatment delivery, and follow-up in ECSRT. As the topic of imaging using all available techniques is extensive, and many tumor sites can be treated with stereotactic radiotherapy, this chapter will only focus on three key target areas, i.e., lung, liver, and vertebral lesions, in order to highlight the main principles.

APPROPRIATE SELECTION OF PATIENTS

ECSRT is a labor-intensive process and appropriate patient selection is required in order to identify patients who are most likely to benefit from this approach. Patients with small primary tumors or limited metastatic disease are the key candidates for ECSRT, and an important aspect of imaging studies for patient selection is the exclusion of patients who have more extensive or rapidly progressing disease. In the absence of data from prospective randomized clinical trials of ECSRT for metastatic disease, the surgical literature may offer useful pointers for patient selection criteria (1–6). In general, patients who have controlled primary tumors with a limited number of metastases (3 or less) that are restricted to a single organ system, and have a good performance score, can be considered candidates for ECSRT.

Staging accuracy for patients with cancer has been improved substantially by the availability of PET. PET has the ability to detect cancer on the basis of biochemical and molecular processes within tumor tissues, and can provide quantitative information, not only on metabolic activity but also on perfusion (7,8), oxygenation (9–11), and proliferation (12–14). A literature review suggests that [18]FDG-PET is between 10% and 20% more accurate than conventional imaging for diagnosing, staging, and restaging of many tumor types (15), including tumors of the lung (16–23), colorectal cancer (24–26), head and neck cancer (27), breast cancer (28,29), and melanoma (30,31).

In the following sections, the aspects of imaging in the patient selection will be highlighted separately for three tumor sites, namely, lung cancer, hepatic malignancies, and vertebral metastases.

The Role of Imaging in the Selection of Patients with Lung Cancer

Local control rates of only 30–55% have been reported for conventionally fractionated radiotherapy for stage I non-small cell lung cancer (NSCLC) (32,33). In contrast, local control rates as high as 80–90% have been reported for hypofractionated ECSRT (34–37). However, accurate staging is essential as ECSRT would be an inappropriate treatment if occult hilar or mediastinal nodal metastases were present. After a clinical diagnosis of stage I NSCLC using conventional staging procedures, only around 65–71% of patients will have the same pathological stage, with upstaging to stage II in 15%, stage III in 16%, and stage IV in 4% of patients (17,38).

[18]FDG-PET has been shown to be superior to conventional CT scans in the staging of patients with NSCLC (16,18–23,39,40). However, as false-positive findings may occur in granulomatous disease such as tuberculosis or sarcoidosis (41,42), [18]FDG-PET uptake alone is not a sufficient basis to select patients with solitary pulmonary lesions. Similarly, false-negative findings have been reported for broncho-alveolar carcinoma, carcinoid, and in NSCLC measuring less than 1 cm (43), and histological or cytological confirmation is advisable prior to ECSRT regardless of the findings on [18]FDG-PET scans. As ECSRT is usually restricted to either medically inoperable patients with early stage lung cancer or patients refusing surgery, mediastinoscopy is rarely performed and staging is confined to non-invasive methods. [18]FDG-PET scans are more reliable than CT scans for the detection of mediastinal or hilar lymph node metastases, with a mean sensitivity and specificity of $79\% \pm 3\%$ and $91\% \pm 2\%$ for PET and $60\% \pm 2\%$ and $77\% \pm 2\%$, respectively, for CT (39). The accuracy of nodal staging can be increased even further using co-registration of CT and PET scans, or an integrated PET-CT (44–46).

In patients with early-stage NSCLC, endobronchial ultrasound (EBUS) can be useful in excluding metastases to mediastinal and hilar nodes (47). In addition, EBUS may also have a role in the assessment of patients with peripheral nodules in whom no definite histological diagnosis is available (48). In such patients, EBUS permits the visualization of the internal structure of peripheral pulmonary lesions, information that appears to correlate with histology of the lesion.

The Role of Imaging in the Selection of Patients with Hepatic Malignancies

The suitability of local treatments for liver metastases has traditionally been based upon their number, distribution, and size using anatomical imaging studies such as contrast-enhanced CT scans, MRI, and ultrasonography. The sensitivity of transabdominal ultrasonography is relatively poor in comparison to intraoperative ultrasonography, in particular due to the failure to detect smaller metastases (49–51). In a series of 157 patients with liver metastases, 247 out of a total of 290 lesions found with intraoperative ultrasound, intraoperative palpation, and histopathologic examination had been correctly identified by helical CT, yielding an overall detection rate of 85% (52). The high positive predictive value of 96% indicates that histological or cytological confirmation prior to ECSRT is required only for equivocal lesions on contrast-enhanced CT scans. [18]FDG-PET scanning improves the selection of candidates for local treatment of liver metastases from colorectal cancer by identifying extrahepatic disease sites, (53) and in detecting unresectable disease (54–57). However, anatomical imaging studies remain superior for identifying small liver metastases, as the detection rate for lesions of 1 cm or smaller was only 25% with FDG-PET scans, compared to 85% for lesions larger than 1 cm (55,58). The low sensitivity for detection of smaller liver metastases is partly a result of the high hepatic background activity produced by the high metabolic activity of normal hepatocytes.

The Role of Imaging in the Selection of Patients with Vertebral Metastases

The appropriateness of ECSRT for vertebral metastasis is determined by the multiplicity of bone metastases. While determination of the number of involved sites is usually based on conventional technetium-99m methylene diophosphate (Tc-99m MDP) whole body bone scans, several authors have reported a substantially higher sensitivity and a better accuracy of [18]FDG-PET scans in the detection of bone metastases (59–62). In addition, [18]FDG-PET revealed more metastatic lesions than bone scanning, independent of the type of cancer or location of bone involvement (63). Thin-section CT scans can be used to determine the local extension of vertebral metastases, and coronal and sagittal multiplanar reconstructions can assist in determining the local extent of bony destruction and provide detailed information about infiltration and potential spinal instability. The visualization of the local extension of vertebral metastases, particularly with respect to the epidural and paravertebral regions and the relation to the spinal cord, is superior using gadolinium-enhanced multiplanar MRI scans (64).

GENERAL PRINCIPLES OF TARGET DEFINITION

The steep dose-gradients, characteristic of ECSRT, imply that the accurate definition of target volumes is of utmost importance in order to avoid marginal misses. To ensure that representative target volumes are generated for ECSRT treatment planning, imaging techniques will have to be used that reflect the method of treatment delivery. For instance, if treatment delivery is performed during abdominal compression or respiratory gating, planning CT scans should also be performed under identical conditions. In addition, an imaging procedure of a lung tumor lasting a few minutes may not provide representative target volumes if the lesion is treated with respiration-gated single fraction SRT which may take up to 2 hours (65,66).

The small margins used for ECSRT dictate that careful attention must be paid to limiting variations and inconsistencies in contouring GTVs. Interobserver variability in contouring target volumes appears to be a major factor contributing to geometric inaccuracy (67). In addition, with respect to the critical dose distributions in ECSRT, variations in contouring adjacent normal tissues, which can also be substantial (68,69), should be taken into account. Although some residual interobserver variability remains inevitable, measures to diminish such variations, including standard contouring protocols, the use of standardized optimal window-level settings for contouring, thin slice planning CT scans, and multimodality image registration techniques are of paramount importance (70,71). The development of reliable segmentation software tools may in the future also decrease the impact of human error.

Although only minimal acute toxicity has been reported after ECSRT, late toxicity may become important in patients who are treated with curative intent. A significant risk of late radiation-induced Grade 3–5 complications has been reported after high-dose irradiation or chemoradiotherapy of the thorax (72). While these findings were reported after fractionated conventional radiotherapy, it indicates that doses to normal tissues should be minimized in ECSRT by using optimal techniques, and these doses should be carefully documented. In view of the large fraction sizes used in ECSRT, establishing the actual dose delivered to critical normal tissues is important in order to derive normal tissue tolerance doses. The ICRU Report 62 recommends drawing margins around organs at risk to produce planning organ at risk volumes (PRVs) to account for geometric uncertainty in the radiotherapy treatment process (73). The use of such PRVs requires that data on organ mobility and systematic uncertainties in patient setup are available. However, this is generally not the case at present.

Occasionally, ECSRT is performed for residual disease after induction chemotherapy, e.g., for metastatic disease or T2N0M0 primary NSCLC. There are presently no recommendations available as to whether to irradiate the pre- or postchemotherapy target volumes. Only a careful study of disease recurrence patterns will show if treatment of postchemotherapy volumes is acceptable. Whenever the choice is made to irradiate the prechemotherapy volume, the use of multimodality fusion can aid in an accurate reconstruction of this volume (70).

GENERATING REPRESENTATIVE PLANNING CT SCANS

The challenge of generating representative target volumes for mobile organs has most extensively been addressed for lung lesions. The following section aims to describe potential solutions for this tumor site, although not all solutions are suitable for other mobile tumor sites.

Individualized assessment of mobility, instead of using "standard" margins, is required for ECSRT, as an analysis of the mobility of peripheral lung tumors has revealed that no clear correlation exists between the anatomical location of lung tumors and the extent of mobility (74).

It is commonly assumed that the correct, or at least the mean, position of a normal organ is captured by a single planning CT scan, and that this position is reproduced throughout the treatment. However, planning CT scans may show considerable artifacts due to internal mobility during the generation of the scans (Fig. 1). In addition, fast spiral CT scans will generate a random "snapshot" position of both target volumes and normal tissues, and dose distributions calculated in such a static model are unlikely to represent the actual dose distribution (75). A study in which an abdominal CT scan was performed in a patient who was breathing quietly and freely, and was followed by a CT scan with breath-holding at normal inhalation and normal exhalation, showed that the absolute volume of the liver varied by as much as 12% between studies, due to sampling error. The

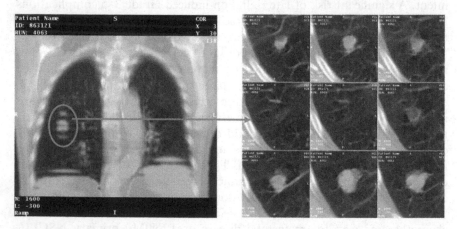

Figure 1 Movement of a solitary lung nodule during CT scanning (1 second/slice) results in discontinuous imaging of the lesion, as seen on a digitally reconstructed radiograph (*left panel*) and consecutive CT slices (*right panel*).

normal tissue complication probabilities (NTCP) calculated from static exhale and inhale studies in six patients varied randomly from 3% to 44% for doses that resulted in a 15% NTCP on the free-breathing studies (76).

As standard imaging techniques are lacking in information on the time factor, several approaches have been used to ensure adequate target coverage, including:

1. a full characterization and incorporation of internal mobility,
2. restriction of respiration-induced mobility during both pretreatment imaging and treatment delivery,
3. respiration-gated planning CT scan and gated treatment delivery,
4. real-time tumor tracking.

Full Characterization and Incorporation of Internal Mobility

Characterization and incorporation of all intrafractional tumor mobility, although time consuming, represents the simplest of measures to deal with the problem of internal mobility. An obvious disadvantage of this approach is that an unnecessarily larger volume will be irradiated, particularly if extremes of mobility are incorporated. For an adequate dosimetric analysis, the full incorporation of internal mobility should not only include the target volume, but also adjacent normal structures in order to integrate all time-weighted changes in anatomy.

Fluoroscopy is not an appropriate method for characterizing mobility in high precision radiotherapy, as only limited mobility data can be generated (if at all) on superior–inferior and medio-lateral movements (77,78). More importantly, the observed mobility cannot be accurately linked to the geometry of planning CT scans.

The fusion of target volumes generated on "two-phase" CT scans, obtained at either deep or quiet inspiration and expiration, has also been used to characterize internal mobility (78–81). However, summation of target volumes generated at deep inspiration and deep expiration will not only lead to an overestimation of the actual target volume (82), but the reproducibility of such target volumes is questionable (66). However, it has been argued that "two-phase" planning, by removing the need for large symmetric, population-based margins, allows for a reduction in the amount of irradiated normal tissue, and could thereby improve the reliability of patient data for DVH modeling (81). An alternative method of obtaining an individualized internal target volume (ITV) is the summation of target volumes generated on multiple rapid planning CT scans (Fig. 2). The exact number of CT scans needed for generating an optimal ITV is unknown, and as the fusion of multiple "snapshot" positions is unlikely to cover the full range of mobility, a small additional "internal" and "setup" margin for generating planning target volumes (PTVs) will be required.

Another method that is restricted for use in lung tumors is the generation of "slow" CT scans that are performed with a CT revolution time of

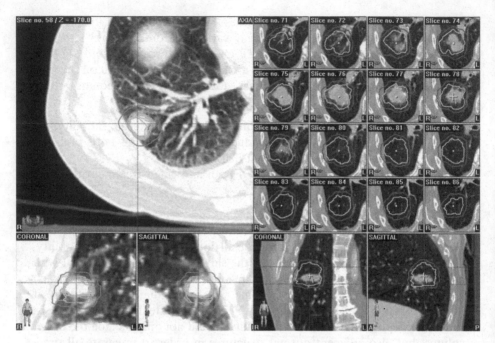

Figure 2 Generating target volumes for a stage I lung tumor. The ITV (*orange contour on left panel*) encompasses all GTVs contoured on six consecutive multi-slice CT scans (*light yellow contours on left and right panel*). The ITV was expanded with a 3 mm margin to derive the PTV (*red contour on right panel*). (*See color insert.*)

4 sec/slice (83,84). The GTVs generated from single slow CT scans are generally located in a central position relative to an "optimal CTV" generated using six separate CT scans during quiet respiration. Being centrally located, GTVs generated using slow CT scans can enclose the 6-scan volume by applying a symmetrical 3D margin of 5 mm (85). A complete breathing cycle in patients with lung cancer has been reported to range between 1.5–3.5 sec and 3.6 ± 0.85 sec (86,87), and the need for an additional margin (of 5 mm) may reflect factors such as minor variations in mobility between respiratory cycles and contouring variations. This 5 mm margin reflects the "internal margin" only; additional margins to account for patient-setup are required as well. As symptomatic radiation pneumonitis is very uncommon in patients irradiated for stage I NSCLC (33), the modest increase in PTV for a plan based upon a slow CT scan with an additional margin is not clinically relevant.

Minimizing Respiratory Motion

A simple and frequently used method for restricting respiration-induced tumor mobility is the application of abdominal pressure, both during pretreatment imaging and treatment delivery, for decreasing the mobility of both lung and liver lesions (88–91).

SRT during patient breath-holding, usually at end-inspiration, has been used as a method for minimizing the mobility of targets in the lung and liver (92,93). Although theoretically attractive, this method has a number of practical disadvantages. Cooperative patients have to be coached thoroughly in order to generate reproducible results, and an individualized assessment is required for each patient. In addition, a considerable number of medically inoperable patients with compromised respiratory function cannot tolerate breath-holding (65,92,94). When performing breath-holding, some residual mobility persists due to variations in breath-holding and cardiac action, and this movement must also be incorporated. In addition, tumor drifts have been reported during treatment, which is particularly relevant for SRT in view of the long fractional treatment time (95).

Recently, Onishi et al. (96) described a self-breath-holding system, which is based on the control of the radiation beam by patients themselves. Planning CT scans during patients' self-breath-holding were repeated three times, and the tumor positions on these scans showed that the technique was reproducible within a 2 mm distance. In addition to patient-controlled breath-holding, several authors have reported minimizing mobility using active breathing control (ABC) (97,98), or even using general anesthesia and high-frequency ventilation (34).

Respiratory Gating

Respiratory gating constitutes an attractive alternative to the breath-holding techniques, although advanced gating equipment at the CT scan and linear accelerator is mandatory. The approach of "prospective gating," i.e., performing respiration-triggered CT scans for radiotherapy planning, has major limitations (99). Firstly, CT sessions will have to be long, as only one slice is acquired at each table position per breathing cycle, and multiple scans of similar duration would be required if many respiratory phases are to be imaged. The long image acquisition time for each CT set increases the likelihood of patient movement during the scanning process. Another drawback is the fact that the respiratory phase at which the scan is to be performed has to be predetermined before image acquisition.

A major recent advance in CT scanning technology has been the use of multi-slice CT scans to characterize the 4D position, which includes the time factor, of tumors or normal organs from co-registered respiratory signals. This requires multiple CT slices to be performed at each relevant table position ("over-sampling") for at least the duration of one full respiratory cycle, while simultaneously recording signals which are generated using a respiratory motion monitoring system (100). Each image from such a scan is sorted into an image bin that corresponds with the phase of the respiratory cycle in

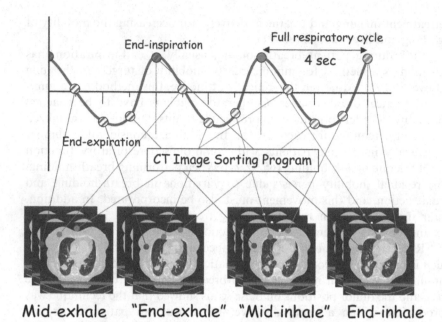

Figure 3 A 4D CT dataset is derived by performing multiple CT slices at each table position ("over-sampling"), while simultaneously recording respiratory signals. Each image is then sorted into a bin that corresponds with the phase of the respiratory cycle at which the image was acquired.

which the image was acquired ("retrospective gating"). The complete set of such image bins accumulated over a respiratory cycle constitutes a 4D data-set (Fig. 3). Motion artifacts are significantly reduced in the 4D dataset compared to 3D images, and reconstruction volumes match those expected on basis of stationary-phantom scans to within 5% in all cases (101). The initial reports concerning the use of 4D CT scanning for radiotherapy planning described the use of a single-slice spiral CT and mainly phantom studies (100,101), but clinical experience in a single patient with lung cancer was also reported (112).

Tumor Tracking Radiotherapy

One of the most advanced methods for coping with the problem of mobile target volumes is fluoroscopic real-time tumor-tracking radiation therapy (RTRT). Prior to performing a planning CT scan, radio-opaque gold markers are inserted in or near the tumor. This is performed using broncho-scopic insertion for peripheral lung lesions, transcutaneous insertion for liver lesions, or cystoscopic or percutaneous insertion for the prostate. The robustness of the treatment plan is dependent upon a constant relationship between the fiducials and tumor isocentre. Using fluoroscopic tracking, the system triggers the linear accelerator to commence and stop irradiation only when the marker(s) are located within a predetermined coordinate-range.

The method has a number of limitations, however. The accurate insertion of markers in tumors can be difficult or may be contraindicated. Bronchoscopic implantation of markers in centrally located lung tumors is often unsuccessful due to problems with early displacement (102,103), and the insertion of markers is restricted into small peripheral bronchi in or adjacent to the tumor (103). The difficulty in inserting any marker into lung tumors was highlighted by a report in which it was only possible to insert markers in the proximity of tumors in five (of seven) patients with T1 lung tumors (87). Transthoracal insertion of markers for lung lesions is associated with a substantial risk for pneumothorax (37), a complication that may be life-threatening in patients with compromised pulmonary function.

Ideally, four fiducial markers are required in order to accurately detect tumor rotation and volumetric changes during treatment (104). In patients with prostate cancers, a reduction in the distance between markers that was consistent with tumor regression has been observed during treatment (103,105). Preliminary data suggests that marker migration does not appear to be a major problem in lesions of the liver and prostate (106).

REPEATED TREATMENT PLANNING IN BETWEEN FRACTIONS

Interfractional variation in location of target volumes may play an important role in hypofractionated SRT, in particular when the overall-treatment time is longer than a few days, but may also be relevant for single fraction treatment when the time between imaging and actual treatment delivery is substantial. For hypofractionated SRT, the geometrical accuracy can be improved by irradiating a "target of the day," which relies on image guidance that identifies the target volume position before each fraction. This can be performed in instances when a change in size or position of the tumor or normal tissues is anticipated during treatment, using ultrasound imaging, radiographic imaging of implanted radio-opaque markers, or CT imaging. The general principle of this approach is to adapt the treatment fields to the daily position of the target as detected by each imaging procedure. While attractive, the use of markers only accounts for variations in the spatial position of the target volume and cannot correct for (radiation-induced) changes in volume and shape of the target volume. Data on potential volumetric changes during the course of radiotherapy, including both radiation-induced enlargement and tumor shrinkage, are required to assess the importance of such volumetric changes on dosimetry. Volumetric measurements and beam adjustments may become feasible with the implementation of cone-beam CT scanners, which are linked to the linear accelerator. In instances where volumetric changes can be expected to be present, or

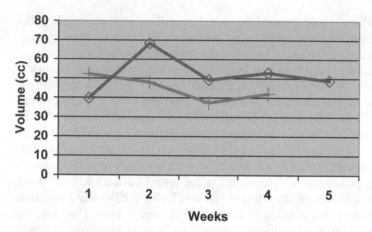

Figure 4 Changes in ITVs seen on weekly CT scans in two patients with peripheral lung tumors when five fractions of stereotactic radiotherapy were delivered in 5 weeks (12 Gy/fraction). (*See color insert.*)

in situations where markers cannot be used, repeated imaging and treatment planning in order to re-establish both the PTV and PRV before subsequent fractions may be warranted.

The reproducibility of target volumes has been studied using repeated CT scans prior to each of three fractions of SRT in 60 CT-simulations for lung targets, and 58 CT-simulations for hepatic targets (91). This analysis showed that had all treatments been based upon a plan derived from the initial scan, an adequate (95% or greater coverage of the target volume by the reference isodose) was only attained in 91% of lung tumors, and 81% of liver tumors. The authors suggested that pulmonary targets with "increased breathing mobility" and liver tumors exceeding 100 cm^3 should undergo repeated evaluation of sufficient margins

Preliminary data from our series in general showed stable ITVs during the 3–5 weeks course of ECSRT; however, an occasional transient but significant increase in ITV after the first fraction of ECSRT was observed (Fig. 4). Additional investigations into the magnitude and impact of time-trends during the course of hypofractionated SRT are awaited.

SITE SPECIFIC COMMENTS

Table: Site-Specific Aspects of Imaging for ECSRT

- Spiral CT-scanning (Fig. 5) should be performed during either the late arterial or portal venous phase (scanning delay 45–80 sec) for optimal visualization of both hypovascular and hypervascular liver metastases (107,108).

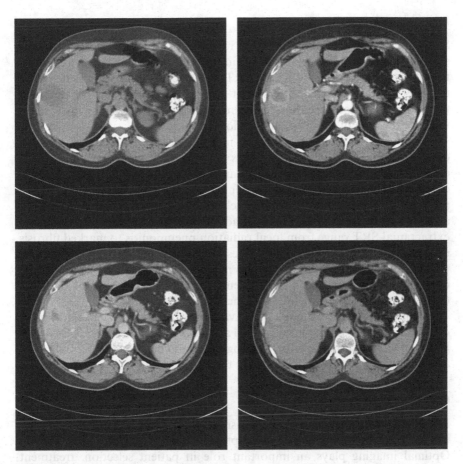

Figure 5 Four-phase hepatic CT scans showing a liver metastasis in the right lobe. The hypodense region seen on the scan without contrast (*upper left panel*) shows distinct contrast enhancement in the late arterial phase (*upper right panel*) and to a lesser degree in the portal venous phase (*lower left panel*). The contrast enhancement has disappeared in the late venous phase (*lower right panel*).

- A trans-abdominal ultrasound-based stereotactic guidance system that accurately localizes the prostate and hepatic lesions is a rapid and direct method to correct for patient position and organ-motion error (109,110).
- Magnetic resonance spectroscopy (MRS) has been used to identify tumor-bearing regions on the basis of an elevated choline/citrate ratio (111,112). Co-registration of this information may permit a "biological target volume" to be generated. However, the spatial resolution of MRS is modest.

FOLLOW-UP IMAGING

Sequential posttreatment imaging is required in order to characterize the sites of disease recurrence and to optimize the planning margins and dose-fractionation schemes used for ECSRT. No elective irradiation is delivered using ECSRT, and some centers omit using separate margins for potential microscopic tumor extension in stereotactic radiotherapy, which could increase the rate of marginal and regional failures.

Volumetric measurements using images after stereotactic radiotherapy can be misleading, as early changes may arise from treatment-induced edema. Transient increases in volume and/or changes in patterns of contrast enhancement have been reported after SRT for brain metastases (113,114), pituitary adenomas (115), vestibular schwannomas (116,117), gliomas (118), and craniopharyngiomas (119). The radiological findings reported following extracranial SRT range from local radiation pneumonitis to marked fibrosis or atelectasis (36,120,121). Difficulties in differentiating between residual tumor and radiation-induced changes mean that the absence of progression on serial studies may be a better denominator of local control than the disappearance of abnormalities on imaging (122).

There is currently limited data available on the indications and timing of PET scans in assessing local control after ECSRT. However, ^{18}FDG-PET has been shown to be superior to using anatomic imaging during follow-up after radiofrequency ablation of liver tumors (123,124).

CONCLUSIONS

ECSRT is a relatively new high-precision treatment modality, and optimal imaging studies are essential for optimizing the technique and results. Optimal imaging plays an important role in patient selection, treatment planning, and verification and follow-up.

REFERENCES

1. Davidson RS, Nwogu CE, Brentjens MJ, et al. The surgical management of pulmonary metastasis: current concepts. Surg Oncol 2001; 10:35–42.
2. Friedel G, Pastorino U, Ginsberg RJ, et al. Results of lung metastasectomy from breast cancer: prognostic criteria on the basis of 467 cases of the International Registry of Lung Metastases. Eur J Cardiothorac Surg 2002; 22:335–344.
3. Headrick JR, Miller DL, Nagorney DM, et al. Surgical treatment of hepatic and pulmonary metastases from colon cancer. Ann Thorac Surg 2001; 71: 975–979.
4. Porte H, Siat J, Guibert B, et al. Resection of adrenal metastases from non-small cell lung cancer: a multicenter study. Ann Thorac Surg 2001; 71:981–985.
5. van Halteren HK, van Geel AN, Hart AA, et al. Pulmonary resection for metastases of colorectal origin. Chest 1995; 107:1526–1531.

6.   Wedman J, Balm AJ, Hart AA, et al. Value of resection of pulmonary metastases in head and neck cancer patients. Head Neck 1996; 18:311–316.

7.   Hoekstra CJ, Stroobants SG, Hoekstra OS, et al. Measurement of perfusion in stage IIIA-N2 non-small cell lung cancer using H(2)(15)O and positron emission tomography. Clin Cancer Res 2002; 8:2109–2115.

8.   Lodge MA, Carson RE, Carrasquillo JA, et al. Parametric Images of Blood Flow in Oncology PET Studies Using [150] Water. J Nucl Med 2000; 41:1784–1792.

9.   Bentzen L, Keiding S, Nordsmark M, et al. Tumour oxygenation assessed by 18F-fluoromisonidazole PET and polarographic needle electrodes in human soft tissue tumours. Radiother Oncol 2003; 67:339–344.

10. Dehdashti F, Mintun MA, Lewis JS, et al. In vivo assessment of tumor hypoxia in lung cancer with 60Cu-ATSM. Eur J Nucl Med Mol Imaging 2003; 30:844–850.

11. Hoebers FJ, Janssen HL, Olmos AV, et al. Phase 1 study to identify tumour hypoxia in patients with head and neck cancer using technetium-99m BRU 59–21. Eur J Nucl Med Mol Imaging 2002; 29:1206–1211.

12. Barthel H, Cleij MC, Collingridge DR, et al. 3′-deoxy-3′-[18F]fluorothymidine as a new marker for monitoring tumor response to antiproliferative therapy in vivo with positron emission tomography. Cancer Res 2003; 63:3791–3798.

13. Dittmann H, Dohmen BM, Paulsen F, et al. [(18)F]FLT-PET for diagnosis and staging of thoracic tumours. Eur J Nucl Med Mol Imaging 2003; only internet version yet.

14. Wells P, Gunn RN, Alison M, et al. Assessment of proliferation in vivo using 2-[(11)C]thymidine positron emission tomography in advanced intra-abdominal malignancies. Cancer Res 2002; 62:5698–5702.

15. Gambhir SS, Czernin J, Schwimmer J, et al. A tabulated summary of the FDG PET literature. J Nucl Med 2001; 42(suppl 5):1S–93S.

16. Bury T, Dowlati A, Paulus P, et al. Whole-body [18]FDG positron emission tomography in the staging of non-small cell lung cancer. Eur Respir J 1997; 10:2529–2534.

17. D'Cunha J, Herndon JL, Herzan DL, et al. Poor correlation between clinical and pathological staging in stage I non-small cell lung cancer: results from CALGB 9761, a prospective trial. Lung Cancer 2005; 48:241–246.

18. Fritscher-Ravens A, Bohuslavizki KH, Brandt L, et al. Mediastinal lymph node involvement in potentially resectable lung cancer: comparison of CT, positron emission tomography, and endoscopic ultrasonography with and without fine-needle aspiration. Chest 2003; 123:442–451.

19. Pieterman RM, van Putten JW, Meuzelaar JJ, et al. Preoperative staging of non-small-cell lung cancer with positron-emission tomography. N Engl J Med 2000; 343:254–261.

20. Schmid RA, Hautmann H, Poellinger B, et al. Staging of recurrent and advanced lung cancer with 18F-FDG PET in a coincidence technique (hybrid PET). Nucl Med Commun 2003; 24:37–45.

21. Scott WJ, Gobar LS, Terry JD, et al. Mediastinal lymph node staging of non-small-cell lung cancer: a prospective comparison of computed tomography and positron emission tomography. J Thorac Cardiovasc Surg 1996; 111:642–648.

22. Steinert HC, Hauser M, Allemann F, et al. Non-small cell lung cancer: nodal staging with FDG PET versus CT with correlative lymph node mapping and sampling. Radiology 1997; 202:441–446.

23. von Haag DW, Follette DM, Roberts PF, et al. Advantages of positron emission tomography over computed tomography in mediastinal staging of non-small cell lung cancer. J Surg Res 2002; 103:160–164.

24. Kalff V, Hicks RJ, Ware RE, et al. The clinical impact of (18)F-FDG PET in patients with suspected or confirmed recurrence of colorectal cancer: a prospective study. J Nucl Med 2002; 43:492–499.

25. Lonneux M, Reffad AM, Detry R, et al. FDG PET improves the staging and selection of patients with recurrent colorectal cancer. Eur J Nud Med Mol Imaging 2002; 29:915–921.

26. Valk PE, Abella-Columna E, Haseman MK, et al. Whole-body PET imaging with [18F]fluorodeoxyglucose in management of recurrent colorectal cancer. Arch Surg 1999; 134:503–511.

27. Kresnik E, Mikosch P, Gallowitsch HJ, et al. Evaluation of head and neck cancer with 18F-FDG PET: a comparison with conventional methods. Eur J Nucl Med 2001; 28:816–821.

28. Siggelkow W, Zimny M, Faridi A, et al. The value of positron emission tomography in the follow-up for breast cancer. Anticancer Res 2003; 23:1859–1867.

29. Vranjesevic D, Filmont JE, Meta J, et al. Whole-body (18)F-FDG PET and conventional imaging for predicting outcome in previously treated breast cancer patients. J Nucl Med 2002; 43:325–329.

30. Gambhir SS, Czernin J, Schwimmer J, et al. A review of the literature for whole-body FDG PET in the management of patients with melanoma. Q J Nucl Med 2000; 44:153–167.

31. Swetter SM, Carroll LA, Johnson DL, et al. Positron emission tomography is superior to computed tomography for metastatic detection in melanoma patients. Ann Surg Oncol 2002; 9:646–653.

32. Lagerwaard FJ, Senan S, van Meerbeeck JP, et al. Has 3D conformal radiotherapy (3D CRT) improved the local tumour control for stage I non-small cell lung cancer? Radiother Oncol 2002; 63:151–157.

33. Qiao X, Tullgren O, Lax I, et al. The role of radiotherapy in treatment of stage I non-small cell lung cancer. Lung Cancer 2003; 41:1–11.

34. Hof H, Herfarth KK, Munter M, et al. Stereotactic single-dose radiotherapy of stage I non-small-cell lung cancer (NSCLC). Int J Radiat Oncol Biol Phys 2003; 56:335–341.

35. Lee S, Choi EK, Park HJ, et al. Stereotactic body frame based fractionated radiosurgery on consecutive days for primary or metastatic tumors in the lung. Lung Cancer 2003; 40:309–315.

36. Uematsu M, Shioda A, Suda A, et al. Computed tomography-guided frameless stereotactic radiotherapy for stage I non-small cell lung cancer: a 5-year experience. Int J Radiat Oncol Biol Phys 2001; 51:666–670.

37. Whyte RI, Crownover R, Murphy MJ, et al. Stereotactic radiosurgery for lung tumors: preliminary report of a phase I trial. Ann Thorac Surg 2003; 75:1097–1101.

38. Hoffmann H. Invasive staging of lung cancer by mediastinoscopy and video-assisted thoracoscopy. Lung Cancer 2001; 34(suppl 3):S3–S5.

39. Dwamena BA, Sonnad SS, Angobaldo JO, et al. Metastases from non-small cell lung cancer: mediastinal staging in the 1990s—meta-analytic comparison of PET and CT. Radiology 1999; 213:530–536.

40. Vansteenkiste JF, Stroobants SG, De Leyn PR, et al. Lymph node staging in non-small-cell lung cancer with FDG PET scan; a prospective study on 690 lymph node stations from 68 patients. J Clin Oncol 1998; 16:2142–2149.

41. Lee J, Aronchick JM, Alavi A. Accuracy of F-18 fluorodeoxyglucose positron emission tomography for the evaluation of malignancy in patients presenting with new lung abnormalities; a retrospective review. Chest 2001; 120:1791–1797.

42. Pitman AG, Hicks RJ, Binns DS, et al. Performance of sodium iodide based (18)F-fluorodeoxyglucose positron emission tomography in the characterization of indeterminate pulmonary nodules or masses. Br J Radiol 2002; 75:114–121.

43. Marom EM, Sarvis S, Herndon JE 2nd, et al. T1 lung cancers: sensitivity of diagnosis with fluorodeoxyglucose PET. Radiology 2002; 223:453–459.

44. Aquino SL, Asmuth JC, Alpert NM, et al. Improved radiologic staging of lung cancer with 2-(18F)-fluoro-2-deoxy-D-glucose-positron emission tomography and computed tomography registration. J Comput Assist Tomogr 2003; 27:479–484.

45. Lardinois D, Weder W, Hany TF, et al. Staging of non-small-cell lung cancer with integrated positron-emission tomography and computed tomography. N Engl J Med 2003; 348:2500–2507.

46. Poncelet AJ, Lonneux M, Coche E, et al. PET-FDG scan enhances but does not replace preoperative surgical staging in non-small cell lung carcinoma. Eur J Cardiothorac Surg 2001; 20:468–474.

47. Okamoto H, Watanabe K, Nagatomo A, et al. Endobronchial ultrasonography for mediastinal and hilar lymph node metastases of lung cancer. Chest 2002; 121:1498–1506.

48. Kurimoto N, Murayama M, Yoshioka S, et al. Analysis of the internal structure of peripheral pulmonary lesions using endobronchial ultrasonography. Chest 2002; 122:1887–1894.

49. el Mouaaouy A, Naruhn M, Becker HD. Diagnosis of liver metastases from malignant gastrointestinal neoplasms; results of pre- and intraoperative ultrasound examinations. Surg Endosc 1991; 5:209–213.

50. Machi J, Isomoto H, Kurohiji T, et al. Accuracy of intraoperativee ultrasonography in diagnosing liver metastasis from colorectal cancer: evaluation with postoperative follow-up results. World J Surg 1991; 15:551–556.

51. Rafaelsen SR, Kronborg O, Larsen C, et al. Intraoperative ultrasonography in detection of hepatic metastases from colorectal cancer. Dis Colon Rectum 1995; 38:355–360.

52. Valls C, Andia E, Sanchez A, et al. Hepatic metastases from colorectal cancer: preoperative detection and assessment of resectability with helical CT. Radiology 2001; 218:55–60.

53. Strasberg SM, Dehdashti F, Siegel BA, et al. Survival of patients evaluated by FDG PET before hepatic resection for metastatic colorectal carcinoma: a prospective database study. Ann Surg 2001; 233:293–299.

54. Desai DC, Zervos EE, Arnold MW, et al. Positron emission tomography affects surgical management in recurrent colorectal cancer patients. Ann Surg Oncol 2003; 10:59–64.

55. Fong Y, Saldinger PF, Akhurst T, et al. Utility of 18F-FDG positron emission tomography scanning on selection of patients for resection of hepatic colorectal metastases. Am J Surg 1999; 178:282–287.

56. Rydzewski B, Dehdashti F, Gordon BA, et al. Usefulness of intraoperative sonography for revealing hepatic metastases from colorectal cancer in patients selected for surgery after undergoing FDG-PET. Am J Roentgenol 2002; 178:353–358.

57. Topal B, Flamen P, Aerts R, et al. Clinical value of whole-body emission tomography in potentially curable colorectal liver metastases. Eur J Surg Oncol 2001; 27:175–179.

58. Rohren EM, Paulson EK, Hagge R, et al. The role of F-18 FDG positron emission tomography in preoperative assessment of the liver in patients being considered for curative resection of hepatic metastases from colorectal cancer. Clin Nucl Med 2002; 27:550–555.

59. Hsia TC, Shen YY, Yen RF, et al. Comparing whole body 18F-2-deoxyglucose positron emission tomography and technetium-99m methylene diophosphate bone scan to detect bone metastases in patients with non-small cell lung cancer. Neoplasma 2002; 49:267–271.

60. Ohta M, Tokuda Y, Suzuki Y, et al. Whole body PET for the evaluation of bony metastases in patients with breast cancer: comparison with 99Tcm-MDP bone scintigraphy. Nucl Med Commun 2001; 22:875–879.

61. Wu HC, Yen RF, Shen YY, et al. Comparing whole body 18F-2-deoxyglucose positron emission tomography and technetium-99m methylene diphosphate bone scan to detect bone metastases in patients with renal cell carcinomas—a preliminary report. J Cancer Res Clin Oncol 2002; 128:503–506.

62. Yang SN, Liang JA, Lin FJ, et al. Comparing whole body (18)F-2-deoxyglucose positron emission tomography and technetium-99m methylene diphosphonate bone scan to detect bone metastases in patients with breast cancer. J Cancer Res Clin Oncol 2002; 128:325–328.

63. Nakamoto Y, Osman M, Wahl RL. Prevalence and patterns of bone metastases detected with positron emission tomography using F-18 FDG. Clin Nucl Med 2003; 28:302–307.

64. Godersky JC, Smoker WR, Knutzon R. Use of magnetic resonance imaging in the evaluation of metastatic spinal disease. Neurosurgery 1987; 21:676–680.

65. Hara R, Itami J, Kondo T, et al. Stereotactic single high dose irradiation of lung tumors under respiratory gating. Radiother Oncol 2002; 63:159–163.

66. Ozhasoglu C, Murphy MJ. Issues in respiratory motion compensation during external-beam radiotherapy. Int J Radiat Oncol Biol Phys 2002; 52:1389–1399.

67. Weiss E, Hess CF. The impact of gross tumor volume (GTV) and clinical target volume (CTV) definition on the total accuracy in radiotherapy theoretical aspects and practical experiences. Strahlenther Onkol 2003; 179:21–30.

68. Collier DC, Burnett SS, Amin M, et al. Assessment of consistency in contouring of normal-tissue anatomic structures. J Appl Clin Med Phys 2003; 4:17–24.

69. Fiorino C, Vavassori V, Sanguineti G, et al. Rectum contouring variability in patients treated for prostate cancer: impact on rectum dose–volume histograms and normal tissue complication probability. Radiother Oncol 2002; 63:249–255.

70. Lagerwaard FJ, van de Vaart PJ, Voet PW, et al. Can errors in reconstructing pre-chemotherapy target volumes contribute to the inferiority of sequential chemoradiation in stage III non-small cell lung cancer (NSCLC)? Lung Cancer 2002; 38:297–301.

71. Senan S, van Sornsen de Koste J, Samson M, et al. Evaluation of a target contouring protocol for 3D conformal radiotherapy in non-small cell lung cancer. Radiother Oncol 1999; 53:247–255.

72. Anscher MS, Marks LB, Shafman TD, et al. Risk of long-term complications after TFG-betal-guided very-high-dose thoracic radiotherapy. Int J Radiat Oncol Biol Phys 2003; 56:988–995.

73. International Commission on Radiation Units and Measurements. ICRU Report 62: Prescribing, Recording and Reporting Photon Beam Therapy (suppl to ICRU Report 50), Bethesda MD, 1999.

74. van Sornsen de Koste JR, Lagerwaard FJ, Nijssen-Visser MR, et al. Tumor location cannot predict the mobility of lung tumors: a 3D analysis of data generated from multiple CT scans. Int J Radiat Oncol Biol Phys 2003; 56:348–354.

75. Booth JT, Zavgorodni SF. Modelling the dosimetric consequences of organ motion at CT imaging on radiotherapy treatment planning. Phys Med Biol 2001; 46:1369–1377.

76. Balter JM, Ten Haken RK, Lawrence TS et al. Uncertainties in CT-based radiation therapy treatment planning associated with patient breathing. Int J Radiat Oncol Biol Phys 1996; 36:167–174.

77. Halperin R, Pobinson D, Murray B. Fluoroscopy for assessment of physiologic movement of lung tumors, a pitfall of clinical practice? [abstr]. Radiother Oncol 2002; 65:Sl.

78. Stevens CW, Munden RF, Forster KM, et al. Respiratory-driven lung tumor motion is independent of tumor size, tumor location, and pulmonary function. Int J Radiat Oncol Biol Phys 2001; 51:62–68.

79. Aruga T, Itami J, Aruga M, et al. Target volume definition for upper abdominal irradiation using CT scans obtained during inhale and exhale phases. Int J Radiat Oncol Biol Phys 2000; 48:465–469.

80. Onimaru R, Shirato H, Shimizu S, et al. Tolerance of organs at risk in small-volume, hypofractionated, image-guided radiotherapy for primary and metastatic lung cancers. Int J Radiat Oncol Biol Phys 2003; 56:126–135.

81. Yamada K, Soejima T, Yoden E, et al. Improvement of three-dimensional treatment planning models of small lung targets using high-speed multi-slice computed tomographic imaging. Int J Radiat Oncol Biol Phys 2002; 54:1210–1216.

82. Senan S, Lagerwaard FJ, Nijssen-Visser MR. Incorporating lung tumor mobility in radiotherapy planning. Int J Radiat Oncol Biol Phys 2002; 52: 1142–1143.

83. Lagerwaard FJ, Van Sornsen de Koste JR, Nijssen-Visser MR, et al. Multiple "slow" CT scans for incorporating lung tumor mobility in radiotherapy planning. Int J Radiat Oncol Biol Phys 2001; 51:932–937.

84. van Sornsen de Koste JR, Lagerwaard FJ, Schuchhard-Schipper RH, et al. Dosimetric consequences of tumor mobility in radiotherapy of stage I non-small cell lung cancer—an analysis of data generated using "slow" CT scans. Radiother Oncol 2001; 61:93–99.

85. van Sornsen de Koste JR, Lagerwaard FJ, de Boer HC, et al. Are multiple CT scans required for planning curative radiotherapy in lung tumors of the lower lobe? Int J Radiat Oncol Biol Phys 2003; 55:1394–1399.

86. Chen QS, Weinhous MS, Deibel FC, et al. Fluoroscopic study of tumor motion due to breathing: facilitating precise radiation therapy for lung cancer patients. Med Phys 2001; 28:1850–1856.

87. Seppenwoolde Y, Shirato H, Kitamura K, et al. Precise and real-time measurement of 3D tumor motion in lung due to breathing and heartbeat, measured during radiotherapy. Int J Radiat Oncol Biol Phys 2002; 53:822–834.

88. Herfarth KK, Debus J, Lohr F, et al. Extracranial stereotactic radiation therapy: set-up accuracy of patients treated for liver metastases. Int J Radiat Oncol Biol Phys 2000; 46:329–335.

89. Lax I, Blomgren H, Naslund I, et al. Stereotactic radiotherapy of malignancies in the abdomen. Methodological aspects. Acta Oncol 1994; 33:677–683.

90. Negoro Y, Nagata Y, Aoki T, et al. The effectiveness of an immobilization device in conformal radiotherapy for lung tumor: reduction of respiratory tumor movement and evaluation of the daily setup accuracy. Int J Radiat Oncol Biol Phys 2001; 50:889–898.

91. Wulf J, Hadinger U, Oppitz U, et al. Stereotactic radiotherapy of extracranial targets: CT-simulation and accuracy of treatment in the stereotactic body frame. Radiother Oncol 2000; 57:225–236.

92. Murphy MJ, Martin D, Whyte R, et al. The effectiveness of breath-holding to stabilize lung and pancreas tumors during radiosurgery. Int J Radiat Oncol Biol Phys 2002; 53:475–482.

93. O'Dell WG, Schell MC, Reynolds D, et al. Dose broadening due to target position variability during fractionated breath-held radiation therapy. Med Phys 2002; 29:1430–1437.

94. Barnes EA, Murray BR, Robinson DM, et al. Dosimetric evaluation of lung tumor immobilization using breath hold at deep inspiration. Int J Radiat Oncol Biol Phys 2001; 50:1091–1098.

95. Murphy MJ, Chang SD, Gibbs IC, et al. Patterns of patient movement during frameless image-guided radiosurgery. Int J Radiat Oncol Biol Phys 2003; 55:1400–1408.

96. Onishi H, Kuriyama K, Komiyama T, et al. A new irradiation system for lung cancer combining linear accelerator, computed tomography, patient self-breath-holding, and patient-directed beam-control without respiratory monitoring devices. Int J Radiat Oncol Biol Phys 2003; 56:14–20.

97. Balter JM, Brock KK, Litzenberg DW, et al. Daily targeting of intrahepatic tumors for radiotherapy. Int J Radiat Oncol Biol Phys 2002; 52:266–271.

98. Wong JW, Sharpe MB, Jaffray DA, et al. The use of active breathing control (ABC) to reduce margin for breathing motion. Int J Radiat Oncol Biol Phys 1999; 44:911–919.

99. Ford EC, Mageras GS, Yorke E, et al. Evaluation of respiratory movement during gated radiotherapy using film and electronic portal imaging. Int J Radiat Oncol Biol Phys 2002; 52:522–531.

100. Vedam SS, Keall RJ, Kini VR, et al. Acquiring a four-dimensional computed tomography dataset using an external respiratory signal. Phys Med Biol 2003; 48:45–62.

101. Ford EC, Mageras GS, Yorke E, et al. Respiration-correlated spiral CT: a method of measuring respiratory-induced anatomic motion for radiation treatment planning. Med Phys 2003; 30:88–97.

102. Harada T, Shirato H, Ogura S, et al. Real-time tumor-tracking radiation therapy for lung carcinoma by the aid of insertion of a gold marker using bronchofiberscopy. Cancer 2002; 95:1720–1727.

103. Shirato H, Harada T, Harabayashi T, et al. Feasibility of insertion/implantation of 2.0-mm-diameter gold internal fiducial markers for precise setup and real-time tumor tracking in radiotherapy. Int J Radiat Oncol Biol Phys 2003; 56:240–247.

104. Murphy MJ. Fiducial-based targeting accuracy for external-beam radiotherapy. Med Phys 2002; 29:334–344.

105. Pouliot J, Aubin M, Langen KM, et al. (Non)-migration of radiopaque markers used for on-line localization of the prostate with an electronic portal imaging device. Int J Radiat Oncol Biol Phys 2003; 56:862–866.

106. Kitamura K, Shirato H, Seppenwoolde Y, et al. Three-dimensional intrafractional movement of prostate measured during real-time tumor-tracking radiotherapy in supine and prone treatment positions. Int J Radiat Oncol Biol Phys 2002; 53:1117–1123.

107. Francis IR, Cohan RH, McNulty NJ, et al. Multidetector CT of the liver and hepatic neoplasms: effect of multiphasic imaging on tumor conspicuity and vascular enhancement. AJR 2003; 180:1217–1224.

108. Gualdi GF, Casciani E, D'Agostino A, et al. Triphasic spiral computerized tomography of the liver: vascular models of non-cystic focal lesions. Radiol Med 1998; 96:344–352.

109. Lattanzi J, McNeeley S, Donnelly S, et al. Ultrasound-based stereotactic guidance in prostate cancer—quantification of organ motion and set-up errors in external beam radiation therapy. Comput Aided Surg 2000; 5:289–295.

110. Trichter F, Ennis RD. Prostate localization using transabdominal ultrasound imaging. Int J Radiat Oncol Biol Phys 2003; 56:1225–1233.

111. Mizowaki T, Cohen GN, Fung AY, et al. Towards integrating functional imaging in the treatment of prostate cancer with radiation: the registration of the MR spectroscopy imaging to ultrasound/CT images and its implementation in treatment planning. Int J Radiat Oncol Biol Phys 2002; 54:1558–1564.

112. Zaider M, Zelefsky MJ, Lee EK, et al. Treatment planning for prostate implants using magnetic-resonance spectroscopy imaging. Int J Radiat Oncol Biol Phys 2000; 47:1085–1096.

113. Huber PE, Hawighorst H, Fuss M, et al. Transient enlargement of contrast uptake on MRI after linear accelerator (linac) stereotactic radiosurgery for brain metastases. Int J Radiat Oncoi Biol Phys 2001; 49:1339–1349.

114. Peterson AM, Meltzer CC, Evanson EJ, et al. MR imaging response of brain metastases after gamma knife stereotactic radiosurgery. Radiology 1999; 211:807–814.

115. Tung GA, Noren G, Rogg JM, et al. MR imaging of pituitary adenomas after gamma knife stereotactic radiosurgery. AJR Am J Roentgenol 2001; 177: 919–924.

116. Nakamura H, Jokura H, Takahashi K, et al. Serial follow-up MR imaging after gamma knife radiosurgery for vestibular schwannoma. Am J Neuro radiol 2000; 21:1540–1546.

117. Szeifert GT, Massager N, DeVriendt D, et al. Observations of intracranial neoplasms treated with gamma knife radiosurgery. J Neurosurg 2002; 97(suppl 5):623–626.

118. Bakardjiev AI, Barnes PD, Goumnerova LC, et al. Magnetic resonance imaging changes after stereotactic radiation therapy for childhood low grade astrocytoma. Cancer 1996; 78:864–873.

119. Chung WY, Pan DH, Shiau CY, et al. Gamma knife radiosurgery for craniopharyngiomas. J Neurosurg 2000; 93(suppl 3):47–56.

120. Choi EK, Lee S-W, Ahn SD, et al. Stereotactic body frame based fractionated radiosurgery on consecutive days for intrathoracic tumors: preliminary results of a phase I/II study. Lung Cancer 2003; 41(suppl 2):S10.

121. Fuss M, Salter BJ, Selva M, et al. Intensity-modulated hypofractionated radioablation for lung lesions. Lung Cancer 2003; 41(suppl 2):S10–S11.

122. Green MR, Ginsberg R, Ardizzoni A, et al. Induction therapy for stage III NSCLC: a consensus report. Lung Cancer 1994; 11(suppl 3):9–10.

123. Anderson GS, Brinkmann F, Soulen MC, et al. FDG positron emission tomography in the surveillance of hepatic tumors treated with radiofrequency ablation. Clin Nucl Med 2003; 28:192–197.

124. Langenhoff BS, Oyen WJ, Jager GJ, et al. Efficacy of fluorine-18-deoxyglucose positron emission tomography in detecting tumor recurrence after local ablative therapy for liver metastases: a prospective study. J Clin Oncol 2002; 20:4453–4458.

7

Radiobiological Considerations of Stereotactic Body Radiotherapy

Steve P. Lee and H. Rodney Withers

*Department of Radiation Oncology, UCLA Medical Center,
Los Angeles, California, U.S.A.*

Jack F. Fowler

*Department of Human Oncology, University Hospital,
Madison, Wisconsin, U.S.A.*

INTRODUCTION: CLINICAL RADIOBIOLOGY AS A FOUR-DIMENSIONAL PROBLEM

Cancer radiotherapy works via biological mechanisms rather than by physically eradicating tumors as practiced by surgeons. That is, radiation therapy is bona fide *biological* therapy—more akin to the craft practiced by medical oncologists using systemic chemotherapy. Furthermore, radiation therapy is done with precise quantification of dosage deposited at the patient's anatomic site of interest. This is feasible because ionizing radiation particles are several orders of magnitude smaller than their subcellular biological targets, so that the probability of such interaction is rare enough to permit a straightforward, albeit simplified, biophysical interpretation. Equipped with a consistent way of measuring the dose, one can analyze the effect of radiation upon living cells after quantifying the resulting biological changes, of which the end-point is often defined operationally as clonogenic cell survival. Various quantitative models have been proposed to explain the observed survival probability as a function of dose. Among

131

these models, the linear-quadratic (LQ) theory has gained wide popularity over the past few decades (1). In addition, a versatile theoretical framework based on the LQ theory has been developed to correlate biological effects of radiation treatments using a variable range of dose rates or fractionation schemes (2,3). Perhaps it suffices to say that the problem of analyzing radio-biology along the *time* domain, as specified by any "unconventional" frac-tionation protocol, has been solved in its most general form. What is left is the problem in the *space* domain, otherwise known as the "volume effect," elicited due to heterogeneous dose distribution in three-dimensional space. In real life, the complexity arising from combined temporal–spatial varia-tion of radiation dose could significantly dictate the practical application of radiation biology in the clinical setting.

The organization of this chapter is structured to follow a thread of synthesis of central ideas rather than a verbatim literature survey. We will first review the fundamental principles in clinical radiation biology along the temporal domain. Specifically, utilization of the LQ theory to quantify biological effects will be discussed. This will lead to the topic of the so-called "double-trouble" effect for which clinical application would call for biolo-gical "correction" despite precise physical dosimetry in three-dimensional space, representing an inevitable problem encountered in the spatial domain. Then, when ultra precision oriented therapy such as stereotactic irradiation (whether single-dose or fractionated) or intensity-modulated radiation therapy (IMRT) is introduced, heterogeneous dose distribution often surfaces to exacerbate the problem of the volume effect and must be considered. This is currently still at the forefront of clinical radiobiological research, but some relevant practical issues will be discussed to hopefully help readers gain insight into what they might face in clinical practice using high-tech driven treatment technologies. Interested readers outside the radiation oncology specialty are urged to consult teaching texts such as Hall (4) or Withers and Peters (5) for a detailed review of basic radiobiology prin-ciples. For on-going research topics in quantitative radiation biology, there are excellent collections of articles in *Seminars in Radiation Oncology* (issues 9:1, 11:3, 12:3, and 14:1) and other major radiation oncology or medical physics journals.

The fact that clinically relevant radiobiology issues can be visualized as a space–time problem should be distinguished from what medical physicists currently describe as "four-dimensional" radiation therapy. The former will be dealt with in detail in this chapter, while the latter pertains to dosimetric problems arising from motion uncertainties due to intra-fractional as well as inter-fractional movements of radiotherapy targets and normal tissues. For extracranial stereotactic radiation treatments, all these issues are of relevance and should be considered in order to devise rational treatment strategy for each patient.

RADIOBIOLOGY PROBLEM ALONG THE TEMPORAL DOMAIN: TIME, DOSE, AND FRACTIONATION

A clinical phenomenon early radiotherapists observed was that the best therapeutic result can be realized by fractionation rather than single-dose treatment (6). However, the biological effect of radiation does not appear to be linearly additive when a course of treatment is split into multiple fractions of smaller doses, each given separately in time. That is, some biological processes seem to occur during the time interval in-between the fractions, such that the final biological effect of these fractions is not equivalent to that of a treatment using the total sum of the doses in one single fraction. We might view this phenomenon—that biological effect of radiation depends on dose fractionation in *time*—as the problem of radiobiology along the temporal domain.

The 4 *R*s of Fractionation Radiobiology

Over the past several decades, we have gained more insights into the biological processes occurring in-between the treatment fractions. They have been summarized by Withers (7) conveniently as the "4 *R*s of fractionation radiobiology": reoxygenation, repopulation, repair, and redistribution.

Reoxygenation

The damage of tissues by radiation depends largely on the formation of hydroxyl radicals, which in turn depends on the availability of oxygen molecules in close proximity. Fractionation allows oxygen to diffuse into the usually hypoxic center of an expanding tumor during the interval between fractions, and thus enables more tumor cell killing during the subsequent treatment. This mechanism, first described by Thomlinson and Gray (8), essentially equates fractionation as an effective hypoxic tumor radiation sensitizer (like some chemicals designed for the similar purpose).

Repopulation

All living cells have the potential to repopulate in number by mitotic growth of clonogens. During the time of a radiation treatment course, both normal tissue progenitor cells and malignant cells may repopulate, and the outcome of such competing processes may influence the therapeutic efficacy significantly. Moreover, Withers et al. have described a phenomenon of "accelerated repopulation" for irradiated cells, which is stimulated by such therapeutic intervention (9). This identifies the overall treatment time as an important clinical variable affecting the chances of tumor control and acute normal tissue reaction. As malignant cells quickly repopulate, protraction of overall treatment time is therapeutically disadvantageous when the dose-limiting normal tissue is not rapidly repopulating. In order to combat this potential bottleneck for tumor control, clinicians sometimes employ the strategy of "accelerated fractionation," i.e., delivering a conventional level of total dose but shortening the overall treatment time with more intensely fractionated patterns (10).

Repair

Cells can be equipped with repair machinery to reverse partial damage caused by a small fraction of radiation dose. They would die if such damage fails to be repaired sufficiently and is exacerbated by further radiation insults. Elkind and Sutton in 1959 described one possible contributing mechanism called "sublethal damage (SLD) repair" (11). By splitting a single dose into two fractions, and observing the amount of dose required for the second fraction to result in the same level of final cell survival as a function of the interfractional time interval, they demonstrated the capability of cells to repair such radiation injury. Furthermore, this repair process proceeds roughly exponentially in time with a typical half-time of about 1–2 hr for clinically relevant tissues. A corollary is that if the dose per fraction is decreased and the interfractional time interval is long enough to allow for complete SLD repair, the total dose required to achieve a fixed level of cell death would be higher. Fractionation thus spares cells from radiation damage in comparison with single-dose irradiation. If normal cells repair better than tumor cells, there would be therapeutic gain by fractionation, and vice versa. Other types of radiation damage repair mechanisms have been proposed (12).

Redistribution

Cells exhibit differential sensitivities towards radiation at different phases of the cell cycle. Most mammalian cells are more sensitive at the junction between G2 and M phases. After an initial fraction of dose, the cells at a more resistant phase (e.g., late S) may survive but then proceed in time eventually to the sensitive phases, thus subjecting themselves to more efficient killing during the next fraction. One can thus appreciate why fast cycling cells like skin or mucosal cells are more prone to radiation killing than slow or dormant ones such as muscle or skeletal cells, a phenomenon realized by investigators in the first decade of radiation oncology history and enshrined as the *Law of Bergonie and Tribondéau* (13).

Empirical Power–Laws

Once early investigators realized the significance of radiobiological effects due to fractionation, some sort of quantitative guideline was clearly desirable. Initially, however, clinicians have for a long while relied mainly on empirical approaches. The first was published in 1944 by Strandqvist (14). In attempting to theorize a quantitative relationship between the total radiation dose needed to achieve a certain clinical effect (e.g., skin reaction) and the extent of fractionation (in the early days often paraphrased as "protraction in time" resulting from the often ultra-low intensity of the radiation sources), Strandqvist borrowed rather empirically the popular *Schwarzschild's Law of Photochemistry* (15): Given that the intensity of light (i.e., dose per time), I, should be inversely proportional to the time of exposure, T, for a certain degree of photochemical exposure (i.e., isoeffect), one might express the following simple isoeffect relationship:

$$I \cdot T^p = \Psi \tag{1}$$

where Ψ is a constant characterizing the desired effect, and the exponent p is a parameter characterizing such a "power–law" relationship $(0 \leq p \leq 1)$. Because the dose, D, is equivalent to $I \cdot T$, then:

$$D \equiv I \cdot T = \Psi \cdot T^{1-p} \tag{2}$$

One can readily see that such an equation predicts a linear curve on a log D versus log T display[a] for the same effect Ψ, with the slope of the line dictated by the parameter p.

Although Strandqvist's approach has been criticized mainly due to the lack of reliable clinical data needed to construct his log–log graph, the methodology was nevertheless a useful endeavor many found easy to emulate. The empirical nature of such an approach necessitated constant revisions, depending on the particular clinical scenario or biological tissue from which useful data were extracted to fit the curves. Various quantitative schemes were invented over several decades to interpret complex clinical observations, yet the approaches largely followed the original framework of Strandqvist, i.e., utilizing phenomenologically oriented entities with empirical assumption of the power–laws. First, after laboratory and clinical investigations showed the importance of the *number* of fractions, Ellis added a fractionation factor to the power–law and created the nominal standard dose (NSD) (16). This concept soon encountered a problem: the entity, NSD, was not linearly additive. That is, there was no easy way to sum the effects of several partial treatments to predict a net effect. To account for the effect at each "subtolerance" dose level, Kirk et al. extended the concept of NSD and devised the term cumulative radiation effect (CRE) (17). Orton and Ellis then developed, after some cumbersome algebra, a linearly additive quantity called the time dose fractionation (TDF) factor (18). Despite the mathematical obscurity, clinicians have generally welcomed the use of TDF in treatment planning, since it and its power–law predecessors represented the only quantitative guidelines available then, and because look-up tables or graphs were readily available.

---

[a] Unless specified otherwise, all logarithmic expressions used in this work (including formulas and figures) pertain to the *natural* logarithm, for which both abbreviations, "log" and "ln," are used interchangeably.

For example, tissue-specific entities termed "Neuret" (19) and "Optic-neuret" (20) were proposed later for the treatment of central nervous system tumors.

As more is learned about the underlying mechanisms of radiation effect on living cells and tissues, the phenomenological guidelines based on power–laws have slowly been replaced by more mechanistically-sound biological principles. More importantly, as wider variability is incorporated into the worldwide practice of fractionation radiotherapy, it has become quite difficult to gather universally applicable empirical guidelines based solely on one's preferred treatment regimens.

The power–laws have been given yet another chance for resurrection when contemporary researchers use the similar phenomenologic approach to model the biology of heterogeneous dose distribution in space, i.e., radiobiology problem in the spatial domain, to be described later in the section on Equivalent Uniform Dose (EUD).

Mechanistic Models and Cell Survival Curves

As implied earlier, a salient feature of radiobiology, in contrast to the pharmacologic principle behind chemotherapy, is the relative ease of quantifying biological effect as a function of radiation dose. This results primarily from the feasibility of measuring the input (radiation dose) and output (cell survival fraction) of a biological process fairly accurately, with the intervening mechanism interpreted readily using biophysical models. The basic assumption is that there exist within each cell critical targets, which when hit by ionizing radiation particles in a *random* fashion may lead to consequential loss of cellular reproductive integrity. This is the essence of the so-called "target-cell hypothesis" or "hit theory" (21).

Desauer was perhaps the first to conceive a mechanistic interpretation of radiation action, suggesting in 1923 a "point-heat" theory that describes radiation effects as resulting from electron impact on protein molecules with microscopic energy absorption and local temperature elevation (22). The discovery of the nature of the generic material three decades later then led to the identification of the most probable targets as chromosomes or DNA molecules. Meanwhile, many experimentally obtained in vitro and in vivo cell survival curves were published, the first ever mammalian survival curve being reported by Puck and Marcus (23). When plotted as a semi-log graph of log SF (survival fraction) versus radiation dose D, most revealed a very similar shape with a "curvy shoulder" at the low-dose region in contiguity with a relatively linear tail towards the high-dose region (Fig. 1A). Evidently, at least two biophysical mechanisms seemed to be operating simultaneously to produce such a result. Various biophysical models have been proposed since, and a clear champion is the LQ model (1). Before we embark on its detailed description, it is perhaps pedagogically sound to introduce another less popular model: the single-hit, multitarget killing model.

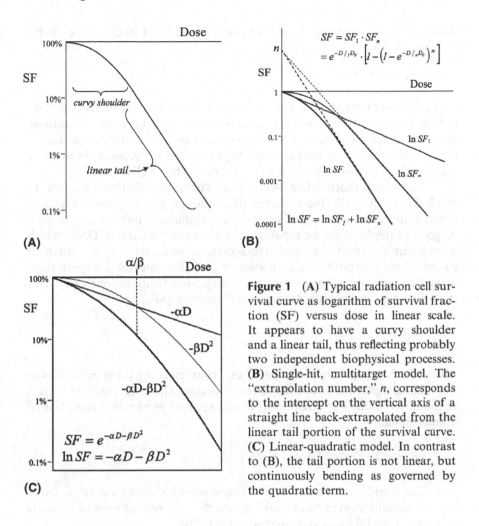

Figure 1 (A) Typical radiation cell survival curve as logarithm of survival fraction (SF) versus dose in linear scale. It appears to have a curvy shoulder and a linear tail, thus reflecting probably two independent biophysical processes. (B) Single-hit, multitarget model. The "extrapolation number," n, corresponds to the intercept on the vertical axis of a straight line back-extrapolated from the linear tail portion of the survival curve. (C) Linear-quadratic model. In contrast to (B), the tail portion is not linear, but continuously bending as governed by the quadratic term.

The Single–Hit, Multitarget Killing Model

This model adequately describes the shape of a typical radiation survival curve with the assumption of two independent components of cell killing (5,21). The first, or *single-hit*, component comes from a straightforward theorization based on a Poisson process[b] of radiation action on a critical target within each cell, which after being hit by the ionizing particle alone will cause irreversible cell death. A conceivable example might be double-strand break of a DNA molecule. Interested readers may refer to the "raindrops in the bucket"

---

[b] This is a ubiquitous stochastic process used by physical scientists to model many natural or artificial phenomena, each with a probability of occurrence that is fundamentally rare.

analogy (5), and appreciate the expression for survival fraction due to this process (SF$_1$) as

$$SF_1 = e^{-D/_1D_0}$$

where D is the radiation dose, and $_1D_0$ is the dose at which the survival fraction becomes e^{-1} ($\sim$37%) of its original value (i.e., a parameter defining the intrinsic radiation sensitivity) which translates *on the average* to one lethal hit per target. On a survival curve presented as a semi-log plot of log SF versus D, the negative reciprocal of $_1D_0$ yields the slope of the expected straight line (Fig. 1B).

The second independent mode of cell killing by radiation is thought to result from cell death due to cumulative (though not necessarily synchronous) injuries elicited at *all* of several, say, n, multiple intracellular targets. A good example might be repairable single-strand breaks of DNA which would require repeated similar damages to consolidate into a permanent chromosome aberration; in such case, $n \geq 2$. By repeated interpretations using Poisson process for each of the n target-inactivations, one can derive the following expression for the survival fraction (SF$_n$):

$$SF_n = 1 - \left(1 - e^{-D/_nD_0}\right)^n$$

where $_nD_0$ is another biological parameter characterizing the effectiveness of the radiation particle to inactivate these targets. Thus, the combined effect of radiation in this two-component model appears to be rather complicated mathematically:

$$SF = e^{-D/_1D_0}\left[1 - \left(1 - e^{-D/_nD_0}\right)^n\right] \tag{3}$$

The semi-log plot based on the above equation shows a survival curve with an initially convex "shoulder" at low dose range, but eventually tends to nearly a straight line as D increases (Fig. 1B).

The Linear-Quadratic (LQ) Model

Based on this model, the survival fraction after a single treatment of radiation dose D can be characterized by the following equation (1,2,24):

$$SF = e^{-\alpha D - \beta D^2} \tag{4}$$

where α and β are tissue-specific parameters governing intrinsic radiation sensitivity. The survival curve takes on a continuously bending downward trend rather than becoming nearly a straight line at high dose range (Fig. 1C). The ratio, α/β, which has a dimension of dose (Gy), can be found algebraically to correspond to the dose at which the linear (α-) and the quadratic (β-) components contribute equally to cell killing. The linear component might be seen as result from the single-hit mechanism described above. While the mechanistic origin of the quadratic component has been somewhat controversial (25,26)—some may argue that the quadratic term is the consequence of fixation between *two* otherwise repairable DNA single strand breaks or damaged chromatids into permanent chromosome aberration—the LQ model is nevertheless useful because of its simplicity and the fact that it does describe the shape of the survival curves adequately (at least from α/β values of about 1–10 Gy).

One of the most attractive roles of the LQ model stems from its ability to explain the differential sensitivities of the so-called *acute-* versus *late-* responding tissues to fractionated radiotherapy (Fig. 2A), thus establishing the theoretical rationale of fractionation when treating acutely-responding malignant tumors embedded within late-responding normal tissues (27).

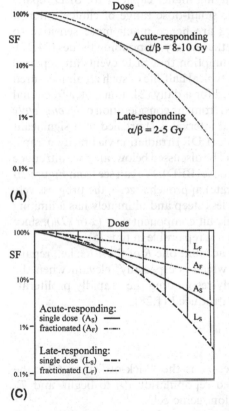

(A)

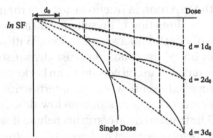

(B)

Figure 2 (A) Distinct shapes of survival curves between acutely-responding and late-responding tissues. The former is characterized by larger α/β ratio and dominated by the linear component, the latter by a smaller α/β and dominated by the quadratic component. (B) Fractionation effect and survival curve. Here the effects of three fractionation schemes are shown, with respective dose per fraction of d_0, $2d_0$, and $3d_0$. Upon fractionation, the initial portion of the single-dose curve is repeated successively, provided that near-completion of sublethal damage repair occurs in-between the fractions. Clearly, the smaller the dose per fraction, the less cell lethality, thus more sparing of the tissue. (C) Differential sparing effects of fractionation upon acute- vs. late-responding tissues. Fractionation spares the late-responding tissue more because of the "curvier" shape of its survival curve (L_s cf. L_F), while the acutely-responding tissue is spared relatively less (A_s cf. A_F).

Indeed, for a fractionated radiotherapy course with n fractions of dose per fraction, d, the overall effect is given by

$$SF = e^{-n(\alpha d + \beta d^2)}. \tag{5}$$

On the survival curve plot, this amounts to repeating by n times the initial fractional amount of cell survival resulting from dose d, each picking up successively where it ends from the previous treatment after complete repair of SLD during the interfractional interval (Fig. 2B). The net result is the sparing of the irradiated tissues, with an "effective slope" of an essentially linear overall survival curve becoming less steep the more fractionated the treatment is. Furthermore, it is seen that by fractionation the late-responding tissue is spared relatively more than the acutely-responding tissue due to its "curvier" shape (signifying higher capacity for SLD repair) of its single-dose survival curve in the small-dose range of clinical interest (Fig. 2C). The late-responding tissues are hence much more sensitive to the variation in fractionation size than the acutely-responding tissues (24,27).

Equation (5) results from the assumption that SLD events are repaired sufficiently in-between fractions. With a typical half-life of such repair measured in hours, the condition is usually satisfied for a daily (24-hour) inter-fractional interval. A useful corollary can be derived from the consideration of *incompletely* repaired events when the interfractional interval is shortened to a significant degree or during continuous low-dose rate (LDR) irradiation via brachytherapy. The mathematical construct behind it will be discussed below, after we introduce a useful concept of biologically effective dose (BED). We can see from Figure 2B that, as the dose per fraction (or dose rate) approaches zero, the progressively more "spared" survival curve becomes less steep and ultimately has a limiting effective slope characterized by the single-hit component only (α or $_1D_0$), since this is the component of damage that is not repairable in time (5).

Note that Eq. (5) only takes into account one R of the 4 Rs: i.e., repair. To account for repopulation of cells which is especially relevant when the tissue under consideration is an acutely-responding (i.e., rapidly proliferating) type, a treatment time factor is introduced (1,28):

$$SF = e^{-n(\alpha d + \beta d^2) + \frac{\ln 2 (T - T_k)}{T_p}} \tag{6}$$

where T is the overall treatment time, T_k is the "kick-off" time after the treatment starts and before accelerated repopulation (9) to begin, and T_p is the effective doubling time of the clonogenic cells.

Finally, since both redistribution and reoxygenation essentially result in sensitizing cells for radiation killing upon fractionation, it is not surprising that these two Rs have been grouped together and named "resensitization" for the purpose of conceptual simplification when using mathematical models (29).

Biologically Effective Dose (BED)

The negative of the exponent in the expression of Eq. (6), denoted E, where $SF \equiv e^{-E}$, can be visualized as a quantitative measure of the "effectiveness" of radiation cell-killing, since it directly reflects how steep the effective slope is on a semi-logarithmic survival curve. Thus,

$$E = n(\alpha d + \beta d^2) - \frac{\ln 2(T - T_k)}{T_p}$$

Based on the LQ model, Barendsen (30) and Fowler (1) have suggested a quantity termed biologically effective dose (BED) (for Barendsen, it was called extrapolated response dose, ERD) which proved to be very convenient in quantifying radiobiological effects and even enabled sensible comparisons among various clinical trials using different fractionation schemes (31). With a dimension of dose (Gy), it is defined (1,30) as:

$$\text{BED} \equiv \frac{E}{\alpha} = nd\left(1 + \frac{d}{\alpha/\beta}\right) - \frac{\ln 2(T - T_k)}{\alpha \cdot T_p} \tag{7}$$

For late responding tissues only, the treatment time factor (i.e., repopulation) can be neglected, and

$$\text{BED} \equiv \frac{E}{\alpha} = nd\left(1 + \frac{d}{\alpha/\beta}\right) \tag{8}$$

This abstract quantity can perhaps be conceptualized best by its representation on the multi-fractionation survival curves (Fig. 3A). One can see that the numerical value of BED for any fractionation scheme is equivalent to the total physical dose needed to cause the same degree of biological effect (cell survival) using an "ultrafractionated" regimen in which d approaches zero and n approaches infinity ($d \rightarrow 0$, $n \rightarrow \infty$) such that the product, nd, equals the given total dose, D (30,32).

Using the single-hit, multitarget killing model, Withers and Peters (5) have analyzed in detail the change in the effective slope of the multifraction survival curve, $D_{0(eff)}$, as the size of dose per fraction changes. Such a cell survival plot—although more complicated mathematically [Eq. (3)]—shows a limiting maximal (least steep) slope characterized by the single-hit mechanism only ($_1D_0$) as the dose per fraction (or dose rate) approaches zero. It is thus analogous to the ultrafractionation scheme of which the total dose is equivalent to the BED for a given biological effect, using the LQ model (Fig. 3A). This supports the notion that BED is indeed a mechanistically sound quantity measuring the isoeffect dose for any fractionation scheme with respect to a particular process of radiation killing (i.e., single-hit or the linear component in the LQ theory), which represents the non-repairable damage to the chromosome that results directly in cell lethality (25,33). Thus, given any fractionation regimen delivering a total dose D, its corresponding

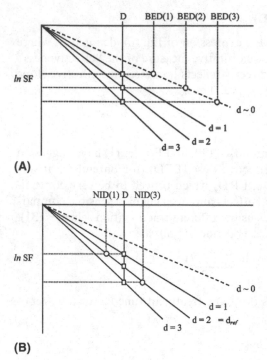

Figure 3 (**A**) Concept of biologically effective dose (BED) as depicted on survival curves. Only late effects are considered. Each line from the origin represents the effective survival curve for a multifraction regimen using dose per fraction, *d*. For a given total physical dose, *D*, a BED as a function of *d*, BED(*d*), can be visualized as the isoeffective total dose of a regimen in which d approaches zero asymptotically. (**B**) Concept of normalized isoeffective dose (NID) as depicted on cell survival curves. As in (A), except here NID(*d*) refers to the isoeffective total dose of an arbitrarily chosen reference scheme in which *d* is 2 Gy. *Source*: Redrawn from Ref. 34.

BED is a unique entity quantifying the equivalent biological effect and free from any arbitrarily chosen "reference" fractionation scheme.

To use BED for clinical application, we may intuitively correlate BED at a given anatomical location with total physical dose deposited at that point, because BED also has a unit of dose (Gy). Furthermore, since BED represents the negative exponent of an exponential function governing the cell-survival curve on a semi-log plot, the quantity is linearly additive for combination of multiple independent treatment schemes. Because of the mathematical simplicity, one might construct a computer algorithm enabling BED "isodose" (or iso-BED) display on commercial treatment planning system (34). However, one should remember that BED varies with the radiosensitivity parameters (i.e., α and β values) specific for the structure in question. Fowler (1) advocated using a subscript to make such a distinction, e.g., Gy_3 for BED based on α/β of 3 Gy, and Gy_{10} for BED with α/β equals 10 Gy.

We can derive readily the isoeffect conversion relation for two fractionation regimens with respective total doses, D_1, D_2; doses per fraction, d_1, d_2; and overall treatment times, T_1 T_2. For isoeffect, $BED_1 \equiv BED_2$; then, from Eq. (7),

$$D_1 = D_2 \frac{(d_2 + \alpha/\beta)}{(d_1 + \alpha/\beta)} - \frac{\ln 2(T_2 - T_1)}{\beta T_p(d_1 + \alpha/\beta)} \tag{9}$$

Note that the second term involving the treatment time factor is no longer dependent in T_k and can be ignored entirely when T_1 equals T_2 or when considering late-responding tissues only (35):

$$D_1 = D_2 \frac{(d_2 + \alpha/\beta)}{(d_1 + \alpha/\beta)} \tag{10}$$

To allow oncologists to relate observed radiation treatment effects with their own clinical experiences, they may translate the BED value implicitly to an equivalent quantity based on an arbitrarily chosen fractionation scheme. The resulting biologically oriented entity has been given many names, such as Linear-Quadratic Equivalent Dose based on 2-Gy fraction (LQED2) (36) or Normalized Isoeffective Dose (NID) (34). Figure 3B illustrates the concept of NID as depicted on cell survival curves, similar to Figure 3A except that the reference scheme is now set arbitrarily at d equals to 2 Gy (thus numerically also equivalent to LQED2). We should emphasize that these are derived merely through a process of normalization to the chosen reference scheme, using the mathematical formula based on the general isoeffect conversion relations [Eq. (9) or (10)]. Nevertheless, there seems to be a general consensus among many radiotherapists that a conventional scheme is about 1.8–2 Gy per fraction, five fractions per week. The clinical wisdom regarding tumor-cure dosage or normal-tissue tolerance levels has commonly been based on experiences using such a regimen. On the other hand, many "altered" fractionation schemes have appeared worldwide (1,10,31), and new treatment techniques may also necessitate manipulation of fractionation patterns such as stereotactic radiotherapy vs. radiosurgery (which differ from each other depending on whether one fractionates the treatment or not). Hence there is seldom a fractionation regimen now a days which can qualify as the "standard," and BED may prove to be a more versatile clinical tool to be used as the lingua franca in the quantification of biological effects for a given tissue in cancer therapy.

The Incomplete Repair Model

Some radiotherapy techniques may deviate from the conventional daily fractionation scheme, such that the induced SLD may not have sufficiently long (24-hr) inter-fractional interval for adequate repair. In addition, during continuous LDR brachytherapy, there is concurrent competition between repair and continuing radiation damage at a protracted pace. To account for these complex effects in time, the incomplete repair (IR) model may be utilized. It basically assumes that the efficiency of repair follows first-order kinetics, i.e., exponential in time (37,38). The concept of BED (in conjunction with the LQ theory) can then be applied for much generalized use. For example, for brachytherapy:

$$\text{BED} = D\left(1 + \frac{g(\tau) \cdot D}{\alpha/\beta}\right) \tag{11}$$

$$g(\tau) = \frac{2}{\mu\tau}\left[1 - \frac{1}{\mu\tau}(1 - e^{-\mu\tau})\right] \tag{12}$$

where μ is the rate constant for SLD repair, and τ is the time of continuous irradiation (33,38,39). Repair kinetics for many tissues of clinical relevance have been studied, e.g., by split-dose experiment using various range of inter-fractional intervals, with the values μ or $g(\tau)$ inferred and tabulated (40). Comparing with Eq. (8), the additional time-dependent factor, $g(\tau)$, is incorporated in Eq. (11) to modify the value of BED during continuous irradiation, or as the inter-fractional interval is decreased such that the repair becomes less complete. One can see that $g(\tau) \to 1$ for $\tau \to 0$ (i.e., almost instantaneous exposure of radiation such as treatment via daily fractionation) and Eq. (11) reverts to Eq. (8).

   With further extension of the IR model, a generalized theoretical framework has been developed to determine equivalent biological effects of LDR or high dose rate (HDR) brachytherapy (2,3). Indeed, with the property of linear additivity, BED can be used to quantify the overall effects of fractionated teletherapy, brachytherapy, and indeed *any* variable range of dose rates or fractionation schemes (Fig. 4). In this sense, one might say that the problem of analyzing radiobiology in the *temporal* domain (represented by heterogeneous distribution of dose rates along the time axis, with its area under the curve yielding the radiation dose) has been solved in its most general form.

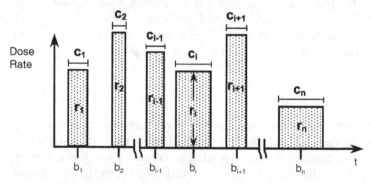

Figure 4   Heterogeneous spread of radiation dose rate along the time (t) axis, with each ith episode of irradiation centering upon b_i, dose rate of r_i, and treatment interval of c_i (thus the dose is r_ic_i). Mathematical theory has been established to quantify this most general form of radiation treatment scheme, whether by irregularly fractionated external beam teletherapy or by brachytherapy of low or high dose rate. *Source*: Adapted from Ref. 2.

TCP and NTCP

It is important to note that BED, despite its versatile theoretical use, does not directly reflect clinical endpoints which can be measured readily in cancer medicine. Clinically, the terms tumor control probability (TCP) and normal tissue complication probability (NTCP) come closer in giving patients a quantitative sense of radiobiological consequence. They are defined, according to Poisson statistics, as:

$$TCP = e^{-M \cdot SF_M} \tag{13}$$

$$NTCP = e^{-N \cdot SF_N} \tag{14}$$

where M is the number of clonogenic cells in the tumor (or "tumorlets"), N is the number of functional subunits (FSUs, at times called tissue rescue units, TRUs) for normal tissue, and SF_M and SF_N are the respective surviving fractions as functions of radiation dose and intrinsic radiation sensitivity [per Eq. (5) or (6)] (5). When plotted against dose (thus termed dose–response curves), both TCP and NTCP present as sigmoid curves. Furthermore, one can show that the number M or N would dictate primarily the location of the curve along the abscissa (dose axis): the higher the number, the more towards the right the steep portion of the curve is located. The slope of either curve at its steepest portion can become "flattened" when heterogeneous distribution of the radiation sensitivity parameters (α, β, etc.) is introduced within a patient population.

It is perhaps worthwhile to discuss here the mathematical expression of the "steepest slope" for these dose–response curves. For the sake of simplicity, we assume that α predominates such that β can be ignored (especially for acutely responding tissues like tumors, or in general by considering the "effective slope" of a multi-fractionation radiation survival curve). Without considering the heterogeneity of α, one can show readily that the steepest slope is given as αe^{-1} and is located at the "inflection point" of the curve where the corresponding probability is e^{-1} or $\sim 37\%$, and the dose, D_{37}, is equal to $\ln M/\alpha$ (for the TCP curve). A more popular entity to associate with the slope of the response curve is the gamma factor, defined as the product between dose and the slope (hence a dimensionless quantity) (41,42). γ-50 is thus related to the slope where the probability is 50%, with the corresponding dose, D_{50}. It is trivial to show that this slope is equal to $\alpha \cdot \ln 2/2$, and

$$\gamma_{50} = D_{50} \cdot \alpha \cdot \ln 2/2 \tag{15}$$

where

$$D_{50} = \frac{-\ln \, (\ln 2/M)}{\alpha}$$

Clinicians often aim for maximum tumor cell killing while minimizing damage to the adjacent normal tissues in order to achieve a better clinical outcome by optimization of the therapeutic ratio, defined rather figuratively as the benefit–risk ratio of TCP over NTCP. In fact, almost all innovative ways to improve the outcome of radiation therapy to date has amounted to widening the gap between TCP and NTCP dose–response curves. A useful concept is the so-called uncomplicated TCP (UTCP), defined as (43):

$$UTCP = TCP \cdot (1 - NTCP)$$

It can be seen that UTCP has a shape of a bell curve, with its peak located at an ideal dose where TCP is nearly maximized and NTCP minimized.

Clinically, the fact that the TCP dose–response curve is sigmoid signifies that dose escalation beyond the steepest portion of the curve rarely pays off when the corresponding NTCP is significant. On the other hand, for a malignancy with relatively high cure rate at a well-established conventional level of dosage, any small amount of underdosage within the tumor may compromise the TCP tremendously. These issues will be explored further when the "volume effect" is also considered (see section on Heterogenous Dose Distribution and TCP).

FROM TEMPORAL PROBLEM TO SPATIAL CONSIDERATION: THE "DOUBLE-TROUBLE" EFFECT

With the development of modern treatment planning systems, radiation dose distributions within patients' bodies are readily available and usually displayed as two- or three-dimensional contour plots. These "isodose" plots represent great assets to clinicians who often need to evaluate the actual dosage deposited at a critical site. The value of dose at such point may be drastically different from the dose *prescribed* originally at any particular site (e.g., the isocenter or somewhere within the tumor target) or any isodose level deemed appropriate by the clinician.

Nevertheless, taking care of the differences among physical dose received at the point of prescription and those at various sites of interest by isodose contour plots may not be sufficient for the clinicians to assess the true biological effects at these points. As described above, the biological effects will depend greatly on *how* the physical dosage is delivered in time, namely, the fractionation scheme. Figure 5 illustrates a hypothetical case of head and neck cancer from which one may appreciate the degree of changes of biological effects on tumor target or normal tissues, depending merely on the way clinicians choose to prescribe the treatment dose (34). When physical doses are compared with what is deposited at the prescription point, one should note that by fractionation, "what gets hot, gets hotter biologically; and what gets cold, gets colder biologically." (Fig. 5, 34). Above all, the magnitude of the deviation between physical and biological doses is more

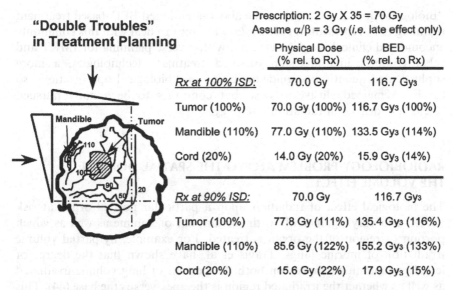

"Double Troubles" in Treatment Planning

Prescription: 2 Gy X 35 = 70 Gy
Assume α/β = 3 Gy (*i.e.* late effect only)

	Physical Dose (% rel. to Rx)	BED (% rel. to Rx)
Rx at 100% ISD:	70.0 Gy	116.7 Gy₃
Tumor (100%)	70.0 Gy (100%)	116.7 Gy₃ (100%)
Mandible (110%)	77.0 Gy (110%)	133.5 Gy₃ (114%)
Cord (20%)	14.0 Gy (20%)	15.9 Gy₃ (14%)
Rx at 90% ISD:	70.0 Gy	116.7 Gy₃
Tumor (100%)	77.8 Gy (111%)	135.4 Gy₃ (116%)
Mandible (110%)	85.6 Gy (122%)	155.2 Gy₃ (133%)
Cord (20%)	15.6 Gy (22%)	17.9 Gy₃ (15%)

Figure 5 The "double-trouble" effect is illustrated here with a display for treatment using an orthogonal pair of wedged photon beams for a hypothetical tumor in the maxillary sinus. When the physical dose at the isocenter (tumor) is set at 100%, the mandible is seen to receive 110%, and the spinal cord only 20%. The results of biological correction using BED are tabulated, with the dose prescribed at the tumor (*top*) and the minimal peripheral dose of 90% (*bottom*), respectively.

pronounced for late-responding tissues than for acutely-responding ones due to the different curvatures of their single-dose cell survival curves (Fig. 2C).

Radiation oncologists thus must consider the biological impact of fractionation on any particular structure of interest, especially the late-responding type. This is neglected on the conventional treatment plans based on physical dosimetry alone. The added complexity due to radiobiology consideration has been described as the "double-trouble" effect by Withers (36): the first trouble comes from the difference between physical dose prescribed and actual dose received at any point (*spatial* heterogeneity of total dose), and the second trouble results from the variation of biological effects with different dose per fraction (*spatial* heterogeneity of dose per fraction). The distinction between these two troubles is a consequence of fractionation (thus a *temporal* problem). The notion of the double-trouble effect represents thus a prelude to treating clinical radiobiology issues as problems existing within a space–time frame of reference, i.e., a four-dimensional domain.

In dealing with the double-trouble effect, conscientious clinicians armed with only physical dose dosimetry plans will often estimate biological effects qualitatively and choose a particular treatment plan accordingly.

"Biological dosimetry," such as the above-mentioned BED-based treatment planning (34), represents a rudimentary attempt to deal with this commonly encountered clinical issue. Nowadays, with inverse planning for IMRT and other complex high-precision oriented treatment technologies, a more sophisticated quantitative guideline based on "biological optimization" so far has remained elusive at best, but continues to be a hotly pursued research endeavor in radiation oncology.

RADIOBIOLOGY PROBLEM ALONG THE SPATIAL DOMAIN: THE VOLUME EFFECT

The biological effect of radiation upon a particular normal organ at risk (OAR) can vary significantly with the amount of volume as well as which portion or region of the organ is treated. For example, by partial volume irradiation of murine lungs, Travis et al. have shown that the degree of lethal pneumonitis depends on both the percent of lung volume irradiated as well as whether the irradiated region is the apex versus the base (44). This is commonly termed the "volume effect" (45,46) and until recently has largely been ignored during treatment planning because the complexity involved would have been rather difficult to deal with. Instead, planning physicists would strive to achieve uniform dose distribution as much as possible. The first step would be to cover the *entire* target volume with homogeneous dose, then an attempt is made to minimize the dose to the OAR to be at least below the perceived tolerance level for the *whole* organ. The cumulative clinical experiences throughout past decades have thus pertained mostly to uniform dose distribution over any structure of interest.

However, with the advancement in treatment technologies like IMRT, one can now manipulate dose distribution relatively at ease, especially via inverse planning algorithm. But such action often results in heterogeneous dose distributions, whether within the tumor or the OARs. Even during forward treatment planning for stereotactic or conformal radiotherapy, while it is feasible to conform tightly the dose coverage for the target tumor, one might wish to push the tolerance dose of the surrounding OAR to the extreme by partial organ irradiation. Conversely, selectively escalating dose within the tumor (i.e., dose painting), especially when directed by functional imaging showing metabolically hyperactive spots, might be perceived to be beneficial. In all these cases, the volume effect may no longer be negligible.

From Eqs. (13) and (14), we note that both TCP and NTCP depend on *size:* i.e., the *number* of tumor cells or FSUs, respectively. First, assume radiation dose is distributed heterogeneously within the tumor target or normal organ but the tumor cells or FSUs are organized *isotropically* uniformly in space, what then might be the effect of partial volume irradiation? One could perhaps appreciate that the total sum of biological effects due to irradiation of a collection of partial volumes with heterogeneous doses may not be equal to the effect of delivering the *averaged* dose to the whole volume homogeneously. That is, the biological effect of partial volume irradiation is not linearly additive. Second, the condition of isotropic organization for tumor cells is perhaps easier to accept since a tumor is usually conceptualized as containing millions to billions of closely packed tumor cells, like identical marbles packed closely in a jar. But for normal tissues this is not a trivial matter since obviously FSUs can be distributed anisotropically for some OARs, thus representing a complex issue to consider for the analysis of the volume effect, namely, tissue organization (see section on Tissue Organization).

Partial Organ Irradiation and Heterogeneous Dose Distribution

Dose Volume Histogram (DVH)

To deal with the effect of partial normal organ irradiation quantitatively, a seemingly straight-forward solution would be to use an empirical approach like the power laws again. A typical example is stereotactic radiosurgery (SRS) for brain tumors. Clinicians performing this technique have used the so-called "Kjellberg's Diagram," which also follows the empirical concept of power–laws (47). Here the amount of volume (related to proton beam diameter) irradiated is assumed to be inversely proportional to the radiation dose for a constant biological effect (e.g., 1% or 99% chance of brain necrosis). It does not take into account dose distribution outside the SRS treatment volume. Flickinger has suggested a more refined approach using the "integrated logistic model" (48) to incorporate the effect of partial brain irradiation (see next section), but it remains to be a variation of the same theme as the power–law model, i.e., empirical approach with statistical fitting of clinical data and applicable specifically for brain irradiation.

The FSUs in OARs like the brain can be considered more or less isotropically organized (although not cranial nerves), and during SRS the volume receiving high dose is typically small relative to the whole brain, with rapid drop-off of dose outside the treatment volume. Thus, using the simple power–law relationship to direct clinical practice is probably acceptable. Having said that, we might point out that dose "homogeneity" is still a debatable issue between specialists doing single dose SRS like Gamma Knife (less homogeneity in general) and those preferring fractionated stereotactic radiotherapy (SRT) (more homogeneity usually), especially when the treatment volume contains fine structures like cranial nerves (49).

However, when dose distribution is grossly heterogeneous across a significant portion of an OAR (relevant when doing extracranial SRS or SRT), the degree of such heterogeneity might need to be addressed. A useful quantitative tool is the dose–volume histogram (DVH). When shown in a *cumulative* (*integral*) rather than a *differential* form, it reveals the cumulative volume of the structure receiving *at least* the corresponding dose on the abscissa. It assumes a monotonically decreasing shape on a plot of fractional volume versus dose. Clearly, for tumors the ultimate ideal situation would be a DVH curve shaped like a rectangle, with 100% of the volume receiving a certain prescribed dose or more. For OARs the ideal situation would be a "spike" at the origin (or "L-shape" with a tail of zero thickness extending along the abscissa), i.e., 100% of the volume receiving no dose at all. The real situation is of course somewhere in-between, since optimizing radiation therapy is by nature a quid pro quo process: whatever one does to make the tumor DVH as rectangular as possible, the corresponding DVH for OARs would as a result deviate from the "L-shape" more, and vice versa. Keeping the "ideal" shapes for both curves in mind can nevertheless help clinicians evaluate treatment plans using DVH displays as criteria of selection.

Since the biological effect of partial volume irradiation is not linearly additive, and clinicians are more familiar with uniformly irradiated *whole*-organ tolerance dose, a natural question to ask is: given a structure of interest with heterogeneous dose distribution, can one find an effectively *uniform* dose, i.e., a hypothetical dose uniformly distributed over the entire organ, which would result in equivalent biological effect? One possible way, at least mathematically, based solely upon dosimetric measures, is to perform "DVH reduction." For example, Lyman and Wolbarst (50,51) proposed the following empirical recipe: by dividing the dose axis into tiny segments, one can successively "reduce" the corresponding volume algebraically from the extreme right end (maximum dose) of the DVH curve step by step until the maximum (100%) volume is reached at a particular dose level, which would essentially be the "effective dose" (D_{eff}). Once the D_{eff} obtained, one can simply look up an available NTCP versus D curve for whole-organ irradiation by assuming the dose to be at D_{eff}. Several other mathematical algorithms have been proposed for DVH reduction (52), depending on the parameters (volume, dose, response, probability of complication, etc.) for which the theorists chose to manipulate the algebra involved.

Even though DVH is a powerful tool to help clinicians handle the problem of heterogeneous dose distribution in space, one must realize that it often cannot be relied upon to reflect the clinical consequences completely. To use a very simple example: assume that the only dose heterogeneity in an otherwise uniformly irradiated structure, say, rectum, arises from 5% of its volume receiving excessive dose. Such a small "hot spot" may result in very distinct clinical sequalae: inconsequential, if the 5% hot spot scatters rather widely within the rectal wall; ulcer, if the hot spot is concentrated at a point; or stricture, if it is distributed circumferentially around a segment of the rectum (53). Needless to mention, the way FSUs are organized in each OAR may be critical.

Another potential problem with the use of DVH is the definition of the baseline volume of the structure of interest, since "volume" as denoted in a DVH is often a fractional (percent) rather than an absolute volume. Thus, different investigators reporting their clinical findings of "5% hot spot in the rectum" may mean 5% of very different structures: rectal volume as defined by multiplying the thickness of the rectal wall by the surface area (whole circumferential versus only the arc portion within the treated volume) cylindrical rectal volume with or without the bowel content, or rectum with a longitudinal length defined differently, etc.

Heterogeneous Dose Distribution and NTCP

Investigators have long realized the importance of quantifying the dependence of NTCP on the amount of partial volume irradiated. Knowing that a NTCP versus D plot, like TCP, should approximate a rising sigmoid curve, several have tackled the problem using the phenomenologic approach. Schultheiss et al. (54) have proposed the logistic model (which gives rise to a sigmoid curve) empirically to describe whole organ irradiation:

$$\text{NTCP}(\nu = 1, D) = \frac{1}{1 + (D_{50}/D)^k} \tag{16}$$

where k characterizes the slope of the sigmoid curve. For radiating only a partial volume ν:

$$\text{NTCP}(\nu, D) = 1 - [1 - \text{NTCP}(1, D)]^\nu$$

This logistic model was also the basis upon which Flickinger (48) constructed his "integrated logistic formula" to model the normal tissue effect of brain radiosurgery.

A sigmoid curve can also be visualized as an integral of a bell curve (i.e., normal or Gaussian function). Thus, Lyman (55) proposed the integrated normal model:

$$\text{NTCP} = \frac{1}{\sqrt{2\pi}} \int_{-\infty}^{t} e^{-x^2/2} dx \tag{17}$$

Where

$$t = \frac{D - D_{50}(\nu)}{m D_{50}(\nu)}$$

$$D_{50}(\nu) = \frac{D_{50}(\nu = 1)}{\nu^n}$$

D_{50} is the dose giving rise to 50% NTCP, and $D_{50}(\nu)$ is the D_{50} for irradiating partial volume ν. One can see that the parameter m would characterize the slope of the NTCP curve, and n is an index ($0 \leq n \leq 1$) for an assumed power–law relationship between dose and irradiated volume.

For heterogeneous dose distribution, one may use the "effective volume method" of Kutcher and Burman (56) to perform the DVH reduction first. It differs from the Lyman and Wolbarst scheme of finding the D_{eff} by reducing the differential DVH sequentially to arrive at a single effective volume, ν_{eff}, which receives the maximum dose of D_1 uniformly, according to the following summing formula:

$$\nu_{\text{eff}} = \sum_{i=1} \nu_i \left(\frac{D_i}{D_1}\right)^{1/n} \tag{18}$$

where n is again the index for the power–law as defined above. The value of ν_{eff} can be used to substitute for ν in the Lyman equation [Eq. (17)]. To assess the corresponding NTCP, one would need to refer to a NTCP versus D curve for the particular amount of volume, ν_{eff}.

By differentiating Eqs. (16) and (17) to find the slope at D_{50}, one can show that the logistic model and the integrated normal model are equivalent when

$$k = \frac{4}{\sqrt{2\pi} \cdot m} \tag{19}$$

Furthermore, using the definition of the gamma factor [Eq. (15)], one can find:

$$\gamma_{50} \equiv D_{50} \cdot \frac{\partial \text{NTCP}}{\partial D}\bigg|_{D=D_{50}} = \frac{1}{\sqrt{2\pi} \cdot m} = \frac{k}{4} \tag{20}$$

The interplay among the three variables NTCP, dose, and volume can best be represented as a three-dimensional plot (Fig. 6). Using Lyman's empirical model, Burman et al. (57) fit the data collected by clinicians (58) and provided useful reference plots for assessing the effect of partial volume irradiation for many critical organs. In particular, the empirical parameters, D_{50}, m, and n can be inferred from these data. One can also see that, among several different normal tissues, the change in the NTCP curves as partial volume changes can display distinct behavioral patterns. For example, as the irradiated volume decreases, some organs show the NTCP curves to become "flatter," while those for others tend to shift to the right with relatively the same slope. The reason for such a phenomenon may be attributed to the different way various normal tissues are organized (to be discussed in Section on Parallel vs. Series structures).

Heterogeneous Dose Distribution and TCP

In contrast to the empirical formulation of NTCP as a function of irradiated volume and dose, TCP can be expressed in a more mechanistically oriented fashion because Eq. (13) involves the term *SF* which can be formulated based on the LQ theory, and tumors are inherently organized more or less

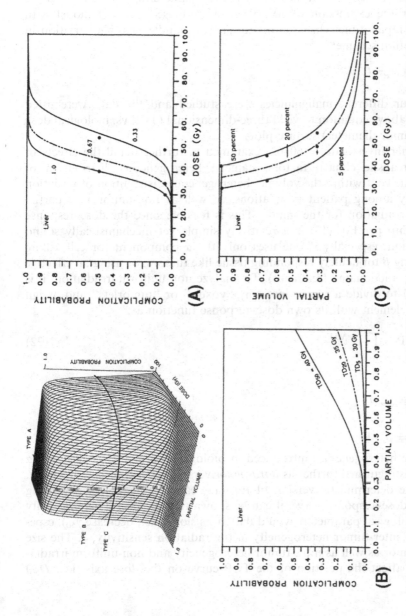

Figure 6 A display of the three-dimensional relationships among normal tissue complication probability (NTCP), dose, and partial volume irradiated. *Source:* From Ref. 57.

isotropically such that the volume effect becomes easier to handle intuitively. Thus, one may write:

$$\text{TCP} = e^{-\rho V \cdot \text{SF}} \tag{21}$$

where ρ is the density of clonogenic cells (typically on the order of 10^8–10^9 per cm^3), and V is the tumor volume. For the sake of simplicity, tumors can be assumed to be spherical with diameter d; hence, $V = \pi d^3/6$.

For the expression of SF, Brenner (59) used the LQ model with an SLD repair function, g, as in Eq. (12) to handle possible variation in fractionation scheme:

$$\text{SF} = e^{-\alpha D - g\beta D^2}$$

Four different malignancies were studied and the data were fitted with the above equation to yield three-dimensional (TCP vs. biological dose versus tumor diameter) surface plots.

Other investigators (60–62) examined in further detail the effects of several realistic clinical factors: namely, heterogeneous distribution of clonogenic cells within the volume, heterogeneous distribution of radiation sensitivity among patient populations, as well as non-uniform or partial volume irradiation for the tumor. This is feasible since the dose–response relationship per Eq. (13) is a relatively simple yet mechanistically sound formulation, especially if one uses only the α component for cell killing (neglecting β for acutely responding tissue like tumors, or using an effective slope for fractionated treatment). To analyze non-uniform irradiation, it is proposed to divide a tumor into tiny "voxels" or "tumorlets" and assign each ith element with its own dose–response function as:

$$\text{TCP} = \prod_{i=1} e^{-N_i \text{SF}_i} \tag{22}$$

where

$$\text{SF}_i = e^{-\alpha D_i}$$

$$N_i = \rho_i \cdot V_i$$

The heterogeneities introduced in biological parameters like ρ and α can be distinguished further as *intra-tumor* versus *inter-tumor* heterogeneity. While the deterministic version of Eq. (13) can result in a sharply rising sigmoid dose–response curve, it can be shown that in general heterogeneity in the biological parameters would flatten its slope (i.e., decrease γ_{50}), especially for inter-tumor heterogeneity in the radiation sensitivity, α. The size of the tumor as well as intra-tumor heterogeneity and non-uniform irradiation can affect the position of the TCP curve on the dose axis (i.e., D_{50}) (61,62).

To illustrate the effects of heterogeneous dose distribution on TCP at least qualitatively, Withers discussed in detail the dependency of TCP on the magnitude of tumor underdosage or overdosage, as well as the fractional volume of the tumor affected (63,64). After comparing with the theoretical prediction of the TCP for an otherwise uniformly irradiated tumor, Withers made the following points regarding tumor *underdosage* (i.e., "cold spots") (Fig. 7):

1. The magnitude of the underdosage is the most powerful determinant of TCP.
2. The fastest rate of decline in TCP occurs when the volume underdosed is still small.

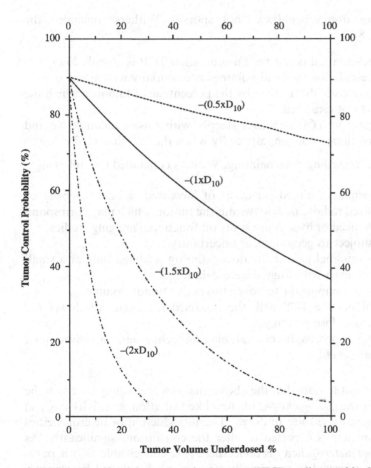

Figure 7 The effect of tumor underdosage on TCP as discussed by Withers (63) and Withers and Lee (64). The key points based on this graph are listed in the text. *Source*: From Ref. 63.

3. Significant inhomogeneity, especially to small volumes, is likely to occur when high precision radiation treatment (e.g., IMRT) is applied to mobile tumors.
4. Single dose treatment (e.g., SRS) can have a very tight margin of error.
5. The rate of decline in TCP is greater in the midrange of the TCP (i.e., the steep portion of the sigmoid curve, between 15 and 80%) achieved with homogeneous irradiation.
6. The planning tumor volume (PTV) may contain lower densities of clonogens, and while it may frequently be underdosed, there may not be a rapid early decline in TCP with small volumes of underdosage.

For tumor *overdosage* (i.e., "hot spots"), Withers concluded the following (Fig. 8):

1. Dose escalation is not very useful when TCP is already high.
2. Dose escalation to small volumes is essentially worthless.
3. TCP is mostly determined by the percentage of tumor in which the dose is not escalated.
4. The gain in TCP increases steeply with dose escalation beyond 50% of tumor volume, especially when the baseline TCP is low.

Therefore, regarding dose painting, Withers concluded the following:

1. It is primarily aimed for areas of increased clonogen density or decreased radiosensitivity within the tumor, which may correspond to enhanced or hypodense spots on functional imaging studies.
2. It is subject to geographical uncertainty.
3. It has minimal gain if the dose painting is aimed only at a small volume, even with huge dose escalation.
4. It is more important to cover the entire tumor volume.
5. The higher the TCP with the standard treatment, the lower the gain from dose painting.
6. It needs expensive functional imaging techniques, but for minimal clinical benefit.

It is important to note that the above analyses are mainly based on the assumption that the biological parameters like radiation sensitivity (e.g., α) or clonogenic density (ρ) are uniform. The introduction of heterogeneities into these parameters is expected to alter the conclusions significantly. As far as *inter-tumor* heterogeneity is concerned, it is conceivable that a parameter like α be subjected to a normally (Gaussian) distributed heterogeneity. Accordingly, what Withers has described represents essentially the mean, or deterministic, behavior and thus remains clinically relevant. However, the

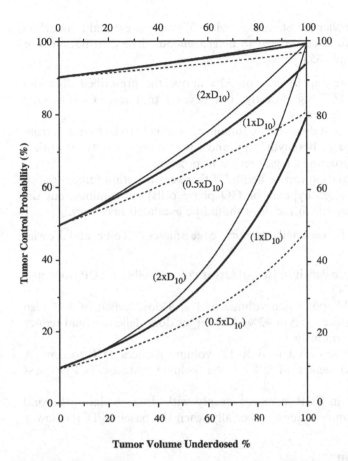

Figure 8 The effect of tumor overdosage on TCP as discussed by Withers (63) and Withers and Lee (64). The key points based on this graph are listed in the text. *Source*: From Ref. 63.

possible existence of *intra-tumor* heterogeneity for parameters like ρ makes it difficult for one to conjure up any a priori form of spatial distribution.[c] When advocating dose painting guided by functional imaging, for example, it might be prudent to know whether the metabolically or pharmacokinetically active spots within the target volume actually correspond to radiosensitive/resistant or highly clonogenic spots. In such a way, selective dose escalation at these sites might be more meaningful beyond what Withers has implied.

---

[c] A potentially even more complicated source of heterogeneity would be in *time*: that is, the biological parameters such as α or ρ might fluctuate randomly in time during the course of radiation treatment.

Tome and Fowler (65,66) and Fowler (67) have presented a modeling scheme to deal with issues related to heterogeneous dose distribution. For *hot spots*, they found (65,67):

1. Boost doses up to 20% or 30% above the prescribed dose can increase TCP significantly, but beyond that level (~30%–50%) the effect saturates.
2. Peak or boost doses inside tumors are unlikely to be harmful, from experience in brachytherapy and SRT, unless it falls on critical normal structures, e.g., urethra in prostate.
3. Dose escalation can be helpful if there exists within tumors radio-resistant (e.g., hypoxic or GO phase cells) subvolumes, but the amount by which the dose should be escalated may vary.

For *cold spots*, especially tumor "edge misses," Tome and Fowler described (66,67):

1. A 10% dose deficit in 10% of target volume reduces TCP from 50% to about 43%.
2. If the cold spot has a volume of 1%, a dose deficit of 20% also would reduce TCP to 43%. Any larger dose deficits would reduce TCP precipitously.
3. A 50% dose deficit in only 1% volume reduces TCP to zero. A 25% dose deficit in 2% of the volume reduces TCP to less than 30%.
4. The gain in TCP increases steeply with dose escalation beyond 50% of tumor volume, especially when the baseline TCP is low.

Tissue Organization

Flexible vs. Hierarchical Structures

Factors relating to the variations in tissue organization play a significant role in repair and repopulation, and may thus contribute to the observed radiation effect, especially for normal tissues. Michalowski and Wheldon first proposed the distinction between the so-called type-H (hierarchical) and type-F (flexible) tissues (68,69). Type-H tissues (e.g., bone marrow, skin, and gastrointestinal tract) contain stem cells which are destined to mature in a stepwise fashion into functional cells. As they lose clonogenicity in the process, these cells become radioresistant because only the rapidly proliferating stem cells are likely to be sensitive to radiation killing. In contrast, type-F tissues (e.g., lung, liver, and kidney) contain cells which can simultaneously maintain their proliferation capacity (thus remaining radiosensitive) as well as serve their normal physiological function. The mathematical models used to analyze the behaviors of these two tissue types are based on physiological and cellular kinetics reasoning, and aided by using time-dependent differential equations. The results predict that type-F tissues can exhibit a dose-dependent kinetics-of-damage expression—the higher the dose, the earlier the time of expression—while that of type-H tissues is relatively independent of the dose. These predictions are in general agreement with clinical observations. Even though this theory is not easily integrated into clinical practice due to the mathematical complexity, it is somewhat more mechanistically sound. Unfortunately, while the physiological and radiobiological behaviors in *time* of critical cells under radiation exposure are considered, no *spatial* variable is introduced to analyze the possible effect of different tissue organization in three-dimensional space, i.e., the volume effect. What may need to happen, if radiation oncologists wish to stick with the flavor of following mechanistic principles, is to advocate quantitative research into the realm of radiation pathophysiology and integrate such knowledge into clinical radiation treatment planning. Using the rectum (a predominantly type-H structure) as an example again, one might wish to know whether its FSUs (stem cells) are organized roughly radially or circumferentially, or what a typical microscopic migratory distance and the associated kinetics for these FSUs happen to be in order to repopulate in a radiation denuded area.

Parallel vs. Series Structures

To take care of the spatial orientation of normal tissue organization, Withers et al. (45) first suggested that a separation be made between *parallel* and *series* structures. The former are typified by kidney, liver, and lung (as well as tumors), while the later include nerves, spinal cord, and peritoneal sheath. From modeling viewpoint, *parallel* tissues have been modeled along the so-called "critical volume" argument (70), namely that the total amount of volume irradiated has direct impact on the chance of complication. The smaller the degree of partial organ irradiated (or the more volume spared within the organ as the functional reserve), the more the dose response curve is shifted to the right, i.e., the higher the dose needed to result in the same complication rate. However, the slopes of these sigmoid curves may remain relatively unchanged. When NTCP is plotted against partial volume irradiated at a constant dose, it is seen that there is a "threshold" volume above which the NTCP rises sharply (67). On the DVH, one sees that irradiating a significant volume of such tissue, even if with moderate doses, would be more detrimental than giving an extremely high dose but to only a small volume of the organ (Fig. 9). Some would thus loosely state that parallel structures demonstrate more significant "volume effect," meaning the bulk of the volume irradiated does matter significantly.

On the other hand, tissues in *series* have "critical elements" arranged in chains upon which irradiating even a small volume of the structure to a sufficiently high dose might incur a complication (71). The prime example would

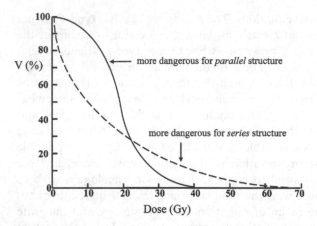

Figure 9 Dose volume histogram (DVH) showing qualitative difference of risk assessment based on whether the structure of the normal organ is *parallel* or in *series*.

be spinal cord, which needs only a hot spot at a given segment to manifest transverse myelitis. On the DVH, a long tail extending to the high dose region might be relatively more serious than when most of the volume receives a moderate dose, in contrast with parallel structures (Fig. 9). One can appreciate that the incidence of a complication increases in proportion to the volume of serially arranged FSUs irradiated. The dose–response curve might shift to the left as more volume (the number of FSUs) is irradiated, with the slope of the NTCP curve becoming steeper. On the NTCP versus volume curve, however, no threshold volume is observed, while the rapidity (slope) of the increase in NTCP as volume increases depends largely on the initial level of response, i.e., intrinsic radiation sensitivity per volume element (67).

Most normal tissues have mixed characteristics of both parallel and series structures. Thus, a concept of relative seriality has been proposed based on the perceived organization of FSUs (42). Figure 10 illustrates such a concept and the corresponding values for various structures of interest (72). The dose–response curves for several organs, each with different degree of partial organ irradiation, are shown as well. It can be seen that tumors are ideal parallel structures, and liver, kidney, and lung are organized in an analogous fashion with relative seriality close to zero. The gastrointestinal tract and the nervous tissues are organized more in series and thus have higher values of relative seriality.

Using the rectum as an example, it might be seen that when a precision-oriented radiotherapy such as IMRT is used for prostate cancer and only treats the anterior wall of the rectum instead of treating the whole circumference, it essentially converts a series type of injury to a parallel type (67).

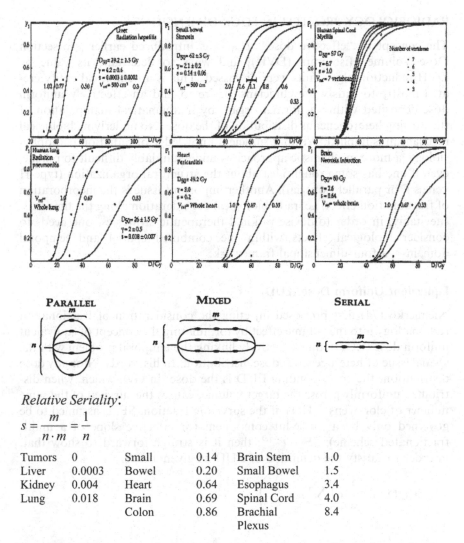

Figure 10 NTCP curves for various structures, showing effects of partial organ irradiation. The concept of relative seriality is shown, with the value tabulated for tumor and various normal tissues. *Source*: From Ref. 72.

The NTCP models based on the consideration of tissue organization are more mechanistically sound than empirical formulations like the Lyman model. It can be shown, however, that the critical element scheme proposed by Niemierko and Goitein (71) gives rise to the same prediction as the Lyman and Wolbarst (LW; 52,53) model at low levels of NTCP (73), which is applicable in usual clinical settings. It can predict D_{eff} in the LW scheme and v_{eff} in the Kutcher and Burman (KB; 56, 73) model.

RADIOBIOLOGY PROBLEM IN FOUR-DIMENSIONS

The concept of "effective dose," D_{eff}, was introduced earlier [see section Dose Volume Histogram (DVH)] and ways to determine its value by DVH reduction algorithms were discussed. This is an empirical entity created mostly to satisfy the clinicians' desire to find an effectively uniform dose deposited within a normal organ, by mathematical manipulation of the existing heterogeneous distribution of the dose. No underlying biological mechanism is implied. Without sufficient knowledge of radiation pathophysiology, a more mechanistic approach is understandably difficult to pursue, even if one has some rough idea about the structural organization (type-H versus F or parallel vs. serial). Another important issue is the incorporation of fractionation effect, i.e. radiobiological consideration along the time axis. Inevitably, in order to devise rational therapeutic strategies, one needs to consider biological effects within the combined spatial and temporal domains—a four-dimensional framework.

Equivalent Uniform Dose (EUD)

Niemierko (74) first proposed injecting the consideration of fractionation radiobiology into the volume effect by formulating the concept of equivalent uniform dose (EUD), thus effectively linking the temporal problem with the spatial issue of heterogeneous dose distribution. In his words: "For any dose distribution, the corresponding EUD is the dose (in Gy), which, when distributed uniformly across the target volume, causes the survival of the same number of clonogens." Thus, if the surviving fraction, SF, is assumed to be governed only by a single-hit component (or effective slope of a multi-fractionated scheme): $SF = e^{-\alpha D}$, then it is straightforward to show that, in order to satisfy the definition of EUD as given above,

$$EUD = -\frac{1}{\alpha}\ln\left(\sum_{i=1}^{N} \nu_i e^{-\alpha D_i}\right) \tag{23}$$

or

$$EUD = -\frac{1}{\alpha}\ln\left(\frac{1}{N}\sum_{i=1}^{N} e^{-\alpha D_i}\right) \tag{24}$$

where N is the number of volume elements (voxels) and ν_i is the volume of the ith voxel with corresponding dose D_i.[d]

---

[d] Note that Niemierko (74) used the term SF2, the surviving fraction after 2 Gy, rather than the parameter α as in Eqs. (23) and (24), to denote the factor pertaining to intrinsic radiosensitivity. The expressions he wrote are algebraically equivalent to, but a bit more cumbersome than, what are shown above. Furthermore, they are tied to a rather arbitrarily chosen reference fractionation regimen (by referring to a 2-Gy per fraction scheme).

Niemierko proceeded to include the effects of variable tumor volumes, non-uniform spatial distribution of clonogens (i.e., intra-tumor heterogeneity), unconventional fractionation schemes [by incorporating Eq. (10)], cell repopulation [by incorporating treatment time factor similar to Eq. (9)], and heterogeneous biological parameters in a patient population (i.e., inter-tumor heterogeneity).

Perhaps because of its mathematical complexity, EUD as depicted in Eq. (23) or (24) has not gained enough popularity among clinicians. Niemierko has thus advocated an alternative approach, though reverting back to the paradigm of using power laws (75). In this version, EUD is defined as:

$$\text{EUD} = \left(\frac{1}{N} \sum_{i=1}^{N} D_i^a \right)^{1/a} \tag{25}$$

The parameter, a, is clearly an empirical parameter to be inferred from retrospective analysis of clinical data. Its values for various structures of interest, including cancers, have been collected and tabulated (75). One might notice that it has negative values for malignant tumors, smaller positive values ($\sim$0.5–3) for commonly considered "parallel" organs like liver and lung, and higher values (10–20) for "serial" structures like spinal cord and gastrointestinal tract. Thus, despite its phenomenological origin, EUD as formulated in Eq. (25) may be linked with more mechanistically oriented quantities as in Eqs. (23) and (24), perhaps by considering factors stemming from structural organization or radiation pathophysiology.

It remains to be seen whether the phenomenological approach of Eq. (25) would gain the attention of clinical practitioners readily. As with all power laws seen in the history of the specialty, such an approach may stir up future controversy, since it is not clear whether some of the major pitfalls associated with empirical laws might surface eventually. Nevertheless, as Niemierko and Mohan pointed out (75), the difficulty of applying a mechanistically oriented model is quite real. Since the development in high-precision oriented treatment technique is here to stay and in fact is flourishing commercially, there is a sense of urgency in trying to implement "biological" optimization. In this regard, empirical guidelines may represent a quick and easy solution, just like what Strandqvist's plot did for dose fractionation more than half a century ago.

Equivalent Uniform Biologically Equivalent Dose (EUBED)

Based on Niemierko's concept of EUD and Barendsen's BED, Jones and Hoban (76) introduced the equivalent uniform biologically effective dose (EUBED), mainly for the need to incorporate a wide variety of fractionation schemes (much like what BED was designed for but EUBED adds the consideration of the volume effect). This represents thus a rather bold step of combining the radiobiological problems in the four-dimensional framework of time and space. Analogous to Eq. (23), and using the definition of BED as in Eq. (8), one can derive the following:

$$\text{EUBED} = -\frac{1}{\alpha}\ln\left(\sum_{i=1}^{N} \nu_i e^{-\alpha\text{BED}_i}\right) \tag{26}$$

where BED_i denotes the value of BED at the ith volume element.

With fractionation, using the term *eud* to denote the equivalent uniform dose *per fraction,* one can write

$$\text{EUBED} = n \cdot \text{eud}\left(1 + \frac{\text{eud}}{\alpha/\beta}\right) \tag{27}$$

which is seen to be entirely analogous to Eq. (8). Furthermore, EUBED is related to EUD by the following:

$$\text{EUBED} = \text{EUD}\left(1 + \frac{\text{eud}}{\alpha/\beta}\right) \tag{28}$$

The clinical applicability of the EUBED concept has been discussed in detail by Jones and Hoban (76), especially with a comparison of the IMRT optimization process between a physical dose-based and an EUBED-based dosimetry (77). They also utilized the concept of integral biologically effective dose (IBED) advocated by Clark et al. (78). The latter group of investigators had used differential DVHs and the IBED concept to analyze the toxicity of hypofractionated stereotactic radiotherapy to brain stem. Specifically, IBED is defined as:

$$\text{IBED} = \sum_i \Delta\text{BED}_i$$

$$= \sum_i nd_i\left(1 + \frac{d_i}{\alpha/\beta}\right)\frac{\Delta\nu_i}{V} \tag{29}$$

where the dose axis on the differential DVH is divided into i dose-bands, each with width of 1% of the maximum dose, and d_i is the dose delivered to the ith band. The volume within each dose-band is denoted as $\Delta\nu_i$ and the total volume is V. The fact that the total biological effect, IBED, can be determined by summing up (integrating) individual BED elements (ΔBED_i) highlights once again the versatility of BED as a linearly additive quantity.

SPECIFIC ISSUES REGARDING SRS AND SRT

Clinicians performing stereotactic radiation typically distinguish between two types of approaches: single-dose (SRS) and fractionated (SRT) treatments. Equipped with the knowledge of the radiobiological principles discussed so far, we might begin to address several issues specific to SRS and SRT.

General Guidelines in Choosing SRS vs. SRT

Based on what we have discussed about the biology of fractionation, i.e., that fractionation spares better late-responding tissues than the acutely-responding type (see section on Mechanistic Models and Cell Survival Curves), certain general guidelines might be appropriate regarding selection of SRS versus SRT. First, whenever an aggressive tumor (thus, acutely-responding) is found located in close proximity to or enclosing a critical late-responding normal tissue, SRT would probably be more beneficial than SRS since the biological advantage of fractionation can be exploited. In this scenario, the stereotactic treatment is truly a form of radiation therapy, i.e., *biological* therapy. On the other hand, if there is not much difference between the tumor (e.g., a benign or low-grade lesion) and the surrounding normal tissue as far as the shapes of their radiation survival curves (that is, α/β) are concerned, it may be legitimate to offer patients SRS treatment, especially when radical excision of the tumor is perceived to be useful but contraindicated due to an unacceptably high operative risk. Stereotactic irradiation used in this way—for a purely tumor-*ablation* purpose—serves just like a surgical tool, hence the appropriate name of radio-surgery. We should emphasize that, since fractionation always spares late-responding tissues better than acute ones, and that tumors generally belong to a more acutely-responding type—with the possible exception of prostate cancer (79)—SRT will in general have a theoretical advantage over SRS. SRS is often favored for logistic reasons rather than biological considerations per se.

Tumor Debulking with SRS vs. Radical Field Coverage

Even though SRS can be used to substitute for real surgical resection, a fundamental tenet in surgical oncology still needs to be observed: that is, partial tumor resection (tumor debulking, equivalent to partial SRS field coverage) is rarely helpful. Accepting the common oncologic notion that a 1 cm diameter of solid tumor nodule harbors about 10^9 cells, then a "90%" debulking still leaves 10^8 cells behind, a "99%" debulking leaves 10^7 cells, etc. Thus, it is important to ensure that the SRS field coverage of the lesion be as radical (complete, with adequate margins) as possible. Radiographic imaging to help clinicians delineate precisely the extent of the tumor is thus crucial. In fact, functional imaging studies like positron emission tomography (PET) or magnetic resonance spectroscopy (MRS) could probably augment the efficacy of high-precision radiation therapy better if they can help detect previously unseen tumor edges rather than, or in addition to, picking out metabolically active spots within a tumor.

Treatment Field Margins

A radiation treatment plan requires judicious choice for margins of field coverage, especially for SRS or SRT, where dose fall-off outside the treatment volume is steep. This is based on the concern for undetectable tumor edge as well as motion uncertainty. In modem treatment planning terminology, the concepts of clinical target volume (CTV) and planning target volume (PTV) are defined precisely for this purpose (80,81). For stereotactic treatment, one of its most advertised virtues is its high precision and the extremely narrow margin achievable such that the surrounding normal tissue can be spared to the fullest extent possible. However, one must be aware that the tight field margin also means that it is much less forgiving if one makes a mistake when delineating the gross tumor volume (GTV) and CTV for treatment planning. A 5% shortage in diameter (e.g., by outlining a 9.5-mm rather than a truly 10-mm diameter of a spherical tumor) at the periphery would translate into about 14% of the volume at the outer "shell" being outside the volume to which the tumor dose is prescribed (Fig. 11). Because SRS acts like surgeon's knife, the 1.4×10^8 cells in the outer portion have a very good chance to be underdosed and survive (in particular if this peripheral region is hypoxic. Furthermore, if the dosimetry is normalized to a prescribed dosage at the edge of the CTV, then, based on the principle of fractionation biology

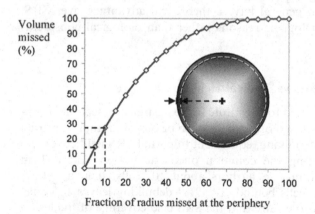

Fraction of radius missed at the periphery

Figure 11 The volume of the outer shell of a missed spherical tumor is plotted against the percent fraction of the radius missed at the periphery, when the radiation is aimed precisely at the inner sphere. For a 5% miss of the radius, the outer shell occupies 14% volume of the original sphere. For a 10% miss of the radius, more than a quarter of the spherical volume would be underdosed.

described above (see the section entitled From Temporal Problem to Spatial Consideration: The Double-Trouble Effect), the "biological" margin is even tighter than what the physical margin would imply, because of the different dose per fraction inside and outside the CTV. This augmentation of change in biological dose in an inhomogeneously irradiated volume is not surprising since inside the CTV the dose *per fraction* is higher than the prescribed level, hence even higher after biological correction, and vice versa (much lower) for dose outside the CTV (Fig. 12).

Unconventional Fractionation for SRT

The technology of SRT, often with removable body-fixation frames, has been developed to overcome the biological disadvantages of single-dose treatment as used in SRS. However, perhaps due to the wide acceptance of SRS, or because SRT is simply a more laborious procedure, clinicians might have a lingering desire to minimize the number of fractions for patient treatment. Thus, rather than following the long-held practice of conventional fractionation by using 1.8–2 Gy per fraction, unconventional fractionation schemes using a significantly higher fractional dose, i.e., hypofractionation, have been tried for SRT (82,83). Brenner and Hall have supported the practice of accelerated fractionation (with decreased overall treatment time) when using SRT, specifically for intracranial lesions (84). They suggested that the spatial sparing of the normal tissues by stereotactic technique alone may suffice to overcome the radiobiological disadvantage of hypofractionation. Certainly, when

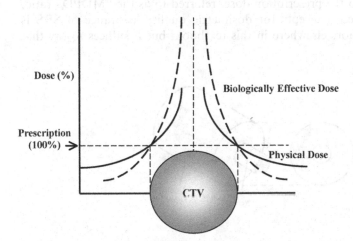

Figure 12 The dose profile across and outside a spherical tumor, with the prescribed dose specified as 100% at the edge of the mass. The rapid drop-off of physical dose, so characteristic for high-precision oriented radiation treatment, in fact translates to an even sharper drop-off after biological correction using, say, biological effective dose (BED).

applying SRT to extracranial disease sites, care must be taken to minimize the toxicity to various acutely-responding normal tissues like skin and mucosa if accelerated treatment is contemplated. For late-responding tissues, both the dose per fraction and the total dose are key factors to consider. The guidelines as outlined in the section on Biologically Effective Dose (BED), with the concept of BED or the isoeffect conversion relations of Eqs. (9) and (10), can be used to compare various fractionation schemes quantitatively (10,31) and provide a starting point for designing treatment protocols.

Coverage, Homogeneity, and Conformality

The effect of geographic miss (or, more correctly, underdosage) at the peripheral edge of a spherical tumor is illustrated in Figure 11, showing inadequate field "coverage." There may also be problems of "conformality" or "conformity" between the intended target volume and the actual irradiated volume. Furthermore, "homogeneity" pertains to the issue of heterogeneous dose distribution, with the associated volume effect discussed above (see section on Partial Organ Irradiation and Heterogeneous Dose Distribution). These entities are well specified in the quality assurance guidelines set forth by the Radiation Therapy Oncology Group (RTOG) for SRS (85): *Coverage* is described as the percent of prescription isodose completely encompassing the target. The *conformity index* is defined as the ratio of the prescription isodose volume to the target volume, referred as the "PITV" ratio. The *homogeneity index* is defined as the ratio of the maximum dose to the prescription dose, referred to as the "MDPD" ratio. Utilization of these concepts for dosimetric quality assurance of SRS is discussed by authors elsewhere in this textbook, but it suffices to say that

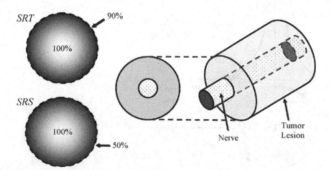

Figure 13 Difference in homogeneity between SRT and SRS for a hypothetical tumor such as acoustic neuroma, which may wrap around the eight cranial nerve. The relatively higher degree of homogeneity achieved in SRT could possibly explain the clinical observation of better hearing preservation. *Source*: From Ref. 49.

the incorporation of radiobiological considerations (especially for SRT) would certainly introduce a higher level of complexity. Hopefully, the theoretical considerations as discussed in this chapter would assist readers to gain some qualitative appreciation of the issues involved. As an example, Figure 13 depicts a clinical scenario regarding the use of SRS versus SRT for an acoustic neuroma, which is hypothesized to contain within its CTV the eighth cranial nerve as a late-responding normal tissue. Because of the higher homogeneity generally achievable by SRT rather than by SRS (thus less differential between the prescribed dose to the tumor and the dose to the cranial nerve, in particular after biological correction using BED, for example), it is anticipated that the patient's sense of hearing might be preserved better by SRT. The preliminary report for a subsetof patients with this disease seems to support such an assertion (49).

NOTE ADDED IN PROOF

Simultaneous Integrated Boost (SIB)

With the advent of IMRT and inverse planning, heterogeneous dose distribution might be planned *on purpose* in an approach called "simultaneous integrated boost" (SIB) (75). The idea of SIB stems from one's desire to simultaneously escalate the dose to the primary tumor while maintaining approximately the same conventional level of dose to the regional structures, e.g., lymphatics, which might harbor subclinical metastases. This is in contrast to the traditional "shrinking-field" technique[e] in which the primary tumor "boost" is done sequentially in time after a bigger treatment volume containing the tumor and the regional lymphatics has been given a dose considered sufficient for the control of subclinical disease. The latter structure might be described as CTV2, to be distinguished from CTV1 which is equivalent to the earlier-defined CTV (see section on Treatment Field Margins) that represents the perceived direct microscopic extension of the malignant tumor beyond the GTV. For example, the shrinking-field technique for most head and neck cancers usually involves a boost to the gross primary tumor and its edges (GTV+CTV1) to about 70 Gy total, *after* such volume and the regional lymphatic (CTV2) have been given approximately 50 Gy. With SIB, the treatment volume would include both the primary and the cervical lymph nodes, each prescribed with different dose level but for the *entire* time duration of the treatment course. Clearly, this treatment volume can be quite extensive, a scenario not encountered often by specialists using SRS or SRT for intracranial tumors. From the consideration of both the double-trouble effect and the treatment time factor as discussed earlier, the application of biological dosimetry for SIB technique may prove to be more complicated. Some empirical guidelines have been extracted from a few clinical reports[f] (75). Recommendation from RTOG seems to dwell upon delivering the conventional 2 Gy per fraction to the CTV1, higher (2.2 Gy)

---

[e] Fletcher GH. Clinical radiation therapy. In: Fletcher GH, ed. Textbook of Radiotherapy. 3rd ed. Philadelphia: Lea and Febiger, 1980:228.

[f] Blanco AI, Chao C. Principles & Practice of Radiation Oncology Updates, 3(3). Philadelphia: Lippincott, 2002.

for the GTV (hence equivalent to a form of *accelerated fractionation* strategy), and lower (1.8 Gy) for CTV2 (75).

Dose Response for Subclinical Disease

Both CTV1 and CTV2, by definition, are perceived to harbor undetected—or sub-clinical—tumor cells. However, they have quite distinctive bases for their dose-response relationship. For CTV1, the importance to cover tumor edges with adequate margins has been emphasized previously. Its dose-response depends directly on the amount of malignant cells present within the irradiated field (Eq. 13), while the ulti-mate chance of cure for the patient can also be hindered by those cells missed "geo-graphically" during a planned precision-oriented treatment. On the contrary, the subclinical disease confined within the CTV2 arises from the probabilistic dissemina-tion and establishment of metastases. The dose-response curve for these subclinical metastases has been reported to resemble a linear rather than a sharply rising sigmoid shape as for bulky primary tumors.[g] A biophysical model based on the kinetics of primary tumor growth and the probability of subsequent metastatic colony forma-tion and growth has been proposed[h] in order to provide a more mechanistic way of interpreting the clinical observations.

The Role of Ultra-Precision Oriented Radiation Therapy in Cancer Medicine

With the advent of computer technology, ultra-precision oriented radiotherapy tech-niques like SRS, SRT, or IMRT have certainly fulfilled the goal long-held by oncol-ogists to deliver adequate dose for tumor control while minimize toxicity to the normal tissues. Is this however equivalent to finding the "holy grail" in cancer med-icine—as some enthusiastic technophiles so optimistically perceive? The answer is, unfortunately, not quite. One needs to simply look at Table 1 to appreciate that the bottleneck in cancer therapy lies largely in the control of metastatic disease rather than primary tumor control. Clearly, when a malignancy is diagnosed relatively early (i.e., localized), the cure rate (measured roughly as 5-year survival) has been rather satisfactory for most common cancers *even before the days of precision oriented radia-tion therapy*. In contrast, when a patient presents with metastatic disease, the survival outcome is often dismal. This underlies the fundamental tenet of cancer "preven-tion" and screening, that early diagnosis plus early treatment can translate into long survival.

Nevertheless, from Table 1 one can also see that treatment results for some malignancies remain poor despite the fact that the tumor is diagnosed at a localized stage. While this may simply mean that the diagnostic resolution for micrometastases is something to be improved, inadequate local control by curative surgery or radia-tion therapy does represent a significant cause. This is highly conceivable especially when one realizes that these malignancies are often gastrointestinal or pulmonary in origin, for which radiation therapy is often limited in dose due to low tolerance of the surrounding normal structures (small intestine or lungs, respectively) and

---

[g] Withers HR, Peters LJ, Taylor JMG. Dose-response relationship for radiation therapy of subclinical disease. Int J Radiat Oncol Biol Phys 1995; 31:353–359.

[h] Lee S. Ph.D. dissertation, University of California, Los Angeles, 2001.

Table 1 Comparison for Five-Year Survival Rates Between Local and Systemic Stages for Some Common Cancers

Cancer Type	Local (%)	Systemic (%)	All Stage (%)
Prostate	99	30	87
Breast	97	20	84
Uterus	95	26	84
Bladder	93	6	81
Cervix	91	9	69
Colorectum	91	7	61
Stomach	61	2	21
Lung	48	2	14
Esophagus	22	2	11
Liver	13	2	6
Pancreas	13	2	4

Source: U. S. NCI Surveillance, Epidemiology, and End Results Program, 1996

its accuracy hindered by motion uncertainty introduced by breathing movement. The corollary is, if one can introduce high dose to these tumors while minimizing normal tissue damage, then enhancement of local control may translate into higher survival. It may thus be highly productive to invest utilization of precision radiotherapy for these particular cancers. The recent development in respiratory gating technique, or broadly speaking image-guided radiation therapy (IGRT)—to handle what physicists describe as *4-dimensional* treatment, may be justified further in this regard.

Even for prostate cancer, for example, which has enjoyed very high survival rate when early-stage patients are treated with old-standard radiation therapy, dose escalation using conformal or IMRT technique may translates into higher *distant metastasis* control, at least in theory. This phenomenon, that successful local control can impact on distant disease outcome and thus survival, has been reported in a modeling study using Goldie-Codman mechanism to simulate metastatogenesis.[i]

In summary, dose escalation via ultra-precision oriented radiation therapy may not necessarily be the key to solving the cancer problem, in view of the fact that distant metastasis remains to be the bottleneck. *We can kill what we can see, it is often what we cannot see that kills the patient.* In this regard, it is not difficult to see that when the zenith is attained, precision radiotherapy is at most equivalent to bloodless cancer surgery, along with all the oncologic constraints (uncertain tumor margins, uncertain metastasis, etc.) faced by surgeons. However, while we must continue to advocate the importance of early diagnosis and intervention for most cancers, we may also receive great dividend to simultaneously invest efforts in implementing precision radiotherapy techniques such as IGRT for those malignancies which historically have not enjoyed adequate rates of local primary tumor control.

---

[i] Yorke ED, Fuks Z, Norton L, Whitmore W, Ling CC. Modeling the development of metastases from primary and locally recurrent tumors: comparison with a clinical data base for prostatic cancer. Cancer Res 1993; 53:2987–2993.

REFERENCES

1. Fowler JF. The linear-quadratic formula and progress in fractionated radiotherapy. Br J Radiol 1989; 62:679–694.
2. Brenner DJ, Hall EJ. Conditions for the equivalence of continuous to pulsed low dose rate brachytherapy. Int J Radiat Oncol Biol Phys 1991; 20:181–190.
3. Brenner DJ, Huang Y, Hall EJ. Fractionated high dose-rate vei-sus low dose-rate regimens for intracavitary brachytherapy of the cervix: equivalent regimens for combined brachytherapy and external irradiation. Int J Radiat Oncol Biol Phys 1991; 21:1415–1423.
4. Hall EJ. Radiobiology for the Radiologist. 5th ed. Philadelphia: Lippincott, 2000.
5. Withers HR, Peters LJ. Biological aspects of radiation therapy. In: Fletcher GH, ed. Textbook of Radiotherapy, 3d ed. Philadelphia: Lea and Febiger, 1980:103–180.
6. Coutard H. Roentgentherapy of epitheliomas of the tonsillar region, bypopharynx, and larynx fiom 1920 to 1926. Am J Roentgenol 1932; 28:313–331 and 343–348.
7. Withers HR: The 4R's of radiotherapy. Lett JT, Alder H, eds. Advances in Radiation Biology. Vol. 5. New York: Academic, 1975:241.
8. Thomlinson RH, Gray LH. The histological structure of some human lung cancers and the possible implications for radiotherapy. Br J Cancer 1955; 9: 539–549.
9. Withers HR, Taylor JMG, Maciejewski B. The hazard of accelerated tumor clonogen repopulation during radiotherapy. Acta Oncol 1988; 27:131–146.
10. Ang KK, Thames HD, Peters LJ. Altered fractionation schedules. In: Perez CA, Brady LW, eds. Principles and Practice of Radiation Oncology. 3d ed. Philadelphia: Lippincott, 1998:119–142.
11. Elkind MM, Sutton H. Radiation response of mammalian cells grown, in culture I. Repair of X-ray damage in surviving Chinese hamster cells. Radiat Res 1960; 13:556–593.
12. Curtis SB. Lethal and potentially lethal lesions induced by radiation—a unified repair model. Radiat Res 1986; 106:252–270.
13. Bergonié J, Tribondéau L. Comptes Rendus de l'Alcadémie des Sciences 1906; 143:983; Translation of original article: Interpretation of some results of radiotherapy and an attempt at determining a logical technique of treatment. Radiat Res 1959; 11:587–594.
14. Strandqvist M. Studieren über die kumulative Wirkung der Röntgen-strahlen bei Fraktionierung. Acta Radiol 1944; 55(suppl):1–300.
15. Schwarzschild K. On the law of reciprocity for bromide of silver gelatin. Astrophys J 1900; 11:89.
16. Ellis F. Fractionation in radiotherapy. In: Deeley TJ, Woods CAP, eds. Modern Trends in Radiotherapy. Vol. 1. London: Butterworths, 1967:34–51.
17. Kirk J, Gray WM, Watson ER. Cumulative radiation effect. Part I. Fractionated treatment regimens. Clin Radiol 1971; 22:145–155.
18. Orton CG, Ellis F. A simplification in the use of the NSD concept in practical radiotherapy. Br J Radiol 1973; 46:529–537.
19. Sheline GE, Wara WM, Smith V. Therapeutic irradiation and brain, injury. Int J Radiat Oncol Biol Phys 1980; 6:1215–1228.

20. Goldsmith BJ, Rosenthal SA, Wara WM, Larson DA. Optic neuropathy after irradiation of meningioma. Radiology 1992; 185:71–76.
21. Alpen EL. Theories and models for cell survival. In: Alpen EL, ed. Radiation Biophysics 2d ed. SanDiego: Academic Press, 1998:132–287.
22. Desauer F. The cause of the action of X-rays and X-rays of radium upon living cells. J Radiol 1923; 4:411–415.
23. Puck TT, Marcus PI. Action of X-rays on mammalian cells. J Exp Med 1956; 103:653–666.
24. Thames HD, Withers HR, Peters LJ, Fletcher GH. Changes in early and late radiation responses with, altered dose fractionation: implications for dose–survival relationships. Int J Radiat Oncol Biol Phys 1982; 8:219–226.
25. Brenner DJ, Hall EL. The origins basis of the linear-quadratic model. (Letter) Int J Radiat Oncol Biol Phys 1992; 23:252.
26. Yaes RJ, Patel P, Maruyama Y. Response to Brenner and Hall. (Letter) Int J Radiat Oncol Biol Phys 1992; 23:252–253.
27. Withers HR, Thames HD, Peters LJ. Differences in the fractionation response of acute and late responding tissues. In: Karcher KH, Kogelnik HD, Reinartz G, eds. Progress in Radio-Oncology II. New York: Raven Press, 1982:257–296.
28. Travis EL, Tucker SL. Isoeffect models aid fractionated radiation therapy. Int J Radiat Oncol Biol Phys 1987; 13:283–287.
29. Brenner DJ, Hlatky LR, Hahnfeldt PJ, Hall EJ, Sachs RK. A convenient extension of the linear-quadratic model to include redistribution and reoxygenation. Int J Radiat Oncol Biol Phys 1995; 32:379–390.
30. Barendsen GW. Dose fractionation, dose rate and isoeffect relationships for normal tissue response. Int J Radiat Oncol Biol Phys 1982; 8:1981–1997.
31. Fowler JF. Intercomparisons of new and old schedules in fractionated radiotherapy. Sem Radiat Oncol 1992; 2:67–72.
32. Yaes RJ, Patel P, Maruyama Y. On using the linear-quadratic model in daily clinical practice. Int J Radiat Oncol Biol Phys 1991; 20:1353–1362.
33. Lea DE, Catcheside DG. The mechanism of the induction by radiation of chromosome aberrations in *Tradescantia*. J Genet 1942; 44:216–245.
34. Lee SP, Leu MY, Smathers JB, McBride WH, Parker RG, Withers HR. Biologically effective dose distribution based on the linear quadratic model and its clinical relevance. Int J Radiat Oncol Biol Phys 1995; 33:375–389.
35. Withers HR, Thames HD, Peters LJ. A new isoeffect curve for change in dose per fraction. Radiother Oncol 1983; 1:187–191.
36. Withers HR. Biologic basis of radiation therapy. In: Perez CA, Brady LW, eds. Principles and Practice of Radiation Oncology 2d ed. Philadelphia: Lippincott, 1992:64–96.
37. Lea DE. A theory of the action of radiations on biological materials capable of recovery I. The time–intensity factor. Br J Radiol 1938; 11:489–497.
38. Thames HD. An 'incomplete-repair' model for survival after fractionated and continuous irradiations. Int J Radiat Biol 1985; 47:319–339.
39. Oliver R. A comparison of the effects of acute and protracted gamma-radiation on the growth of seedlings of *Vicia faha* II. Theoretical calculations. Int J Radiat Biol 1964; 8:475–488.

40. Thames HD, Hendry JH. Normal tissue tolerance: time, dose, and fractionation. In: Thames HD, Hendry JH, eds. Fractionation in Radiotherapy. London: Taylor & Francis, 1987:218–237.

41. Bentzen SM, Tucker SJ. Quantifying the position and steepness of radiation dose–response curves. Int J Radiat Biol 1997; 71:531–542.

42. Källman P, Ågren A, Brahmes A. Tumor and normal tissue responses to fractionated non-uniform dose delivery. Int J Radiat Biol 1992; 62:249–262.

43. Wambersie A, Hanks G, Van Dam J. Quality assurance and accuracy required in radiation therapy: biological and medical considerations. In: Madhvanath U, Parthasarathy KS, Venkateswaran TV, eds. Selected Topics in Physics of Radiotherapy and Imaging. New Delhi: McGraw-Hill, 1988:1–24.

44. Travis EL, Liao Z-X, Tucker SL. Spatial heterogeneity of the volume effect for radiation pneumonitis in mouse lung. Int J Radiat Oncol Biol Phys 1997; 38:1045–1054.

45. Withers HR, Taylor JMG, Maciejewski B. Treatment volume and tissue tolerance. Int J Radiat Oncol Biol Phys 1988; 14:751–759.

46. Withers HR, Thames HD. Dose fractionation and volume effects in normal tissues and tumors. Am J Clin Oncol 1988; 11:313–329.

47. Kjellberg RN, Hanamura T, Davis KR, Lyons SL, Adams RD. Bragg-peak proton-beam therapy for arteriovenous malformations of the brain. N Engl J Med 1983; 309:269–274.

48. Flickinger JC. An integrated logistic formula for prediction of complications from radiosurgery. Int J Radiat Oncol Biol Phys 1989; 17:879–885.

49. Selch MT, Pedroso A, Lee SP, Solberg TD, Agazaryan N, Cabatan-Awang C, DeSalles AAF. Stereotactic radiotherapy for the treatment of acoustic neuromas. J Neurosurg 2004. Accepted, for publication.

50. Lyman JT, Wolbarst AB. Optimization of radiation therapy 3. A method of assessing complication probabilities from dose–volume histograms. Int J Radiat Oncol Biol Phys 1987; 13:103–109.

51. Lyman JT, Wolbarst AB. Optimization of radiation therapy 4. A dose–volume histogram reduction algorithm. Int J Radiat Oncol Biol Phys 1989; 17:433–436.

52. Hamilton CS, Chan LY, McElwain DLS, Denham JW. A practical evaluation of five dose–volume histogram reduction algorithms. Radiother Oncol 1992; 24:251–260.

53. Mark LB. Challenges defining structures of interest in radiation therapy treatment planning. In: Paliwal BR, Fowler JF, Herbert DE, Mehta MP, eds. Volume & Kinetics in Tumor Control & Normal Tissue Complications. Madison: Medical Phys, 1998:18–31.

54. Schultheiss TE, Orton CG, Peck RA. Models in radiotherapy: volume effects. Med Phys 1983; 10:410–415.

55. Lyman JT. Complication probability as assessed from dose volume histograms. Radiat Res 1985; 104:S13–S19.

56. Kutcher GJ, Burman C. Calculation of complication probability factors for non-uniform normal tissue irradiation: the effective volume method. Int J Radiat Oncol Biol Phys 1989; 16:1623–1630.

57. Burman C, Kutcher GJ, Emami B, Goitein M. Fitting of normal tissue tolerance data to an analytic function. Int J Radiat Oncol Biol Phys 1991; 21:123–135.

58. Emami B, Lyman J, Brown A, Coia L, Goitein M, Munzenrider JE, Shank B, Solin LJ, Wesson M. Tolerance of normal tissue to therapeutic irradiation. Int J Radiat Oncol Biol Phys 1991; 21:109–122.
59. Brenner DJ. Dose, volume, and tumour-control predictions in radiotherapy. Int J Radiat Oncol Biol Phys 1993; 26:171–179.
60. Deasy J. Inter-patient and intra-tumor radiosensitivity heterogeneity. In: Paliwal BR, Fowler JF, Herbert DE, Mehta MP, eds. Volume & Kinetics in Tumor Control & Normal Tissue Complications. Madison: Medical Physics Publishing, 1998:363–381.
61. Webb S, Nahum AE. The biological effect of inhornogeneous tumour irradiation with inhomogeneous clonogenic cell density. Phys Med Biol 1993; 38:653–666.
62. Suit H, Skates S, Taghian A, Okunieff P, Efird JT. Clinical implications of heterogeneity of tumour response to radiation therapy. Radiother Oncol 1992; 25:251–260.
63. Withers HR. Biological aspects of conformal therapy. Acta Oncol 2000; 39:569–577.
64. Withers HR, Lee SL. The biology of IMRT. In: Paliwal BR, Herbert DE, Fowler IF, Mehta MP, eds. Biological & Physical Basis of IMRT & Tomotherapy. Madison: Medical Physics Publishing, 2002:303–311.
65. Tome WA, Fowler JF. Selective boosting of tumor subvolumes. Int J Radiat Oncol Biol Phys 2000; 48:593–599.
66. Tome WA, Fowler JF. On cold spots in tumor subvolumes. Med Phys 2002; 29:1590–1598.
67. Fowler JF. Radiobiological issues in IMRT. In: Paliwal BR, Herbert DE, Fowler IF, Mehta MP, eds. Biological & Physical Basis of IMRT & Tomotherapy. Madison: Medical Physics Publishing, 2002:8–22.
68. Michalowski A. Effects of radiation on normal tissues: hypothetical mechanisms of limitations of in situ assays of clonogenicity. Radiat Environ Biophys 1981; 19:157–172.
69. Wheldon TE, Michalowski A, Kirk J. The effect of irradiation on function in self-renewing normal tissues with differing proliferative organisation. Br J Radiol 1982; 55:759–766.
70. Niemierko A, Goitein M. Modeling of normal tissue response to radiation: the critical volume model. Int J Radiat Oncol Biol Phys 1993; 25:135–145.
71. Niemierko A, Goitein M. Calculation of normal tissue complication probability and dose-volume histogram reduction schemes for tissues with a critical element architecture. Radiother Oncol 1991; 20:155–176.
72. Brahme A. Optimized radiation therapy based on radiobiological objectives. Sem Radiat Oncol 1999; 9:35–47.
73. Webb S. Conformal radiotherapy treatment planning, In: Webb S. In: The Physics of Three-dimensional Radiation Therapy: Conformal Radiotherapy, Radiosurgery and Treatment Planning. Bristol and Philadelphia: Institute of Physics Publishing, 1993:1–38.
74. Niemierko A. Reporting and analyzing dose distributions: a concept of equivalent uniform dose. Med Phys 1997; 24:103–110.
75. Niemierko A, Mohan R. Intenstiy-modulated radiation therapy. Part II. Radiobiological aspects. Refresher Course 303. 44th Annual Meeting of the American

Society of Therapeutic Radiology and Oncology, New Orleans, LA, Oct 6–10,2002.

76. Jones LC, Hoban PW. Treatment plan comparison, using equivalent uniform biologically effective dose (EUBED). Phys Med Biol 2000; 45:159–170.

77. Jones L, Hoban P. A comparison of physically and radiobiologically based optimization for IMRT. Med Phys 2002; 29:1447–1455.

78. Clark BG, Souhami L, Pla C, Al-Amro AS, Bahary J-P, Villemure J-G, Caron J-L, Olivier A, Podgorsak B. The integral biologically effective dose to predict brain stem toxicity of hypofractionated stereotactic radiotherapy. Int J Radiat Oncol Biol Phys 1998; 40:667–675.

79. Brenner DJ, Hall EJ. Fractionation and protraction for radiotherapy of prostate carcinoma. Int J Radiat Oncol Biol Phys 1999; 43:1095–1101.

80. Prescribing, Recording, and Reporting Photon Beam Therapy. Bethesda: International Commission on Radiation Units and Measurements, Report 50,1993.

81. Prescribing, Recording, and Reporting Photon Beam Therapy (Supplement to ICRU Report 50). Bethesda: International Commission on Radiation Units and Measurements, Report 62, 1999.

82. Brada M, Laing RW, Graham J, Warrington AP, Hines F. Fractionated stereotactic radiotherapy in the treatment of recurrent high grade glioma—dose escalation study. Acta Neurochir 1993; 122:151.

83. Pozza F, Colombo F, Chierego G, Avanzo RC, Marchetti C, Benedetti A, Casentini L, Danieli D. Low grade astrocytomas: treatment with unconventional fractionated stereotactic radiation therapy. Radiology 1989; 171:565–569.

84. Brenner DJ, Hall EJ. Stereotactic radiotherapy of intracranial tumors—an ideal candidate for accelerated treatment. Int J Radiat Oncol Biol Phys 1994; 28:1039–1041.

85. Shaw E, Kline R, Gillin M, Souhami L, Hirschfeld A, Dinapoli R, Martin L. Radiation Therapy Oncology Group: radiosurgery quality assurance guidelines. Int J Radiat Oncol Biol Phys 1993; 27:1231–1239.

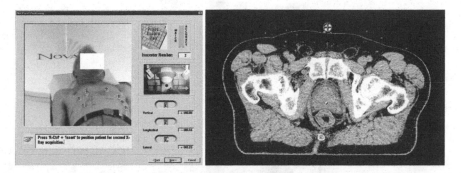

Figure 3-2 *Left*: Patient with IR reflective marker. (Note that the camera system has identified the markers indicated by the circles, and the coincidence with the planned position indicated by the small crosses.) *Right*: CT-image showing IR marker (localized by software), contours of CT, PTV, and rectum, and position of the treatment isocenter.

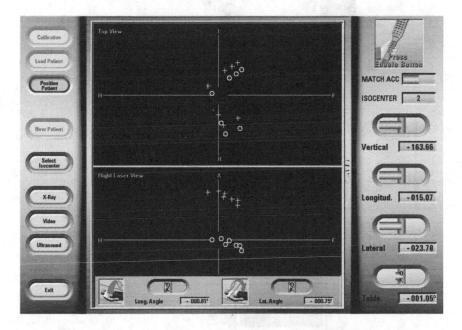

Figure 3-3 Illustration of the graphical interface of ExacTrac 3.0/NOVALIS BODY with the patient on the treatment couch prior to treatment setup. Note the detection of transversal and rotational patient position at the right side and bottom of the image. The circles indicate the actual position and the crosses indicate the planned position where the patient will be moved.

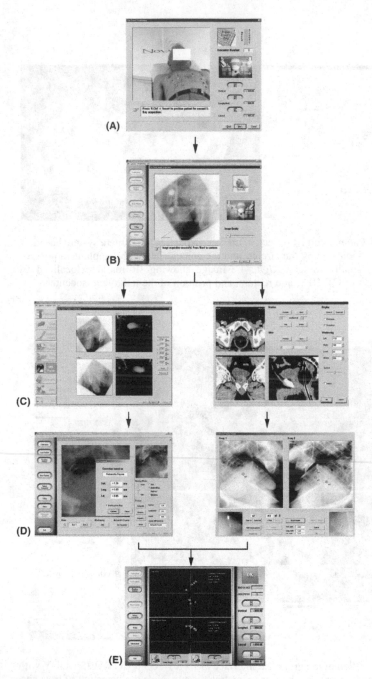

Figure 3-4 Flowchart illustrating the different steps in the positioning procedure using ExacTrac 3.0/NOVALIS BODY. From top to bottom: (**A**) Patient on the treatment couch with IR reflective markers. (**B**) Acquisition of X-rays (only one shown). (**C–D**) Calculation of 3D correction vector based on either automated fusion of X-ray images with DRRs representing the ideal position (*left*) or matching of implanted radio-opaque markers (*right*). (**E**) Automated patient positioning.

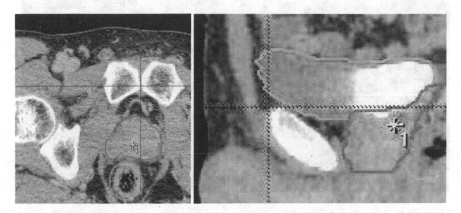

Figure 3-5 Illustration of the distances taken to define the position of the treatment isocenter with respect to bony structures for verification with portal film. The distance of the isocenter to the midline and to the lines tangential to the superior and ventral border of the os pubis are measured according to the dotted line.

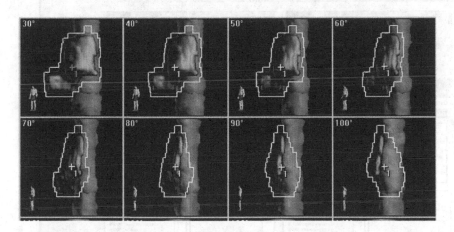

Figure 3-7 Beam's eye views of a dynamic arc (10° gantry steps). The yellow line surrounding the target (green) indicates the conformal field shape created by the multileaf collimator. The spinal cord (magenta) is shown running vertically through each frame. Parameters such as arc length, dose, and the margin between the field edge and the tumor are specified by the user. Dose distributions may be customized using software tools that allow for preferential sparing of organs at risk (OARs) and for graphical editing of field shapes in any BEV.

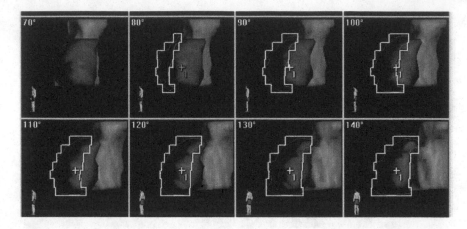

Figure 3-8 Beam's eye view of a dynamic arc with an "organ at risk" (OAR). The field shape (yellow) intentionally blocks part of the target (purple) in order to minimize the dose to the OAR behind it.

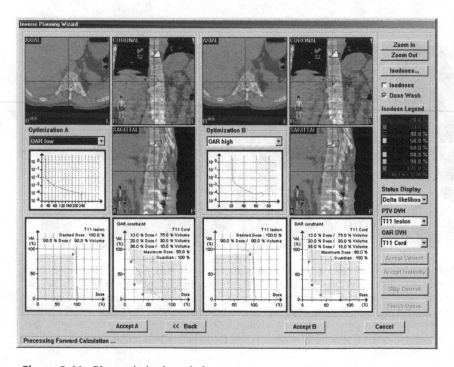

Figure 3-11 Plan optimization window.

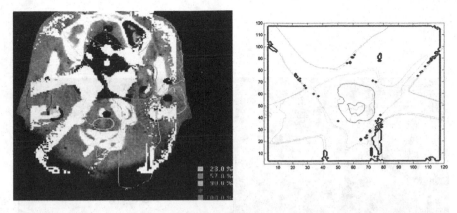

Figure 3-14 The importance of the choice of an appropriate phantom when mapping treatment parameters from a patient treatment to a phantom for verification of dose distribution is illustrated here. The left-hand pane shows the result from mapping into an anthropomorphic phantom; the white "erased" pixels indicate regions where the gamma tolerance (4% DD, 4mm DTA) is not met between measured and calculated dose distributions. The right-hand pane shows the same treatment mapped into a homogeneous cubic phantom; the "bold" pixels indicate regions where the gamma tolerance is not met. The homogeneous mapping does not show possible errors due to tissue heterogeneities and might give a false sense of confidence.

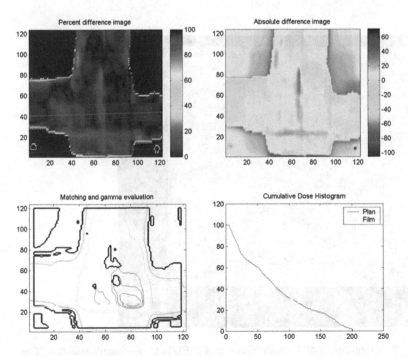

Figure 3-15 Illustration of in-house developed tool for verification of dose distribution (measured and calculated) at the AZ-VUB showing percent difference, absolute difference, and gamma map overlayed with both dose distributions and a cumulative dose histogram.

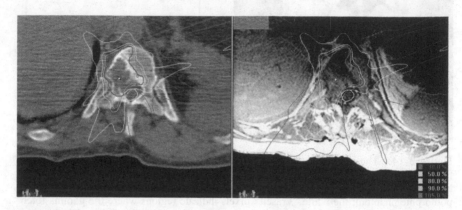

Figure 3-17 Eight-field IMRS dose distribution for T11 metastasis on fused CT/MR. The 30%, 50%, 80%, 90%, and 105% isodose lines are displayed. The maximum dose is 105%.

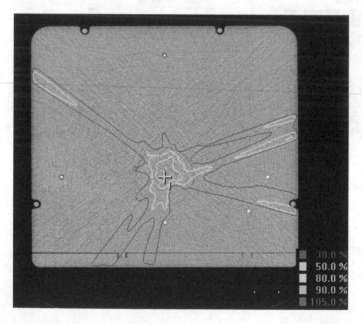

Figure 3-18 Eight-field IMRT plan mapped to a MEDTEC benchmark phantom. The 30%, 50%, 80%, and 90% isodose lines are displayed.

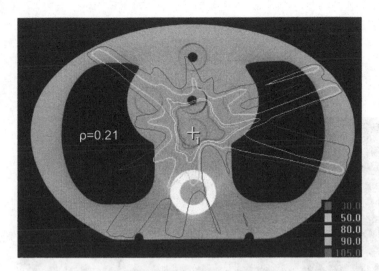

Figure 3-19 Eight-field IMRT plan mapped to a CIRS thorax phantom. The 30%, 50%, 80%, 90%, and 105% isodose lines are displayed.

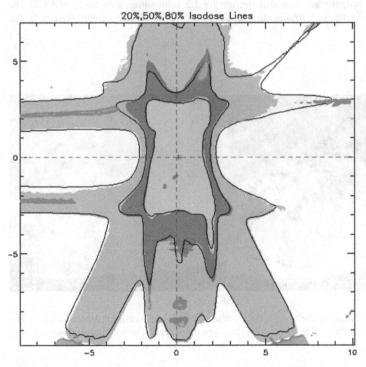

Figure 3-20 Comparison of a film measurement to calculation using gamma-index analysis for an IMRT dose distribution. Solid black lines are the calculated isodose lines; colorwash is the corresponding isodose lines from film. Dark green are the area where the dose criterian was exceeded.

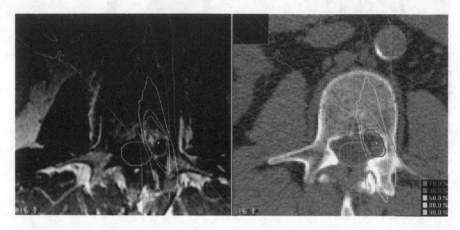

Figure 3-22 Dynamic arc dose distribution for L2 schwannoma on fused MR/CT. The 10%, 30%, 50%, 80%, and 90% isodose lines are displayed. The maximum dose is 100%.

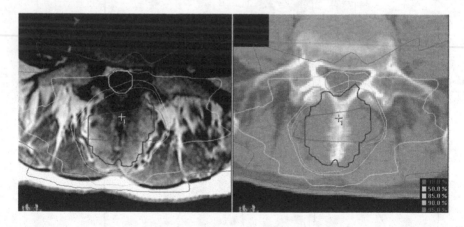

Figure 3-23 Conformal field dose distribution for L5 metastasis on fused MR/CT. The 30%, 50%, 85%, 90%, and 95% isodose lines are displayed. The maximum dose is 100%.

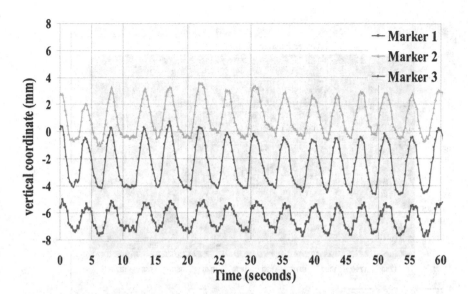

Figure 3-24 Vertical isocenter displacement as a function of time for three markers attached to the anterior surface of one patient. Though data are shown only for the first 60 sec, the pattern repeats over the entire 20 min.

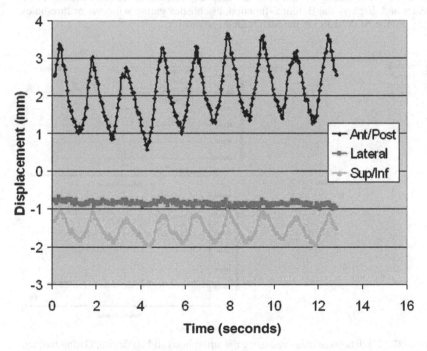

Figure 3-25 Marker displacement as a function of time for a single marker attached to the anterior surface of one patient. The stereophotogrammetry system is capable of reporting marker coordinates at a frequency of up to 10 Hz.

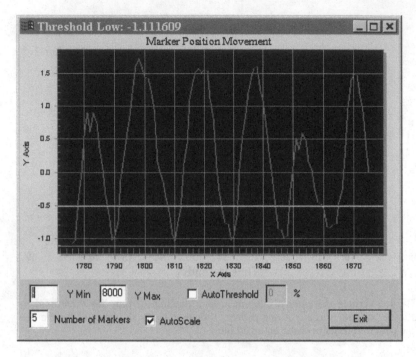

Figure 3-26 The gating control software monitors respiration through the ExacTrac, calculates and displays the Baroni F-function, establishes gating windows or thresholds, and triggers the NOVALIS via the MHOLDOFF/status bit.

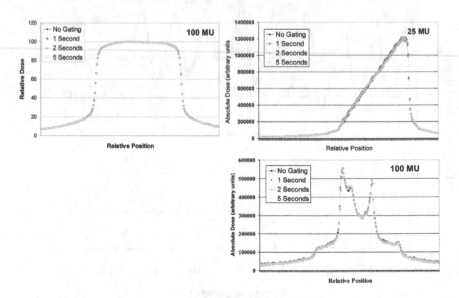

Figure 3-27 2D data were measured using the amorphous silicon device. Gating frequencies of 0.2, 0.5, and 1.0 Hz were used in addition to non-gated conditions. Profiles are shown for an open 10×10 cm^2 square field (*top left*), a dynamic wedge (*top right*), and arbitrary intensity map (*bottom right*).

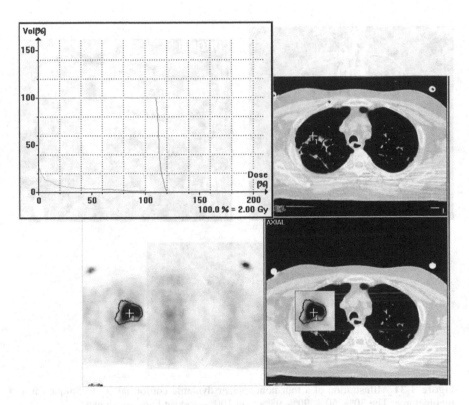

Figure 3-30 Example of target localization for a lung lesion using co-registration information from PET and CT imaging, with cumulative dose–volume histogram resulting from a coplanar dynamic conformal arc treatment.

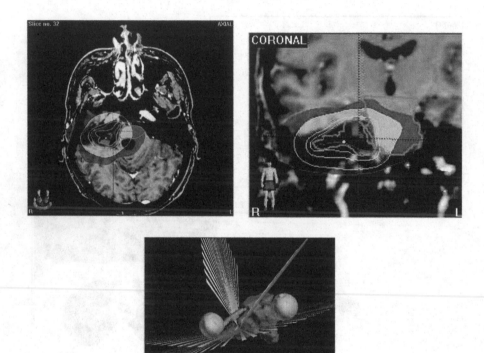

Figure 3-31 Illustration of a four noncoplanar dynamic conformal arc technique for a meningioma. The 30%, 50%, 90%, 98%, and 100% isodose lines are shown.

(A)

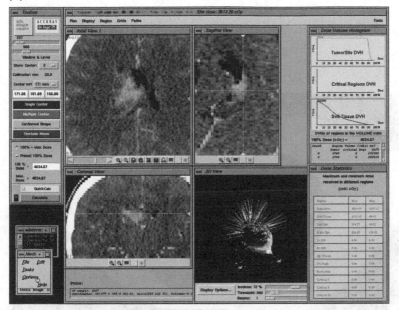

(C)

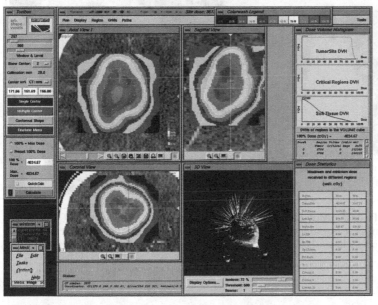

Figure 4-3 (**A**) Manual delineation of the target. Beam directions for optimized treatment of specific tumor shape (up to 1200, *lower left corner*) are computed automatically by the inverse planning system. (**C**) Both beam directions and beam weights are computed automatically, once target and critical regions have been delineated, and upper/lower dose thresholds have been entered.

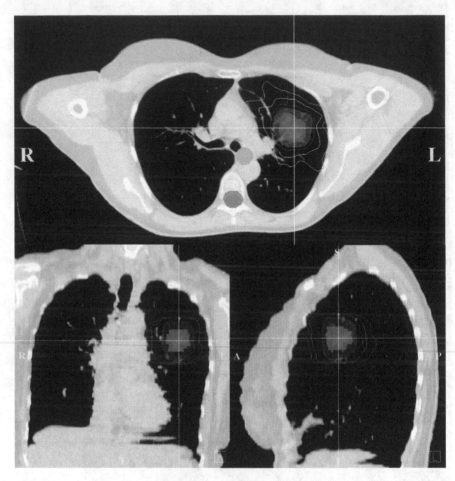

Figure 5-5 Isodose distribution for the case report example. Shown are the CTV (bright red), PTV (darker red), esophagus protection region (green), spinal cord protection region (blue), and isodose lines: 100% (dark blue) 90% (red), 70% (yellow), and 50% (green).

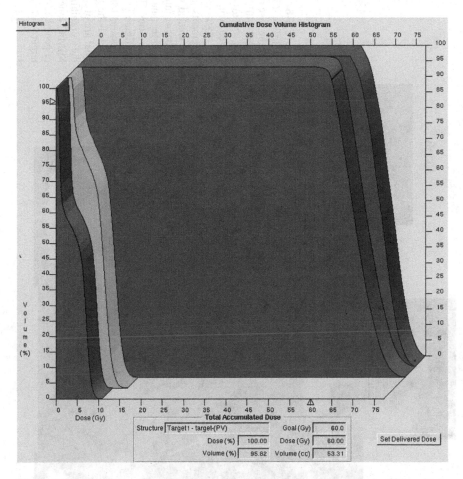

Figure 5-7 Cumulative dose volume histogram for the case report example. Shown (from back to front) are the CTV, PTV, esophagus, and cord.

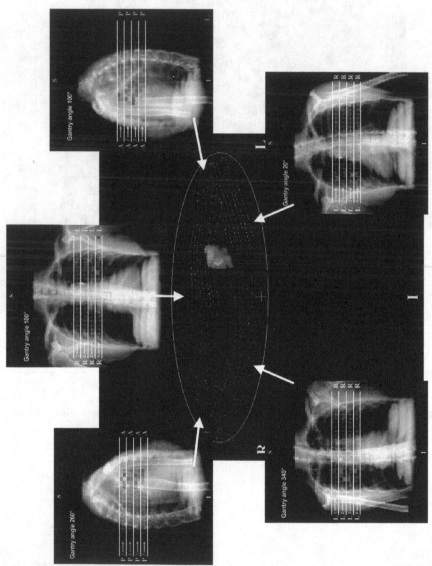

Figure 5-8 Depicting five of the 64 different intensity patterns used for the case report example (gantry angles 340°, 260°, 180°, 100°, and 20°). Note that the patient was treated with a "straight" couch (i.e., 180° Varian), and four couch increments (or treatment slices). The shaded squares represent pencil beam intensities utilized, with brighter shades indicating higher intensities. The central region of the figure graphically depicts pencil beams used, as dots on the surface of the patient. Note that the final arc of the treatment uses only the cranially located row of MIMiC vanes because inferior row of pencil beams does not "see" the target volume.

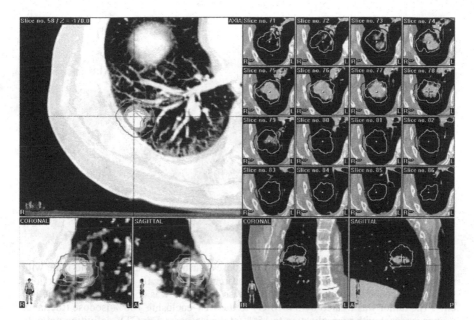

Figure 6-2 Generating target volumes for a stage I lung tumor. The ITV (*orange contour on left panel*) encompasses all GTVs contoured on six consecutive multi-slice CT scans (*light yellow contours on left and right panel*). The ITV was expanded with a 3 mm margin to derive the PTV (*red contour on right panel*).

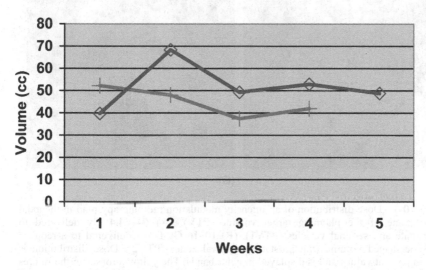

Figure 6-4 Changes in ITVs seen on weekly CT scans in two patients with peripheral lung tumors when five fractions of stereotactic radiotherapy were delivered in 5 weeks (12 Gy/fraction).

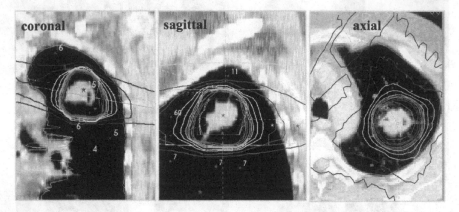

Figure 9-1 CTV-definition and conformal dose distribution in a 43-year-old male with primary lung cancer cT2 cN0 cM0 (adenocarcinoma grade II) in the left upper lobe medically inoperable due to severe heart disease. The CTV was 45 cm^3, the PTV was 100 cm^3. The tumor was treated by 3 × 10 Gy to the PTV-enclosing 100%-isodose (the inner orange isodose) with normalization to 150% at the isocenter. For CTV definition not only the macroscopic tumor but also the small tumor extensions into the periphery have to be included into the target volume (the numbers in the coronal and sagittal reconstruction show the point dose in percent to the prescribed fraction dose of 10 Gy).

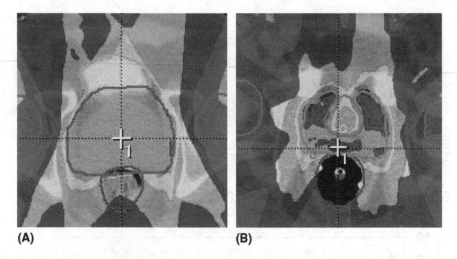

(A)　　　　　　　　　　　　　**(B)**

Figure 10-1 Dose distribution of an intensity modulation radiotherapy plan in the axial central plane of the planning target volume (PTV). (**A**) 64–64.4 Gy delivered to the prostate and seminal vesicles (PTV1); (**B**) 10–16 Gy boost delivered to a reduced horseshoe-shaped volume (the prostate peripheral zone) (PTV2). Dose distribution is given in percent values and is displayed in color bands. The yellow crosses in the figures represent the treatment isocenters for PTV1 and PTV2, respectively.

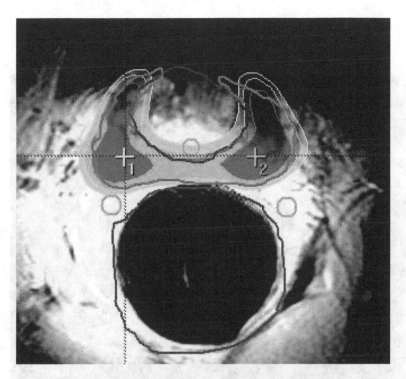

Figure 10-4 Dose distribution overlying the axial central plane of an endorectal MR image of the prostate containing the PTV2 (bilateral prostatic peripheral zone). Isodose bands of 100% or above (*red*), 90–100% (*yellow*), and 80–90% (*green*) are displayed.

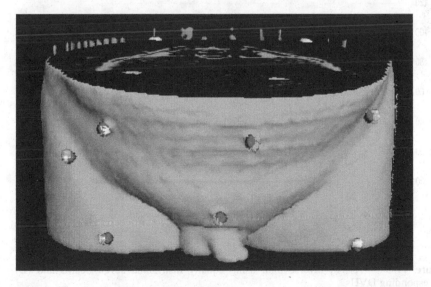

Figure 10-5 Digital volumetric reconstruction to simulate the setup reproducibility with ExacTrac. Infrared marker based registration between the CT at simulation (*red*) and the CT while on treatment (*green*) performed to assess target repositioning quality.

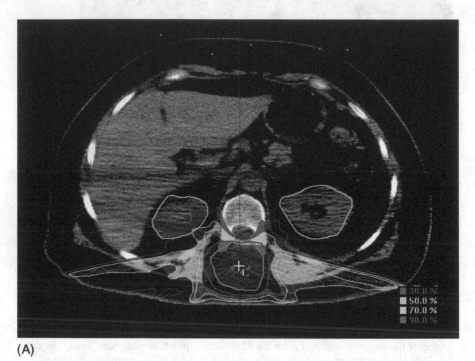

(A)

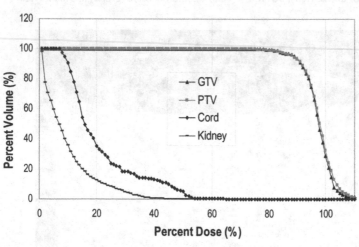

(B)

Figure 11-3 (**A**) An inverse plan using equally distributed seven beams and (**B**) corresponding DVHs.

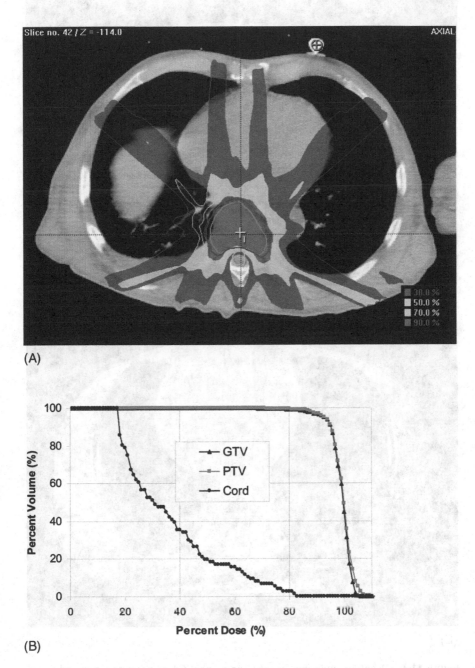

Figure 11-4 (**A**) An inverse plan using five beams and (**B**) corresponding DVHs.

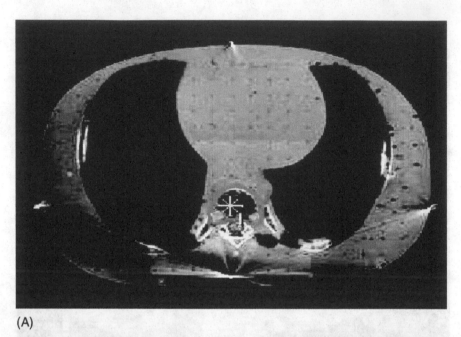

(A)

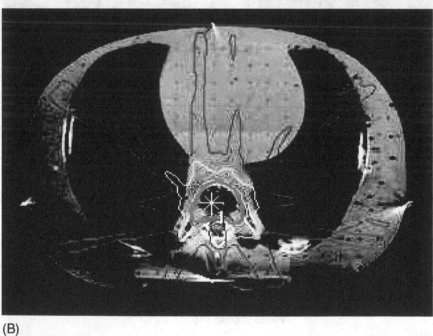

(B)

Figure 11-6 Phantom study images. (**A**) The original CT image with target and spinal cord indicated. (**B**) The planned dose distributions for 90%, 50%, and 30% isodose curves normalized to the isocenter.

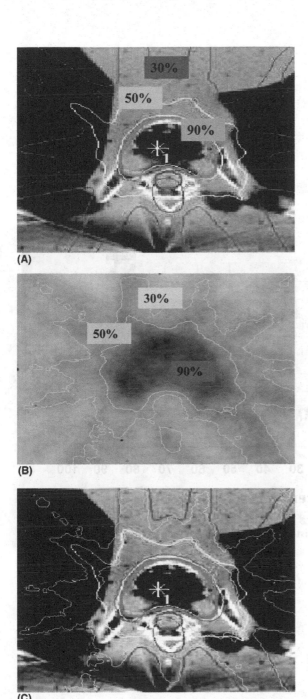

(A)

(B)

(C)

Figure 11-7 Phantom study results. (**A**) The planned isodose distributions in the region where the film was inserted. Solid curves represent planned isodose lines labeled 90%, 50%, and 30% relative to the isocenter. (**B**) The original film dose image with three corresponding isodose curves. (**C**) Both planned and corresponding measured isodose distributions are overlaid on the original CT image.

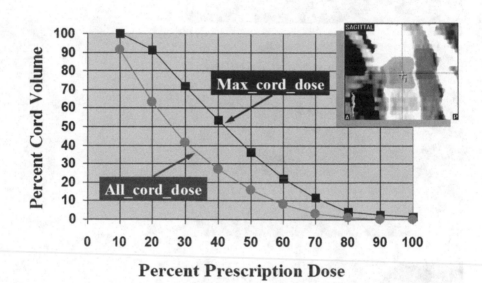

Figure 11-8 Dose–volume histograms (DVHs) for cord doses.

8

Stereotactic Radiation Therapy of Liver Tumors

Klaus K. Herfarth

Department of Radiation Oncology, University of Heidelberg, Germany

Martin Fuss

Department of Radiation Oncology, University of Texas Health Science Center, San Antonio, Texas, U.S.A.

INTRODUCTION

The first reports of successful radiation treatment of liver tumors were published 1954. Philipps et al. treated 36 patients with symptomatic liver metastases with doses of 19–36 Gy. The symptoms were reduced in more than 50% of the cases (1). Since that time, the benefits of palliative whole liver radiation have been confirmed in multiple studies (2–4). However, dose escalation of whole liver radiation from 27 to 33 Gy resulted in a significant increase of liver toxicity (5). Treatment-associated radiation induced liver damage (RILD) as a dose limiting toxicity appears 4–8 weeks after radiation therapy. Clinical symptoms include weight gain, increased abdominal girth, ascites, and a substantial rise in alkaline phosphatase. Ingold et al. (6) first described the clinical picture in 1965. The mortality rate of RILD is approximately 10–20%. The pathophysiological counterpart is veno-occlusive disease (VOD). Reed and Cox were the first to characterize the histological changes of RILD as marked congestion, which involves mainly the central portion of each lobule with atrophy of the inner liver plates (7). The wall of the small veins reveals a large number of fine reticulin fibers that crisscross the lumen of the vein and the adjacent afferent sinusoids (8). Chronic radiation liver damage is characterized by a distortion of the liver architecture: variable distances between the central veins and portal areas, fibrosis of the central veins, and concentric fibrosis of portal areas (9).

The occurrence of RILD is not only dependent on the dose, it is also dependent on the irradiated volume (10,11). Emami et al. estimated a TD 5/5 (tolerance dose with 5% complications in 5 years) of 30 Gy for whole liver radiation. If 1/3 or 2/3 of the liver could be spared, the TD 5/5 was estimated to increase to 35 and 50 Gy, respectively (12). Based on more recent data by the University of Michigan using three-dimensional treatment planning and conformal therapy, Dawson et al. estimated an even more pronounced volume effect with a TD 5/5 of 31, 47, and 90 Gy for whole liver, 2/3 liver, and 1/3 liver radiation, respectively (13). The basis for this calculation was a hyperfractionated (1.5 Gy bid) conformal treatment in conjunction with an intra-arterial FdUrd chemotherapy in 43 patients. The total doses reached 90 Gy (14).

A stereotactic treatment approach for liver malignancies should achieve better normal tissue sparing than conventional or conformal planning and delivery techniques. Therefore, a further dose escalation or hypofractionated dose delivery should be possible. First steps of stereotactic radiation therapy of liver malignancies were performed at the Karolinska Institute in Stockholm, Sweden (15).

Potential targets for stereotactic radiation in the liver are primary and secondary liver tumors. The incidence of these tumors, indications for stereotactic radiotherapy, liver specific difficulties for the treatment, applied doses, and current and future trials are described and discussed in the following sections.

INCIDENCE

There are two major groups of liver tumors: primary liver tumors and secondary liver tumors. Hepatocellular carcinoma (HCC) accounts for about 80–90% of the primary liver tumors. The incidence of the disease is currently approximately 1–3/100,000 in the United States and in Europe, with a recently observed growth of the incidence. The incidence increases with age and is associated with chronic liver damage (cirrhosis), often related to hepatitis C virus infection. Regions with high levels of hepatitis infections (countries in the Far East) have a 100–150 times higher incidence of HCC. Other risk factors are aflatoxins produced by the fungi *Aspergillus flavus*, which is a major cause of HCC in underdeveloped countries. HCCs are often multinodular and multifocal tumors. About 30% of the patients with HCC show distant metastases (mostly in the lungs, peritoneum, adrenal glands, and bones) at the time of diagnosis.

Cholangiocellular carcinoma (CCC) has an incidence of 1–2/100,000. This chapter focuses on the intrahepatic CCC only. CCC affecting the confluence of the right and left hepatic duct is also called a Klatskin tumor. Klatskin have a high tendency of perineural and subendothelial spread. This character-istic makes it difficult to evaluate the whole tumor involvement using imaging studies. About 30–50% of the patients show lymph node involvement at the time of diagnosis. One-third show distant metastasis (liver, lung, and peritoneum) at this time.

Liver metastases, or secondary liver tumors, show up in about 35% of all patients with solid tumors during the course of disease. Even higher numbers are published in organ specific section statistics: the highest incidence for 1008 patients was seen in patients with pancreatic cancer (86%), followed by breast cancer (60%), colorectal cancer (42%), lung cancer (39%), and stomach cancer (34%) (16). Due to the portal vein drainage, the liver is the first site of hema-tological spread of colorectal cancers. Therefore, liver metastases can be seen as a kind of advanced loco regional disease in patients with colorectal can-cer. The median survival for patients with untreated liver metastases varies between 5 and 19 months (17,18). Survival is dependent on the primary tumor and the extent of extrahepatic tumor involvement.

THE ROLE OF STEREOTACTIC BODY RADIATION THERAPY IN THE MULTI-DISCIPLINARY TREATMENT ARSENAL

The current therapeutic gold standard for primary and secondary hepatic tumors is surgical resection. The type of resection varies between an atypical resection, segment resection, hemihepatectomy, extended hemihepatectomy, and liver transplantation.

The resectability rate of HCC depends on the site of the tumor and the existence of accompanying liver cirrhosis. Resection is not recommended for patients with advanced cirrhosis (Child classification B or C). Five-year sur-vival rates of up to 76% have been reported for resected primary HCC in selected studies (19). For large and/or not resectable HCC, locally ablative therapies (e.g., percutaneous ethanol injection, radiofrequency ablation) and also radiation therapy have been described (20–23). Radiation dose depends on the volume of spared normal liver volume and is more limited for patients with liver cirrhosis (see later this chapter). The sparing of normal liver tissue favors a stereotactic approach of radiation therapy in these patients. Blomg-ren et al. treated nine patients with primary HCC using a stereotactic hypo-fractionated radiation approach. They reported no local failure with a median follow-up time of 12 months. However, two patients with cirrhosis developed RILD with non-tractable ascitic fluid and died 1.5 and 2.5 months after therapy. In one of these patients, a very large volume of nearly 300 cm^3 was treated (24). Sato et al. stereotactically treated 18 patients with primary HCC. They combined the radiation treatment with local chemotherapy. No local failure was observed with a median follow-up of 10 months after the frameless hypofractionated stereotactic radiation therapy. Only one patient showed definite deterioration of serum liver function tests (25). The available data on stereotactic radiation therapy of HCC is still very limited and follow-up times are short. However, these limited data show promising results in inoperable patients if enough functional liver tissue can be spared.

For intrahepatic cholangiocarcinomas, 5-year survival rates of up to 44% have been published after surgical resection (26). However, due to the subepithelial spread, only about 50% of the intrahepatic cholangiocarcinomas are suitable for resection (26). Experiences with radiation therapy have not been very promising in non-resectable cholangiocarcinomas (27). Due to the patterns of local tumor spread, only large margins around the gross tumor volume may ensure sufficient local control. Therefore, sufficient sparing of functional normal liver tissue is difficult to achieve, even when a stereotactic approach is used. The number of patients with CCC treated with stereotactic irradiation is very low in published series and follow-up times are typically limited (24,28,29). Therefore, any indication for stereotactic radiation therapy of an intrahepatic primary cholangiocarcinoma should be set on an individual basis.

Primary therapy for metastatic liver disease usually is systemic chemotherapy. However, a local therapeutic approach might also have a curative intention in cases of metastatic colorectal cancer. Surgical resection is the standard therapy in case of solitary secondary liver lesions. Wilson and Adson retrospectively analyzed patients with limited liver metastases of colorectal cancers. About 25% of the resected patients survived 5 years while none of the comparable patients with unresected liver metastases were alive after 5 years (30). Similar observations were made by Adson et al. (18), with 25% 5-year survival in the resected group and 2.5% 5-year survival in the unresected group. Patients with resections of metachronous liver metastases of colorectal cancers have similar 5-year survival rates of 20% after each resection (31–33).

Several minimal-invasive thermo-ablative approaches have been developed for inoperable metastases including radiofrequency ablation (34), laser-induced thermotherapy (35), or cryotherapy (36). However, solitary inoperable liver metastases are also the major indication for the only non-invasive cancer treatment, stereotactic body radiation therapy. Local tumor control rates of 80–100% have been published after stereotactic radiation therapy of liver metastases with low treatment-associated morbidity (24,28,29). Potential advantages compared with thermo-ablative procedures include non-invasiveness, reduced risk of damaging of blood vessels (especially near the liver hilum), and lack of blood flow-mediated temperature transport to distant liver regions. As of today, there are no definite indications for stereotactic radiation therapy of liver metastases since the indications vary between the published series. The major indication was inoperability due to surgical or medical reasons. There is no established contraindication for centrally located tumors, mostly due to the fact that data for high-dose radiation damage to centrally located liver structures is unavailable. One contraindication, however, is close proximity to other organs of the gastro-intestinal tract, i.e., tumors located close to the surface of the liver. Blomgren et al. reported of hemorrhagic gastritis or duodenal ulcers if the stomach or the duodenum were irradiated with more than three times 5 Gy (24). The maximal tumor size suitable for stereotactic body radiation therapy is controversial. While most studies limit eligibility to metastases smaller than 5–6 cm in diameter, other study groups have also successfully treated larger tumors (24,28). The indication for stereotactic body radiation therapy of larger liver tumors depends mostly on the volume of the liver and the chances of sparing enough functional liver tissue from the high dose area.

ORGAN-SPECIFIC DIFFICULTIES

Organ Motion

Liver radiation therapy and, even more so, conformal and stereotactic radiation therapy to targets in the liver have to account for several organ-specific challenges. Organ motion secondary to diaphragm motion with the breathing cycle is obviously the most problematic challenge. Traditionally, planning target volume safety margins are assigned to account for both inter-fraction and intra-fraction liver motion (37–39). While individually the range of liver motion varies, appropriate safety margins range from about 10 mm cranio-caudally to as much as 3 or 4 cm. The addition of such significant safety margins leads to the inclusion of relevant and dose limiting amounts of normal liver and other tissues-at-risk volumes to provide for a high probability of target volume dose coverage during radiation fraction delivery.

Several more or less technologically advanced strategies may be applied to reduce the respiration-dependent liver motion predominantly occurring during fraction delivery. Instructed deep breath-holding, or shallow breathing with support of oxygen via a mask may reduce diaphragm movement in compliant patients (40–42). While the reported clinical experience of instructed breathing relates predominantly to radiotherapy of thoracic tumors (40–47), the resulting tumor immobilization can be directly translated to abdominal targets since liver motion occurs as a function of diaphragmatic motion (13,48). Similar positive experiences have been reported by use of a so-called Active Breathing Coordinator or institution-specific breath-hold valve devices where the patient is coached to inhale to a predetermined depth and to hold this breathing volume for up to 20 sec, during which time frame radiation delivery is enabled (13,49). Similar to shallow breathing instructions, the use of such devices depends on patient compliance, and careful patient monitoring during treatment delivery is required.

More mechanistic approaches to reduce liver motion with inhalation/exhalation depend on abdominal pressure devices attached to the stereotactic body frame (50–52). A plate, often triangular or trapezoid in shape, is pressed onto the upper abdomen in an angle to constrain liver motion. While at least borderline-uncomfortable for the patient, these devices can effectively reduce the respiration dependent liver motion and allow for reduction of PTV margins to at or below 10 mm in the cranio-caudal direction (50).

Most recently, respiratory gating using software-controlled assessment of the anterior abdominal or chest wall breathing-related movement has been implemented at selected centers (40). Typically, camera-based systems track the breathing cycle-related anterior/posterior motion of a small indicator positioned onto the chest or anterior abdominal wall (53–57). The derived breathing amplitude can be used to determine the phases of the breathing cycle, during which the least surface motion occurs, and subsequently this subset of the breathing cycle is defined as the time window for beam delivery. Such approaches may significantly reduce the impact of still-existing organ motion but the associated cost is measured in the increase in time to deliver the prescribed radiation dose. In clinical reality, up to 70% of the breathing cycle has to be disabled for beam delivery, increasing the net treatment delivery time by a factor of two or more. Since typical treatment delivery times for stereotactic body radiation therapy already vary between 30 min and up to 2 hr, such prolongation may become relevant, as treatment delivery time and patient compliance (in terms of patient motion on the table or in the immobilization device) are closely related.

Imaging for Treatment Planning and Setup Assessment Prior to Treatment Delivery

Image data for SBRT planning of liver malignancies are typically based on CT imaging with and/or without intravenous contrast. In order to use any strategy to reduce safety margins for breathing-related motion, any device used must be in place during simulation imaging. Occasionally, this requirement may cause problems with the limited opening diameter of the used CT scanner. Breathing motion during image data acquisition may cause a variety of well-characterized imaging artifacts, which in the best of scenarios may render the target volume larger than its true anatomical size (58–60). However, randomly, a liver lesion may be rendered smaller than its anatomical size in the resulting treatment planning image dataset, with the inherent risk for underestimation of the volume that needs to be treated. The acquisition of a fast (spiral) breath hold scan in addition to slow helical or sequential slice acquisition during free breathing may be helpful in estimating the true target extent.

The use of intravenous contrast media should be mandatory in SBRT treatment planning for liver lesions, although it needs to be appreciated that especially liver metastases show a fill-in phenomenon that may suggest smaller lesion size in post-contrast CT slices than in the corresponding native CT slice. Thus, a combination of a native scan with at least one contrast phase scan is recommended. The addition of a multi-phase liver contrast scan, such as a three-phase liver CT used typically for diagnostic purposes, may further aid in the determination of lesion extent. If the patient setup is controlled immediately before treatment delivery, with the patient repositioned in the body immobilization device, additional application of intravenous contrast may not be feasible due to the associated secondary risk with loading excess contrast media and subsequent renal excretion. Thus, identification of the liver lesions in such control CT data may be compromised, especially when primary liver tumors are the target.

Few experiences have been made with implementing MRI and PET data into the SBRT planning process for liver tumors. The increasing availability of fast abdominal imaging sequences for MRI may prove this imaging modality to be of great aid in delineating the target volumes in the future. The superior soft tissue contrast inherent to MRI over CT may prove especially helpful in the delineation of HCC and CCC targets. The metabolic properties of most primary and secondary liver tumors differ from the surrounding healthy tissue of the liver and image data co-registration may not only aid in the process of target delineation but also in the ultimate tumor response assessment in the foreseeable future. New PET tracers based on amino-acid metabolism rather than glucose consumption may prove to be more specific for proliferating tumor tissues, enabling effective and appropriate biological tumor targeting.

DOSES AND CLINICAL OUTCOME

The development of dose escalation in conformal radiotherapy should be highlighted first since definite conclusions for a hypofractionated stereotactic approach can be drawn from these data, and the analysis of data on partial liver irradiation gives more insight on the effects of dose escalation as it is intended in stereotactic radiotherapy.

Dose Escalation in the Normal Liver

The most extensive experience of partial liver radiation together with or without whole liver radiation and intra-arterial chemotherapy has been achieved at the University of Michigan (14,60–62). A total of 203 inoperable patients with normal liver function had been radiated for HCC ($n = 58$), CCC ($n = 47$), and liver metastases ($n = 98$) from 1987 to 1999. Forty-one patients were treated with whole liver radiation (24–36 Gy), 20 patients were treated with whole liver radiation followed by a boost to a partial liver volume (to 45–66 Gy) and 142 patients were treated with partial liver radiation alone (48–90 Gy) in doses of 1.5–1.65 Gy delivered twice daily (bid). The median dose was 52.5 Gy (range 24–90 Gy). Simultaneously, intra-arterial chemotherapy with 5-FU ($n = 169$) or bromodesoxyuridine (BUdR, $n = 34$) was administered. Treatment plans and total dose were adjusted to an expected level of normal liver toxicity of 10% using a modified

Lyman-NTCP-model (61,62). As predicted, in 19 patients (9%) RILD of RTOG-grade ≥ 3 (treatment required) was observed. Six patients had received whole liver radiation, six whole liver radiation plus local radiation boost, and seven were treated by partial liver radiation alone. The strongest parameter predicting liver toxicity was the mean liver dose. In patients with hepatic toxicity, the mean liver dose was 37 Gy (NTCP 0.17) compared to 31 Gy in patients without RILD (NTCP 0.04), which is in accordance to Emami et al.'s (12) previously published volume-related doses for the whole liver of the TD5/5 at 30 Gy and the TD50/5 at 40 Gy. Using the adjusted Lyman–Kutcher–Burman NTCP model, the risk for RILD increased by 4% for a Gy increase of mean liver dose exceeding 30 Gy. The best fit to clinical data was achieved using a $TD_{50whole\ liver}$ of 43.3 Gy, n (volume effect) of 1.1, and m (steepness of the dose–response curve at $TD_{50whole\ liver}$) of 0.18. The volume effect (expressed by the term n) seems to be most important for toxicity. According to the NTCP model n is close to 0 with low- and close to 1 with high-volume dependence. The authors have adjusted n from 0.32 to 0.69 (61) to now 1.1 as evaluations of a growing number of patients were updated. Analyzing non-dosimetric prognostic factors by logistic regression, Dawson et al. (62) found a significantly increased risk for RILD for hepatobiliary carcinoma (compared to metastases), correlated with the use of BUdR and male gender. In the group receiving 5-FU, male patients with hepatobiliary cancer had the highest risk for RILD. In these subgroups, significantly different parameters for $TD_{50whole\ liver}$, n and m could be derived. Additionally, the results were found to be consistent with the "threshold hypothesis" of Jackson et al. (63), who assumed that the risk for RILD could be kept near 0 if the partial liver irradiation volume could be kept below a threshold volume, regardless of the dose. Dawson et al. discuss that doses as high as 100 Gy might be safely administered for small volumes of normal liver tissue (approximately 1/3 of whole liver). This dose escalation might be beneficial, because the clinical results of the Michigan patients revealed an improved local tumor control with increased dose (14).

Care must be taken if cirrhotic liver is irradiated. All University of Michigan data were collected on patients with a normal liver function. However, when the liver function is impaired, the risk of developing RILD increases, and more liver tissue has to be spared than in healthy liver patients. Seong et al. (64) combined focal liver irradiation in 50 patients with HCC (Child A $n = 38$, Child B $n = 12$) with transarterial-chemo-embolization (TACE). The total dose (30–60 Gy) was determined by the fraction of the non-tumor liver volume receiving more than 50% of the prescribed dose given in 1.8 Gy daily fractions. Six patients were observed with RILD, but unfortunately were not analyzed concerning dose–volume relations. The same group published an analysis of dose–response relation in local radiotherapy for HCC in 158 patients (65). About 90% of patients had liver cirrhosis (Child A 74%, Child B 26%); patients with advanced liver cirrhosis Child C were excluded. The tumor size ranges were <5 cm (11%), 5–10 cm (54%), and >10 cm (35%). The average 3D-conformal planned dose was 48.2 ±7.9 Gy (25.2–59.4 Gy) in daily fractions of 1.8 Gy. While statistic evaluation revealed that the total radiation dose was the only significant factor determining tumor response, hepatic toxicity was also increased with dose. Eleven patients showed RILD: 4.2% ($n = 1$) of all patients in the category of <40 Gy, 5.9% ($n - 3$) from 40–50 Gy and, 8.4% with doses >50 Gy ($n = 7$). Liver cirrhosis of Child B seemed to be a risk factor in development of RILD, but the number of cases was small: 0/16 patients <40 Gy, 2/13 patients 40–50 Gy (15.4%), and 2/20 patients >50 Gy (10%). Nevertheless, the evaluation demonstrates that partial liver irradiation can be performed in considerable large volumes even in patients with impaired liver function. However, the liver function should be evaluated first.

PARTIAL LIVER-RADIATION USING STEREOTACTIC SETUP

Hypofractionation

Blomgren and Lax were the first who published data about stereotactic radiation of liver tumors. Their initial report from 1995 was followed by an update in 1998 (24,50). After having had negative experiences with single-dose therapy, which is discussed later, they mainly used hypofractionated radiotherapy. The fractionation and the overall time of treatment varied greatly. The dose ranged from 2×8 to 3×15 Gy or 4×10 Gy. The dose was prescribed to the PTV encompassing 65% isodose, which resulted in maximal total doses of 20–82 Gy. The treatment time varied between 3 and 44 days (24).

The Swedish group treated 20 primary intrahepatic cancers in 11 patients. The median clinical target volume was 22 cm³ with a range of 3–622 cm³. With a mean follow-up of 12 months, no local failures were observed. However, two fatal cases of RILD in patients with liver cirrhosis were reported. The first patient presented with a 57 cm³ HCC nodule associated with hepatitis C and liver cirrhosis. The tumor was treated with 3×15 Gy to the periphery of the PTV. The patient developed ascites 20 days after completion of the treatment and died the next month. The other patient had a 293 cm³ large HCC treated with 3×10 Gy to the periphery of the PTV. Also, this patient developed nontractable ascites in the first 6 weeks after treatment and died shortly after that. Unfortunately, there is no detailed information about the size of the liver, the degree of pretherapeutic liver impairment, or the mean liver dose. Therefore, no definite conclusions about the risk assessment can be drawn from this published data. Apart from these fatal side effects, patients experienced nausea, fever, or chills for a few hours after radiosurgery.

About 10 patients with 20 metastases were also treated at the Karolinska Institute using the hypofractionated stereotactic regimen. The median CTV was 24 cm^3 with a range of 2–263 cm^3. Tumor response was evaluated after a mean follow-up time of 9.6 months. All tumors showed response to the therapy. One local recurrence was observed 6 months after therapy. Again, patients experienced nausea, fever, and chill a few hours after the procedure. These symptoms were assuaged with a prophylactic treatment with acetaminophen (synonymous with paracetamol in Europe) and anti-emetics later on. One patient suffered from a hemorrhagic gastritis a few weeks after treatment. One-third of the stomach wall had been exposed to 7 Gy for two treatment sessions. Parts of the duodenum were exposed to 4×5 Gy in another patient. This patient developed a duodenal ulcer, which was treated conservatively. These early Stockholm data indicated the feasibility and the possible success rate of a hypofractionated stereotactic treatment for liver tumors. Unfortunately, no dose–volume constrains can be drawn from these data due to the wide range of the applied dose and different fractionation schemes. The Stockholm group has continued to treat patients with hepatic cancer with the stereotactic approach. However, new data have not been published. Wulf et al., from the University of Würzburg in Germany, adopted components of the Stockholm treatment approach (28). They treated 24 patients with liver tumors (one CCC and 23 metastases). The median clinical target volume was 50 cm^3 with a minimum of 9 cm^3 and a maximum of 512 cm^3. All but one patient were treated with 3×10 Gy to the 65% isodose at the periphery of the PTV. One patient was treated by 4×7 Gy, also normalized to the periphery of the PTV. The reason for this altered fractionation schedule was close proximity of the target to the esophagus. The crude local control was 83% at a mean follow-up of 9 months. The actuarial local control after 12 months was reported to be 76%, with a median survival of 20 months. Recurrences occurred 3, 8, 9, and 17 months after treatment. All recurrences were initially treated with 3×10 Gy. Failure of three of these targets occurred marginally. Treatment related morbidity was low: 7/24 patients reported side effects of grade 1 or 2 according to the WHO classification. Side effects were mostly observed following one of three fractions and included fever, chills, and pain, with a typical onset a few hours after irradiation. Additionally, nausea and/or vomiting might occur at the same time. The symptoms ceased spontaneously or could successfully be treated with acetaminophen or prednisolone. Only one patient showed longer lasting fatigue, weakness, and loss of appetite.

Radiosurgery

The term radiosurgery implies a focused single-dose radiation therapy. Most of the stereotactic treatments in the brain were successfully performed using a radiosurgical approach (66,67). Blomgren and Lax also started with a single dose therapy for liver tumors (50). Six tumors in five patients were treated radiosurgically. The median prescribed dose to the periphery of the PTV was

15.5 Gy, ranging from 7.7 to 30 Gy. No recurrences were observed during a median follow-up of 5 months. However, one patient died 2 days after treatment. This patient had a 229 cm³ large HCC in a cirrhotic liver. The tumor was treated with 30 Gy applied to the periphery of the PTV, with a corresponding isocenter dose of 48 Gy. The patient already was icteric and showed signs of ascites at the time of treatment. The other four patients showed marginal recurrences during follow-up as it is mentioned in a later paper of the Stockholm group (24). These two circumstances forced Blomgren and Lax to abandon the radiosurgical approach for large liver tumors.

In 1997, a phase I/II trial was initiated at the German Cancer Research Center in Heidelberg (Germany) proving the feasibility and the clinical outcome of a single-dose radiation therapy of liver tumors (29). The inclusion criteria for the study were non-resectable tumors in the liver. The number of liver lesions should not exceed three tumors (four, if two tumors with less than 3 cm are close together). The size of a single lesion should not exceed 6 cm, and none of the tumors should be immediately adjacent to parts of the gastro-intestinal tract (distance >6 mm). The exclusion criterion was insufficient liver function. Thirty-seven patients were included. A total of 60 tumors were radiosurgically treated at 40 occasions. The targets included four primary hepatic tumors and 56 metastases (mainly colorectal cancer or breast cancer). The median target size was 10 cm³ (1–132 cm³). The dose was prescribed to the isocenter with the 80% isodose encompassing the PTV. The dose was escalated from 14 to 26 Gy based on the liver dose in the dose–volume histogram. After initial dose escalation, an actuarial local tumor control of 81% at 18 months could be achieved with a mean follow-up of 9.5 months. All patients received a prophylactic dexamethasone medication before and after radiation therapy. The actuarial 2 years survival was 59%. Patients with curative treatment intention showed a significant longer survival (actuarial 87% at 2 years) than patients with additional extrahepatic tumor manifestations at the time of treatment (median survival 12 months) (29). An update of these study patients with a mean follow-up of 17 months was published in 2003 (68). Two patients developed late local recurrences 4 years after therapy. The actuarial local control remained unchanged with 81% after 18 months.

As described later in this chapter, a follow-up trial was initiated after these promising initial results. More patients had been radiosurgically treated according to the initial phase II protocol until recruitment of the follow-up trial could be started. A combined total of 78 patients were treated until spring 2003. The mean follow-up was 12 months and the actuarial local tumor control dropped to 72% at 12 months. Analysis of the increased failure rate revealed that patients with metastases of a colorectal cancer showed a significant worse local tumor control than patients with other histologies (68). Of special note, all 11 patients who already had received chemotherapy using CPT-11 or oxaliplatine had shown local recurrences during the first 15 months after therapy. These recurrences were infield and marginal recurrences. Therefore, higher doses and/or larger safety margins should be used especially if colorectal cancer metastases are treated.

Side effects of the treatment were minimal (29). They included mild nausea or loss of appetite for 1–2 weeks in about one-third of the patients. A singultus was observed in two patients and one patient developed fever. There were signs of radiation induced liver disease. All patients who were followed using multiphasic CT scanning showed a sharply demarcated focal radiation reaction. Tumor and radiation reaction could be well differentiated in the portal-venous contrast-enhanced CT scans. Liver vessels ran through the liver reaction and were not displaced, as is seen in case of an expanding tumor. A detailed evaluation and characterization of this focal radiation reaction in 36 of the Heidelberg patients was published in 2003 (69). The area of radiation reaction was hypodense in the majority of the non-enhanced CT scans. Three different types of appearance of the reaction could be defined based on the liver density in the portal-venous and the late phase after contrast agent administration:

- Type 1 reaction: Hypodensity in portal-venous contrast phase, isodensity in the late contrast phase.
- Type 2 reaction: Hypodensity in portal-venous contrast phase, hyperdensity in the late contrast phase.
- Type 3 reaction: Isodensity/hyperdensity in portal-venous contrast phase, hyperdensity in the late contrast phase.

The onset of the reaction was after a median of 1.8 months. While type 1 or 2 reactions were usually observed earlier, type 3 reactions appeared later than the other types. It was also seen that there was a shift of the appearance during follow-up toward type 3 appearances. In addition, the volume of the radiation reaction decreased with follow-up time. The most dramatic shrinkage was observed during the first months after appearance. This lead to the speculation that the whole reaction goes through different radiological stages (type 1, 2, and 3 appearances). The histological basis of these stages was not determined since no biopsies were taken. However, others had reported a type 2 appearance after single-dose radiation therapy and it was histologically confirmed VOD (70).

Based on reconstruction of the dose–volume histograms, the mean threshold dose was 13.7 Gy with a wide range between 8.9 and 19.2 Gy given in a single fraction. One reason for this large variance might be the fact that the volume decreased much between the initial detection and the further follow-up examinations. The examination might have not detected larger reaction volumes and, therefore, the calculated threshold doses might have been overestimated. This was sustained by the significant correlation between the threshold dose and the time of detection (correlation coefficient $r = 0.709$).

Apart from the time factor, other factors that could influence the individual radiation sensitivity (e.g., additional toxic liver agents like alcohol) might have been another reason of the variance. More data are needed to strengthen these threshold doses.

ONGOING STUDIES

As described earlier, there are two different strategies for stereotactic radiation of liver tumors: on one side, a hypofractionated approach with a more or less inhomogeneous dose distribution within the PTV with maximum dose of up to 150% (corresponding to a prescription to the 65% encompassing isodose). On the other side is the radiosurgical approach with a more homogenous dose distribution within the PTV (80% isodose encompassing PTV). The comparison of these two strategies has been the goal of a new phase III trial that was initiated by the two major German groups engaged in stereotactic body radiation therapy of liver targets. The StRaL-trial (Stereotactic Radiation Therapy of Liver Metastases) is a prospective randomized multicenter trial, which has started patient recruitment in March 2003 with a planned enrollment of 276 patients over 5 years. Inclusion criteria are a maximum of three liver metastases, which are surgically inoperable. The maximal size of the tumors is dependent on the number of targets: 5 cm for one target, 4 cm for two targets, and 3 cm for three targets. The primary study goal is the comparison of the local tumor control. Secondary goals are survival, morbidity, and quality of life. The study is designed to prove the equivalence of both treatment arms. Patients in arm A receive a single-dose radiation therapy of 28 Gy normalized to the isocenter with the 80% isodose (22.4 Gy) encompassing the PTV. Patients in arm B receive a hypofractionated therapy with 3×12.5 Gy normalized to the 65% isodose (encompassing the PTV) (Table 1). This increase in dose over published experiences is based on the recent internal updates of the initial phase II data.

In the United States, two active phase I/II multicenter studies are being conducted to determine the optimal dose and the maximally tolerated dose (MTD) for hypofractionated treatment of HCC and liver metastases (71). Both protocols (initiated by investigators from the Universities of Colorado and Indiana) have a similar study design but investigate the two tumor entities separately, secondary to the perceived increased risk of treatment-related toxicity in patients with primary liver malignancies. The initial dose level was 12 Gy delivered three times for a total minimal target dose of 36 Gy in 5–10 days. Dose escalation will be performed in steps of 2 Gy per fraction (6 Gy total dose) up to a total dose of 60 Gy, or upon determination of an MTD. The primary goal of both studies is the determination of the MTD by assessing the dose limiting toxicity (DLT). Secondary endpoints are: 6-month in-field tumor response, failure rate, disease free survival, and overall survival.

Table 1 Target Doses and Normal Tissue Constraints for the German Prospective Randomized Multicenter Trial StRaL

	Arm A 1×28 Gy/isocenter		Arm B 3×12.5 Gy/65% isodose	
	Relative dose/fx (%)	Absolute dose/fx	Relative dose/fx (%)	Absolute dose/fx
Isocenter	100	28 Gy	100	19.2 Gy
Minimum PTV	80	22.4 Gy	65	12.5 Gy
Liver (30% vol.)	43	12 Gy	36	7 Gy
Liver (50% vol.)	25	7 Gy	26	5 Gy
Esophagus (max.)	43	12 Gy	36	7 Gy
Stomach (max.)	43	12 Gy	36	7 Gy
Duodenom (max.)	43	12 Gy	36	7 Gy
Colon (max.)	43	12 Gy	36	7 Gy
Myelon (max.)	43	12 Gy	36	7Gy

A maximum of 15 patients will be enrolled in the phase I portion of each trial (a minimum of three at each dose level), and an additional 13–35 patients will be enrolled in the phase II portion of the studies.

FUTURE RESEARCH

While the methodology and procedural conduct of SBRT for primary and secondary liver malignancies have been well established, the clinical role of or the distinct indications for SBRT in this disease context has not yet been well established. Some of this current shortcoming is certainly related to the fact that SBRT represents a competing treatment modality for local treatment concepts such as RFA, LITT, and cryoablation, and potentially for the present gold standard, surgical resection.

Pending the results of the currently ongoing clinical trials, which are designed to assess the equivalency of single dose and hypofractionated dose scheduling as well as the MTD for three fraction SBRT planning and delivery, the impact of SBRT on disease-specific and overall survival in combination with other established treatment modalities or in comparison with one or more modalities has to be tested. However, in the opinion of the authors it seems especially intriguing to evaluate if combining SBRT with either curative attempt surgery or RFA/LITT can improve upon the local failure rates associated with the use of these modalities and if better local tumor control can result in improved survival rates. A model of combining SBRT with one modality could be to employ SBRT in the waiting phase before liver transplant in small HCC. Thus, SBRT can serve as a desirable bridge-to-transplant, and, depending on the effective time window between SBRT and harvesting of the diseased liver, a histopathological examination can reveal local treatment efficacy in addition to hard outcome endpoints such as disease specific and overall survival rates.

In summary, SBRT has been shown to provide for a feasible and completely non-invasive treatment modality complementing the present armamentarium in the fight against potentially curable localized primary and secondary liver tumors. The acceptance and the ultimate success of this new treatment modality will to a large extent depend upon our willingness to prove its capabilities in the framework of multimodality treatment approaches.

REFERENCES

1. Phillips R, Kamofsky DA, Hamilton LD, Nickson JJ. Roentgen therapy of hepatic metastases. Am J Roentgenol Radiat Ther Nucl Med 1954; 71: 826–834.
2. Borgelt BB, Gelber R, Brady LW, Griffin T, Hendrickson FR. The palliation of hepatic metastases: results of the radiation therapy oncology pilot study. Int J Radiat Oncol Biol Phys 1981; 7:587–591.
3. Leibel SA, Pajak TF, Massullo V, Order SE, Komaki RU, Chang CH, et al. A comparison of misonidazole sensitized radiation therapy to radiation therapy alone for the palliation of hepatic metastases: results of a radiation oncology group randomized prospective trial. Int J Radiat Oncol Biol Phys 1987; 13:1057–1064.
4. Sherman DM, Weichselbaum R, Order SE, Cloud L, Trey C, Piro AJ. Palliation of hepatic metastasis. Cancer 1978; 41(5):2013–2017.
5. Russell AH, Clyde C, Wasserman TH, Turner SS, Rotman M. Accelerated hyperfractionated hepatic irradiation in the management of patients with liver metastases: results of the RTOG dose escalating protocol. Int J Radiat Oncol Biol Phys 1993; 27:117–123.
6. Ingold JA, Reed GB, Kaplan HS, Bagshaw MA. Radiation hepatitis. Am J Roentgenol 1965; 93:200–208.
7. Reed GB, Cox AJ Jr. The human liver after radiation injury. A form of veno-occlusive disease. Am J Pathol 1966; 48:597–611.
8. Fajardo L, Colby T. Pathogenesis of veno-occlusive disease after radiation. Arch Pathol Lab Med 1980; 104:584–588.
9. Lewin K, Millis R. Human radiation hepatitis. A morphologic study with emphasis on the late changes. Arch Pathol 1973; 96:21–26.
10. Haddad E, Le Bourgeois JP, Kuentz M, Lobo P. Liver complications in lymphomas treated with a combination of chemotherapy and radiotherapy: preliminary results. Int J Radiat Oncol Biol Phys 1983; 9(9):1313–1319.
11. Poussin-Rosillo H, Nisce LZ, D'Angio GJ. Hepatic radiation tolerance in Hodgkin's disease patients. Radiology 1976; 121(2):461–464.
12. Emami B, Lyman J, Brown ALC, Goitein M, Munzenrider JE, et al. Tolerance of normal tissue to therapeutic irradiation. Int J Radiat Oncol Biol Phys 1991; 21:109–122.

13. Dawson LA, Brock KK, Kazanjian S, Fitch D, McGinn CJ, Lawrence TS, et al. The reproducibility of organ position using active breathing control (ABC) during liver radiotherapy. Int J Radiat Oncol Biol Phys 2001; 51(5):1410–1421.
14. Dawson LA, McGinn CJ, Normolle D, Ten Haken RK, Walker S, Ensminger W, et al. Escalated focal liver radiation and concurrent hepatic artery fluorodeoxyuridine for unresectable intrahepatic malignancies. J Clin Oncol 2000; 18(11): 2210–2218.
15. Lax I, Blomgren H, Näslund I, Svanström R. Stereotactic radiotherapy of malignancies in the abdomen. Acta Oncol 1994; 33(6):677–683.
16. Bläker H, Hofmann WJ, Theuer D, Otto HF. Pathohistologische Befunde bei Lebermetastasen. Radiologe 2001; 41:1–7.
17. Jaffe BM, Donegan WL, Watson F, Spratt JS, Jr. Factors influencing survival in patients with untreated hepatic metastases. Surg Gynecol Obstet 1968; 127(1):1–11.
18. Adson MA, van Heerden JA, Adson MH, Wagner JS, IIstrup DM. Resection of hepatic metastases from colorectal cancer. Arch Surg 1984; 119(6):647–651.
19. Takenaka K, Shimada M, Higashi H, Adachi E, Nishizaki T, Yanaga K, et al. Liver resection for hepatocellular carcinoma in the elderly. Arch Surg 1994; 129(8):846–850.
20. Matsuura M, Nakajima N, Arai K, Ito K. The usefulness of radiation therapy for hepatocellular carcinoma. Hepatogastroenterology 1998; 45(21):791–796.
21. Matsuzaki Y, Osuga T, Saito Y, Chuganji Y, Tanaka N, Shoda J, et al. A new, effective, and safe therapeutic option using proton irradiation for hepatocellular carcinoma. Gastroenterology 1994; 106(4):1032–1041.
22. Robertson JM, Lawrence TS, Dworzanin LM, Andrews JC, Walker S, Kessler ML, et al. Treatment of primary hepatobiliary cancers with conformal radiation therapy and regional chemotherapy. J Clin Oncol 1993; 11:1286–1293.
23. Seong J, Park HC, Han KH, Lee DY, Lee JT, Chon CY, et al. Local radiotherapy for unresectable hepatocellular carcinoma patients who failed with transcatheter arterial chemoembolization. Int J Radiat Oncol Biol Phys 2000; 47(5):1331–1335.
24. Blomgren H, Lax I, Göranson H, Kræpelien T, Nilsson B, Näslund I, et al. Radiosurgery for tumors in the body: clinical experience using a new method. J Radiosurg 1998; 1(1):63–74.
25. Sato M, Uematsu M, Yamamoto F, Shioda A, Tahara K, Fukui T, et al. Feasibility of frameless stereotactic high-dose radiation therapy for primary or metastatic liver cancer. J Radiosurg 1998; 1(3):233–238.
26. Nakeeb A, Pitt HA, Sohn TA, Coleman J, Abrams RA, Piantadosi S, et al. Cholangiocarcinoma. A spectrum of intrahepatic, perihilar, and distal tumors. Ann Surg 1996; 224(4):463–473.
27. Bowling TE, Galbraith SM, Hatfield AR, Solano J, Spittle MF. A retrospective comparison of endoscopic stenting alone with stenting and radiotherapy in non-resectable cholangiocarcinoma. Gut 1996; 39(96):852–855.
28. Wulf J, Hädinger U, Oppitz U, Thiele W, Ness-Dourdoumas R, Flentje M. Stereotactic radiotherapy of targets in the lung and liver. Strahlenther Onkol 2001; 177(12):645–655.

29. Herfarth KK, Debus J, Lohr F, Bahner ML, Rhein B, Fritz P, et al. Stereotactic single dose radiation therapy of liver tumors: results of a phase I/II trial. J Clin Oncol 2001; 19:164–170.

30. Wilson SM, Adson MA. Surgical treatment of hepatic metastases from colorectal cancers. Arch Surg 1976; 111(4):330–334.

31. Nordlinger B, Vaillant JC, Guiguet M, Balladur P, Paris F, Bachellier P, et al. Survival benefit of repeat liver resections for recurrent colorectal metastases: 143 cases. Association Francaise de Chirurgie. J Clin Oncol 1994; 12(7):1491–1496.

32. Femandez-Trigo V, Shamsa F, Sugarbaker PH. Repeat liver resections from colorectal metastasis. Repeat Hepatic Metastases Registry. Surgery 1995; 117(3):296–304.

33. Herfarth C, Heuschen UA, Lamade W, Lehnert T, Otto G. Rezidiv-Resektionen an der Leber bei primären und sekundären Lebermalignomen. Chirurg 1995; 66(10):949–958.

34. Solbiati L, Goldberg SM, Ierace T, Livraghi T, Meloni F, Dellanoce M, et al. Hepatic metastases: percutaneous radio-frequency ablation with cooled-tip electrodes. Radiology 1997; 205:367–373.

35. Vogl TJ, Müller PK, Mack MG, Straub R, Engelmann K, Neuhaus P. Liver metastases: interventional therapeutic techniques and results, state of the art. Eur Radiol 1999; 9:675–684.

36. Onik GM, Atkinson D, Zemel R, Weaver ML. Cryosurgery of liver cancer. Semin Surg Oncol 1993; 9(4):309–317.

37. Shirato H, Seppenwoolde Y, Kitamura K, Onimura R, Shimizu S. Intrafractional tumor motion: lung and liver. Semin Radiat Oncol 2004; 14(1):10–18.

38. Rosu M, Dawson LA, Baiter JM, McShan DL, Lawrence TS, Ten Haken RK. Alterations in normal liver doses due to organ motion. Int J Radiat Oncol Biol Phys 2003; 57(5):1472–1479.

39. Antolak JA, Rosen, II. Planning target volumes for radiotherapy: how much margin is needed? Int J Radiat Oncol Biol Phys 1999; 44(5):1165–1170.

40. Mageras GS, Yorke E. Deep inspiration breath hold and respiratory gating strategies for reducing organ motion in radiation treatment. Semin Radiat Oncol 2004; 14(1):65–75.

41. Nakagawa K, Aoki Y, Tago M, Terahara A, Ohtomo K. Megavoltage CT-assisted stereotactic radiosurgery for thoracic tumors: original research in the treatment of thoracic neoplasms. Int J Radiat Oncol Biol Phys 2000; 48(2):449–457.

42. Uematsu M, Shioda A, Suda A, Tahara K, Kojima T, Hama Y, et al. Intrafractional tumor position stability during computed tomography (CT)-guided frameless stereotactic radiation therapy for lung or liver cancers with a fusion of CT and linear accelerator (FOCAL) unit. Int J Radiat Oncol Biol Phys 2000; 48(2):443–448.

43. Onishi H, Kuriyama K, Komiyama T, Tanaka S, Sano N, Aikawa Y, et al. A new irradiation system for lung cancer combining linear accelerator, computed tomography, patient self-breath-holding, and patient-directed beam-control without respiratory monitoring devices. Int J Radiat Oncol Biol Phys 2003; 56(1):14–20.

44. Kim DJ, Murray BR, Halperin R, Roa WH. Held-breath self-gating technique for radiotherapy of non-small-cell lung cancer: a feasibility study. Int J Radiat Oncol Biol Phys 2001; 49(l):43–49.

45. Mah D, Hanley J, Rosenzweig KE, Yorke E, Braban L, Ling CC, et al. Technical aspects of the deep inspiration breath-hold technique in the treatment of thoracic cancer. Int J Radiat Oncol Biol Phys 2000; 48(4):1175–1185.

46. Rosenzweig KE, Hanley J, Mah D, Mageras G, Hunt M, Toner S, et al. The deep inspiration breath-hold technique in the treatment of inoperable non-small-cell lung cancer. Int J Radiat Oncol Biol Phys 2000; 48(l):81–87.

47. Hanley J, Debois MM, Mah D, Mageras GS, Raben A, Rosenzweig K, et al. Deep inspiration breath-hold technique for lung tumors: the potential value of target immobilization and reduced lung density in dose escalation. Int J Radiat Oncol Biol Phys 1999; 45(3):603–611.

48. Murphy MJ, Martin D, Whyte R, Hai J, Ozhasoglu C, Le QT. The effectiveness of breath-holding to stabilize lung and pancreas tumors during radiosurgery. Int J Radiat Oncol Biol Phys 2002; 53(2):475–482.

49. Wong JW, Sharpe MB, Jaffray DA, Kini VR, Robertson JM, Stromberg JS, et al. The use of active breathing control (ABC) to reduce margin for breathing motion. Int J Radiat Oncol Biol Phys 1999; 44(4):911–919.

50. Blomgren H, Lax I, Naslund I, Svanstrom R. Stereotactic high dose fraction radiation therapy of extracranial tumors using an accelerator. Clinical experience of the first thirty-one patients. Acta Oncol 1995; 34(6):861–870.

51. Wulf J, Hadinger U, Oppitz U, Olshausen B, Flentje M. Stereotactic radiotherapy of extracranial targets: CT-simulation and accuracy of treatment in the stereotactic body frame. Radiother Oncol 2000; 57(2):225–236.

52. Herfarth KK, Debus J, Lohr F, Bahner ML, Fritz P, Hoss A, et al. Extracranial stereotactic radiation therapy: set-up accuracy of patients treated for liver metastases. Int J Radiat Oncol Biol Phys 2000; 46(2):329–335.

53. Vedam SS, Kini VR, Keall PJ, Ramakrishnan V, Mostafavi H, Mohan R. Quantifying the predictability of diaphragm motion during respiration with a noninvasive external marker. Med Phys 2003; 30(4):505–513.

54. Wagman R, Yorke E, Ford E, Giraud P, Mageras G, Minsky B, et al. Respiratory gating for liver tumors: use in dose escalation. Int J Radiat Oncol Biol Phys 2003; 55(3):659–668.

55. Kubo HD, Hill BC. Respiration gated radiotherapy treatment: a technical study. Phys Med Biol 1996; 41(l):83–91.

56. Keall P. 4-dimensional computed tomography imaging and treatment planning. Semin Radiat Oncol 2004; 14(1):81–90.

57. Tada T, Minakuchi K, Fujioka T, Sakurai M, Koda M, Kawase I, et al. Lung cancer: intermittent irradiation synchronized with respiratory motion—results of a pilot study. Radiology 1998; 207(3):779–783.

58. Chen GT, Kung JH, Beaudette KP. Artifacts in computed tomography scanning of moving objects. Semin Radiat Oncol 2004; 14(l):19–26.

59. Balter JM, Ten Haken RK, Lawrence TS, Lam KL, Robertson JM. Uncertainties in CT-based radiation therapy treatment planning associated with patient breathing. Int J Radiat Oncol Biol Phys 1996; 36(l):167–174.

60. Balter JM, Lam KL, McGinn CJ, Lawrence TS, Ten Haken RK. Improvement of CT-based treatment-planning models of abdominal targets using static exhale imaging. Int J Radiat Oncol Biol Phys 1998; 41(4):939–943.

61. Lawrence TS, Ten Haken RK, Kessler ML, Robertson JM, Lyman JT, Lavigne ML, et al. The use of 3-D dose volume analysis to predict radiation hepatitis. Int J Radiat Oncol Biol Phys 1992; 23:781–788.

62. Dawson LA, Normolle D, Balter JM, McGinn CJ, Lawrence TS, Ten Haken RK. Analysis of radiation-induced liver disease using the lyman NTCP model. Int J Radiat Oncol Biol Phys 2002; 53(4):810–821.

63. Jackson A, Ten Haken RK, Robertson JM, Kessler ML, Kutcher GJ, Lawrence TS. Analysis of clinical complication data for radiation hepatitis using a parallel architecture model. Int J Radiat Oncol Biol Phys 1995; 31(4):883–891.

64. Seong J, Park HC, Han KH, Chon CY. Clinical results and prognostic factors in radiotherapy for unresectable hepatocellular carcinoma: a retrospective study of 158 patients. Int J Radiat Oncol Biol Phys 2003; 55(2):329–336.

65. Park HC, Seong J, Han KH, Chon CY, Moon YM, Suh CO. Dose-response relationship in local radiotherapy for hepatocellular carcinoma. Int J Radiat Oncol Biol Phys 2002; 54(l):150–155.

66. Pirzkall A, Debus J, Lohr F, Fuss M, Rhein B, Engenhart-Cabillic R, et al. Radiosurgery alone or in combination with whole-brain radiotherapy for brain metastases. J Clin Oncol 1998; 16(11):3563–3569.

67. Chen JC, O'Day S, Morton D, Essner R, Cohen-Gadol A, MacPherson D, et al. Stereotactic radiosurgery in the treatment of metastatic disease to the brain. Stereotact Funct Neurosurg 1999; 73(1–4):60–63.

68. Herfarth KK, Debus J. Stereotactic radiation therapy of liver tumors. Radiother Oncol 2003; 68(S1):S45.

69. Herfarth KK, Hof H, Bahner ML, Lohr F, Höss A, van Kaick G, Wannenmacher M, Debus J. Assessment of focal liver reaction by multiphasic CT after stereotactic single-dose radiotherapy of liver tumors. Int J Radiat Oncol Biol Phys 2003; 57:444–451.

70. Willemart S, Nicaise N, Struyven J, van Gansbeke D. Acute radiation-induced hepatic injury: evaluation by triphasic contrast enhanced helical CT. Br J Radiol 2000; 73(869):544–546.

71. Schefter TE, Kavanagh BD, Timmerman RD, Cardenes HR, Baron A, Gaspar LE. A Phase I trial of stereotactic body radiation therapy (SBRT) for liver metastases. Int J Radiat Oncol Biol Phys 2005; 62:1371–1378.

9

Stereotactic Radiotherapy
of Lung Tumors

Robert D. Timmerman

Department of Radiation Oncology, Indiana University School of Medicine,
Bloomington, Indiana, U.S.A.

Jörn Wulf

Department of Radiotherapy, University of Würzburg,
Würzburg, Germany

INTRODUCTION

The purpose of stereotactic irradiation of tumors in the lung is improvement
of local tumor control by escalating the radiation dose. Simultaneously,
acute and late radiation toxicity must be kept to an acceptable level despite
the increased dose. These almost contradictory intentions are matched
together by decreasing the irradiated volume, which is achieved by maximizing efforts to ensure precision of radiation delivery and minimizing breathing mobility of the targets. Therefore, stereotactic irradiation of lung tumors
is best suited for patients who will benefit from increased local tumor
control probability achieved by dose escalation. These criteria are fulfilled
in patients with node negative non-small cell lung cancer (NSCLC) stage I
(cT1-2 cN0 cM0), and in selected cases of stage II (cT3 cN0 cM0 without
central disease but infiltration of a small part of the peripheral thoracic wall)
or patients with solitary or few lung metastases, who usually are selected for
surgical treatment.

Nevertheless a significant number of patients will not be suited for surgery due to confounding medical conditions, or will refuse surgery because of its invasiveness. For these patients, a minimally invasive treatment approach leading to similar local control rates by surgery is required. Unfortunately doses of 60–70 Gy, usually used in conventional fractionated 3D-conformal radiotherapy, lead to local control rates of only 30–50% for stage I disease and therefore could not meet this demand. Retrospective analyses and early data from dose escalation studies support the evidence that increasing the dose will lead to improved local control rates. Compared to dose escalation by conventional 3D-conformal radiotherapy, stereotactic irradiation is performed in one or few fractions, with the advantage that the efforts to achieve maximal setup accuracy and decrease target (breathing) mobility can be feasibly optimized. Furthermore problems such as tumor cell repopulation during a prolonged treatment time, which is often associated with escalating doses by increasing the number of fractions alone, are minimized due to the hypofractionated concept.

Indications

The purpose of stereotactic irradiation of pulmonary targets is local control of circumscribed tumors achieved by very high fraction doses of 20–30 Gy (single dose) or 8×6 Gy to 3×20 Gy (hypofractionation). These tumor ablative doses are ideally restricted to the tumor itself (planning target volume, PTV). Prophylactic or therapeutic irradiation of the loco-regional lymph nodes is not feasible within the stereotactic approach. Due to these methodical restrictions first choice-indications for stereotactic irradiation of pulmonary targets are small primary NSCLC stage I (cT1/2 cN0 cM0) with low risk for lymphatic spread and solitary (or very few) lung metastases (Table 1). Additionally, cT3 cN0 cM0 (stage II) tumors can be considered for stereotactic irradiation if the tumor is peripherally invading the pleura

Table 1 Suggested Indications for Stereotactic Irradiation of Pulmonary Tumors

---

- *First choice*:
NSCLC stage I cT1-2 cN0 cM0
Solitary or <4 lung metastases (with controlled extrapulmonary disease)
- *Second choice*:
NSCLC stage II cT3 cN0 cM0
 (only cT3-tumors with infiltration of the peripheral pleura at the thoracic wall, no central tumors)
Local recurrences of previous irradiated tumors
 (target amenable for localized and volume restricted irradiation)
Stereotactic boost to intrapulmonary primary tumors
 (during conventional RT/RChT of higher stage NSCLC)

---

at the thoracic wall. Centrally growing cT3 tumors should be avoided due to the adverse late radiation response of the mediastinal structures, as discussed later. In general the practice of patient selection should follow the considerations of thoracic surgeons to choose patients for treatment who will benefit from local tumor control quo ad vitam or at least symptomatically (avoidance of bleeding or treatment of pain due to infiltration of the thoracic wall).

In patients with pulmonary metastases, the benefit from local control of a particular metastasis has to be balanced against the risk of further dissemination. One of these beneficial situations in metastasized disease might be observed in patients with isolated lung metastasis after pneumonectomy. In these patients even growth of a single lung metastasis will increase the risk for rapid impairment of lung function.

Second-choice indications might be stereotactic radiotherapy of locally recurrent NSCLC in previously irradiated patients or stereotactic boost irradiation to intrapulmonary tumors, e.g., during primary radio- or radiochemotherapy of advanced stage NSCLC. Under the precondition that organs at risk, such as spinal cord, trachea, and main bronchi or esophagus, can be spared from this additional dose according to the amount of the previous dose, these patients might have a second chance or an increased chance for local tumor control due to a precise and volume sparing therapy.

Patients referred for stereotactic radiation may include individuals with very poor pulmonary function. In these cases, the risk of tumor progression must be carefully weighed against the risk of therapy related pulmonary compromise. Up to now there are no consistent data available on how much even stereotactic radiotherapy is limited by impaired lung function. Theoretically the risk for damage of functional lung tissue should be dependent on the size of the target, location of the tumor (central vs. peripheral), and the assessment of the irradiated volume. In the authors' experience, even patients with a FeV_1 of less than 1 L could be treated without negative impact on lung function. This might be due to the fact that the irradiated volume is restricted to the tumor, which again is not contributing to lung function anymore. Nevertheless there is a risk of about 4% of symptomatic pneumonitis (see below), which mainly affects the functional lung tissue. Therefore some authors restrict stereotactic radiotherapy to patients with a FeV_1 of 1 L and treat patients with a FeV_1 of less than 1 L only exceptionally for very small volumes.

Currently the published results of stereotactic radiotherapy of lung tumors are still based on reports of single institutions with limited target numbers ($n = 17–66$). Therefore at this time surgical treatment should be considered as treatment of first choice in operable patients until larger patient numbers and data from phase-III studies are available. But in patients not amenable to or refusing standard therapy for medical or personal reasons, the stereotactic approach can be offered as a promising treatment modality.

Standard Treatment for Pulmonary Tumors Amenable for Stereotactic Irradiation NSCLC Stage I/II

In most countries lung cancer is the leading cause of cancer deaths in males and one of the leading causes of cancer deaths in females. About 80% of lung cancer is NSCLC. While the mortality rate is slightly decreasing in males, it is continuously increasing in females. In Germany the standardized mortality rate is 42 per 100,000 in males, and 11 per 100,000 in females (year 2000). In the United States the standardized mortality rate is even higher (58/100,000 in males and 25/100,000 in females); in Japan it is lower (30/100,000 in males and 8/100,000 in females). Comparing the incidence rates of 67/100,000 (males) and 9/100,000 (females) reveals that most patients with lung cancer will not be cured (1). A detailed description of incidence and mortality rates and of treatment strategies for different tumor stages in European countries over a period from 1978 to 1997 has recently been published by Janssen-Heijnen and Coebergh (2).

The unfortunate prognosis of patients is mainly due to advanced disease: Most tumors are diagnosed with loco-regional lymph node involvement, infiltration of relevant structures (cT4) or already with distant metastases. Only about 15–30% of tumors are diagnosed with limited disease stage I (cT1-2, cN0, and cM0) or II (cT1-2, cN1 or cT3 cN0, and cM0) (3). Nevertheless these early tumors are treated under curative intention by surgical resection leading to five-year overall survival of 65% for patients with stage I and 41% for patients with stage II disease (4). Five-year overall survival with this therapy ranges from 60% to 90%, with lower survival in the United States and Europe and higher survival in Japan (5–7). Mountain (5) reported 5-year survival rates of 67% for cT1 cN0 cM0, 57% for cT2 cN0 cM0, and 38% for cT3 cN0 cM0. But survival rates depend on the type of surgical resection. In a study comparing limited (wedge or segmental) resection vs. lobectomy or pneumonectomy the survival rates were 59% for limited but 77% for radical resection (8). A randomized trial performed by the Lung Cancer Study Group (9) to compare lobectomy to limited wedge or segmental resection in cT1 cN0 cM0 patients revealed a significant increase of recurrence rate of 75% in the limited surgery group. The overall five-year survival dropped from 65% to 45%. These differences appear to be related to resection line recurrences from inadequate margins associated with less extensive and non-anatomical resections. More recent reports of selected patients treated with wedge resections from Japan, however, would indicate that with modern techniques and staging, the likelihood of close margins is low even with a wedge resection. Indeed, the event-free survival in modern series with wedge resection appears to approach that of lobectomy (7).

Nevertheless in many patients with NSCLC of limited stage the treatment decision will depend on the individual medical condition represented by age, performance status, lung function, and other medical diseases.

According to this assessment and the results of staging procedures including history (weight loss is an important prognostic factor), physical examination, a CT scan of the thorax, abdomen, brain, cardio-pulmonary function tests, and (desirable) a PET scan to detect occult tumor spread, the most appropriate treatment will be defined. If the patient is assumed to be medically inoperable, radiotherapy will be the treatment of choice.

Unfortunately conventional fractionated radiotherapy or 3D-conformal radiotherapy of limited dose <70 Gy has only reached local control and five-year survival rates that are inferior to those achieved by surgery. The cause of this might be partially due to a selection bias choosing the more favorable patients for surgery, but there additionally is evidence that the radiation dose might have been too low. Jeremic et al. (10) published an overview on results achieved by conventionally fractionated radiotherapy: doses of 30–80 Gy to stage I/II NSCLC led to initial/isolated local failure rates of 11–55%. Five-year overall survival ranged between 6% and 45%. The authors concluded that normofractionated doses of at least 65 Gy or equivalent doses of other fractionations are needed to achieve improved local control. Locally uncontrolled tumor was the predominant pattern of failure. A similar analysis of Sibley et al. reviewing publications on tumors treated with a median dose of 60–66 Gy revealed that on average only 15% of patients will be long-term survivors. About 25% will die on intercurrent disease, 30% on distant metastases, and another 30% on locally uncontrolled tumor alone (11,12). From that data the authors derived the importance of dose escalation for further improvement of local tumor control of stage I/II lung cancer in medically inoperable patients. Despite clinical plausibility from these retrospective analyses no clear dose–volume relationship on local control could be derived. Nevertheless there was a trend to superior local control rates for smaller tumors (cT1 vs. cT2).

Starting from that insight several dose escalation protocols have been inaugurated during the last few years. An overview on these studies can be found at Belderbos et al. (13). Because overall treatment time may be a relevant prognostic factor these studies try to increase fraction dose or the number of fractions per time (CHART) to achieve dose escalation up to equivalent doses >80 Gy. While long-term clinical results of these studies are still pending, in all of these approaches volume restriction to achieve an acceptable rate of toxicity is an issue. Therefore in small tumors (stage I) elective irradiation of regional lymph nodes is omitted as supported by reports of Slotman et al. (14), Krol et al. (15), and Bradley et al. (16).

Both strategies of these dose escalation studies—increase of fraction dose to keep a short overall treatment time and decrease of the irradiated volume—are inherent characteristics of the concept of stereotactic radiotherapy. The only restriction of the stereotactic approach compared to normofractionated dose escalation studies is the exclusion of tumors close or adjacent to mediastinal organs at risk due to the very high fraction doses.

Therefore stereotactic irradiation of pulmonary targets is just another concept of dose escalation including all tools available in modem radiotherapy: patient support and external reference systems as stereotactic body frames, 3D-conformal dose calculation and dose distributions achieved by multiple fields shaped by multileaf collimators, breathing control devices and CT verification prior to radiotherapy.

LUNG METASTASES

Oncologically, metastatic disease in the lung defines the systemic spread of the disease and therefore limits the role of local treatment and local tumor control. Nevertheless under certain circumstances patients will benefit even from local control of single metastasis as surgical data show. The clinical results of a large study of the International Registry of Lung Metastases treating 5206 cases from 18 departments in Europe, United States, and Canada with metastasectomy were reported (17). The primary tumor was epithelial in 2260 cases, sarcoma in 2173 cases, germ cell in 363 cases, and melanoma in 328 cases. In 2383 cases single and in 2726 cases multiple metastases were resected, in 88% complete. After a median follow-up of 46 months the 5-, 10-, and 15-year survival was 36%, 26%, and 22% after complete and 13%, 7%, and 0% after incomplete resection. The multivariate analysis showed better prognosis for patients with germ cell tumors, disease-free survival of >36 months after treatment and single metastasis. Nevertheless even in patients with >3 metastases five-year survival was 27% if complete resection could be obtained (17). A recent overview of results of different histologic subtypes is given by Davidson et al. (18), who also describe the criteria for patient selection for metastasectomy:

1. the patient must be able to tolerate the planned procedure,
2. the patient's pulmonary function tests indicate sufficient reserve to compensate for resected lung tissue,
3. the site of the primary tumor must be controlled,
4. no evidence of extrapulmonary disease (or non-uncontrollable extrapulmonary disease), and
5. no better therapy is available.

The last point is the rationale for stereotactic irradiation of lung metastases. It might be superior to metastasectomy because of its non-invasive character and, depending on the size of the target, the sparing of functional lung tissue allowing treatment of patients even with impaired lung function as, for example patients, with lung metastasis after pneumonectomy. Nevertheless stereotactic radiotherapy of pulmonary metastases first has to prove its efficacy to achieve local control rates comparable to those of metastasectomy.

Appropriate thoracic targets are well demarcated and feasibly defined on CT or MRI. Patients with malignant pleural or pericardial effusions or diffuse "miliary" involvement of the lung (e.g., in some disseminated presentations of broncheoalveolar cancer) are not appropriate candidates. There is a controversy over the number of lesions capable of being treated based on both oncological and technical reasons. While treatments may be technically possible, patients with multifocal disease are at greater risk for occult dissemination appearing after treatment, obviating any benefit of controlling existing lesions. Furthermore, dose fall-off from adjacent lesions may overlap creating pockets of substantial unintended dose within normal tissue. As such, treatment-related toxicity of multifocal disease may be supra-additive as compared with toxicity associated with single lesion treatments. With these limitations in mind, extracranial radiation treatment seems best suited for solitary lesions, and few centers will treat more than three to four lesions in total depending on the clinical circumstances.

In summary, as for lung metastases, surgical results for stage I NSCLC underline the importance of local control for prognosis of these patients. Local control can be achieved by sufficiently high radiation doses to the complete tumor volume. The surgical results have important implications toward stereotactic body radiation therapy since tissue destruction for that therapy more closely resembles a wedge resection than a lobectomy. If meaningful doses are delivered, recurrence will be dependent on whether the entire extent of the disease is encompassed at time of treatment. Therefore after careful selection of patients, hopefully the results from stereotactic irradiation will reach equivalency to surgically treated patients.

RADIOBIOLOGY

Normal Tissue Considerations

The primary function of the lung is to exchange oxygen for carbon dioxide between the terminal airways (alveoli) and the blood (respiration). The lung serves to deliver the oxygen-rich air to the alveoli via a series of branching airways. Airflow within these branching airways (bronchi and bronchioles) is powered by pressure gradients generated by the diaphragm and chest wall musculature that are transmitted throughout the lung via the elastic structure of the lung parenchyma. At the level of the alveoli, the lung has a tremendous amount of inherent redundancy, with each neighboring alveoli/blood capillary complex functioning independently and doing basically the same activity (exchanging oxygen for carbon dioxide). The lung is a large organ and most people have a great deal more respiratory capacity than is actually required, constituting a reserve. Throughout life, this reserve may be depleted especially by activities that diffusely damage the parenchyma, like cigarette smoking. Surgeons contemplating a lung resection first try to quantify the amount of reserve in a given patient by measuring surrogate markers (e.g., pulmonary function tests). The surgeon will then determine whether removal of a certain fraction of lung will leave the patient with enough respiratory function to carry on daily activities. All in all, these considerations account for the inherent function of the lung (respiration), the organizational structure of the lung (branching airways leading to terminal alveoli), the redundancy of lung function (e.g., the left lung carries out the same activity as the right lung), and appreciation and quantification of the additional capability (reserve) inherent in the lung. These same considerations are paramount to understanding normal tissue and host responses after irradiation of the lung.

In describing normal tissue changes after therapeutic radiation, Wolbarst et al. (19) described a model where tissue is broken down into relatively small functional subunits (FSU). These FSUs are composed of an organized population of differentiated cells and a smaller population of clonagenic (stem) cells capable of replenishing the differentiated cells. Wolbarst divided FSUs into two general groups: (1) structurally defined units with discrete anatomical structure, and (2) structurally undefined units characterized by a monotonous structure without anatomical boundaries. In this model, damage from radiation was related to cumulative damage of constituent FSUs. According to this model, each alveolus/capillary complex within the lung constitutes a structurally defined FSU. It is presumed that after delivery of radiation, both differentiated and clonagenic cells are damaged, some lethally. In order for surviving clonagens to "rescue" the damaged tissue, they must first migrate to the damaged area and then divide into differentiated cells capable of performing the tissue's function. The migration of rescuing clonagens can occur within an alveolus but not between two adjacent alveoli, even though the two adjacent alveoli are in close proximity. As such, if all clonagenic cells within a single alveolus are damaged, all functional capability of that alveolus will be lost. This is in contrast to a structurally undefined FSU, like the mucosa of the esophagus, where clonagens are free to migrate long distances to rescue damaged epithelium.

Again considering the Wolbarst model, one can identify a threshold dose beyond which all clonagens within a particular structurally defined FSU are incapable of rescue and the FSU will become totally dysfunctional. Moreover, delivering an additional dose beyond the threshold dose within a particular volume containing a defined number of FSUs will not increase the dysfunction since all function is already lost at the threshold dose. For the lung, this threshold dose is probably quite low, in the range of 15–20 Gy given in 2 Gy fractions. The fact that fairly large volumes of lung can be irradiated by these doses without untoward consequences attests by the large functional reserve inherent in the lung.

Tissues that are made up predominantly of structurally defined FSUs are called *parallel functioning tissues* (including peripheral lung, peripheral kidney, peripheral liver, etc.) and occur within organs that are characterized by redundancy of function and large inherent reserves. In contrast, tissues that are made up of predominantly structurally undefined FSUs are called *serially functioning tissues* (including the gastrointestinal tract, large airways, spinal cord, etc.) and occur within organs that involve a "chain" of function. Certainly, some tissues do not fit well into either category (e.g., bone marrow). In treating a lung cancer in the peripheral lung, a parallel functioning tissue, high tumor doses are required to control the clonagenic capability inherent to most lung cancers. Adjacent lung tissue will be exposed to relatively the same dose as the tumor. According to the "critical volume model" proposed by Yeas and Kalend (20), any dose beyond the threshold dose defined above will not add additional toxicity to a given volume. For parallel functioning tissues, the organ will become dysfunctional if a critical volume getting the threshold dose is exceeded. Therefore, according to this model, organ dysfunction is not avoided by limiting the magnitude of *dose* beyond the threshold but rather by limiting the *volume* exposed to any dose beyond the threshold. This critical importance of limiting volume, with more attention than limiting dose, in order to spare organ dysfunction is the hallmark radiobiological principle of extracranial stereotactic radiation therapy.

The biggest shortcoming of both the Wolbarst and Yeas' models relates to the fact that an organ such as the lung is really composed of both parallel and serial tissue entwined in proximity to each other. The actual organization of the lung is similar to a tree or bush with a very large trunk (trachea) branching into large main branches (mainstem bronchi), branching further into smaller branches and twigs (lobar bronchi and bronchioles), and finally into terminal buds or leaves (alveoli/capillary complexes). All of the airways described above are serially functioning tissues since air is being directed along a single path as a chain of function and the clonagens within the airways are situated in the epithelium without anatomical boundaries. In contrast, the alveoli/capillary complexes are parallel functioning tissues with basement membranes and septa separating one alveolus from another limiting clonagen migration.

The type of anatomical arrangement seen in the lung may be referred to as a *branching tubular structure* and is in contrast to organs of the GI tract in which the lumen follows a single straight path known as *linear tubular structure*. An important consideration in relation to extracranial stereotactic radiation therapy between these structures follows because if the dose is intense enough to totally disrupt the function of the serial functioning component (e.g., the bronchus or esophagus), then all downstream functioning tissue will be lost as well (even if they were not irradiated) via collapse of the lumen. In a branching tubular structures, such damage will result in a collapse of the particular branch affected, not the entire organ. The same damage to a linear tubular structure will obstruct all downstream function of the organ (e.g., complete bowel obstruction), a more catastrophic problem for the patient. In the case of lung treatment, with potent doses of radiation delivered to a bronchus or bronchiole, distal collapse or atelectasis will occur which may likely be permanent. As long as the volume lost is less than the organ reserve for the particular individual, no significant symptomatic toxicity will result. If the lost volume is larger than the patient's reserve, the patient will have symptomatic respiratory decline. As such, with potent treatment doses (e.g., ablative doses), the loss of functional lung tissue may be larger than the actual volume irradiated beyond the threshold dose. It may still be reasonable to use such a strategy in order to control tumor proliferation; however, the treating physician must be aware of these two components of lung dysfunction (direct radiation damage to the volume irradiated and subsequent distal collapse of non-irradiated lung) when formulating the treatment plan.

Tumor Control Considerations

According to the models of Douglas and Fowler (21), the logarithm of tumor clonagenic survival as a function of dose may be approximated by a truncated power series known as the *linear–quadratic model*. Various physical explanations have been offered as to why the curve would not be linear, including that double strand DNA damage constitutes an irreparable defect while single strand breaks may be repaired. But, at any rate, with rather low doses per fraction (i.e., up to 6 Gy per fraction), tumors have an enhanced ability to withstand the damaging effects of radiation. Beyond this dose per fraction, tumor kill has an exponential relationship with dose, implying that tumor repair mechanisms are overwhelmed.

In addition to DNA repair as a mechanism for poor local control, radiobiologists have observed the ability of remaining viable tumor cells to increase their rate of cell division after being exposed to radiation. This *accelerated repopulation* is considered to be one of the most significant factors resulting in failure of treatment. Since it takes the cell some time to initiate this response (i.e., many days to weeks), the most viable therapeutic counter to this inherent tumor defense is to deliver all of the radiation very quickly before repopulation is initiated.

Inherent radioresistance is related to many factors. One of the most difficult factors to overcome is tumor hypoxia. Oxygen is required to "fix" damage caused by especially photon radiation. In addition, poorly oxygenated cells are probably not actively dividing, placing them in cell cycle portions less sensitive to radiation. The general strategy in radiation oncology for overcoming tumor hypoxia has been to protract the radiation delivery. The basis for this was that tumors that have "out-grown" their blood supply due to large size would shrink and effectively get closer to a vascular supply. During the later portions of the protracted course, the tumor would theoretically be well oxygenated. Certainly, regardless of the theory behind this strategy, protracted fractionated radiation therapy has not been particularly effective at controlling large necrotic epithelial tumors.

Furthermore, experiments using miniature oxygen probes have indicated that areas of significant tumor hypoxia are not necessarily in the central core of the tumor and, in fact, migrate within the tumor as a result of dynamic vascular changes (22). In this context, lengthy protraction of radiation may not be a viable solution for hypoxia while still a detriment in overcoming repopulation.

Cell cycle effects may also influence radiosensitivity. Certain portions of the cell cycle, like mitosis and G2, are thought to be quite sensitive while other portions, like late S-phase and G0, are considered radioresistant. Again, the general response to overcoming cell cycle effects has been to protract the fractionation of radiation therapy. It is assumed that cells will be committed to moving through the cell cycle. Cells in resistant phases will become sensitive later in the course of radiation according to this theory. The optimal length of protraction of radiation is unclear. Cell cycle times vary, even within a single tumor. At any rate, this feature of radioresistance has implications as to whether a stereotactic treatment regimen should be single fraction vs. a few separated fractions. Further research is needed to resolve this issue.

RADIATION TOLERANCE OF PULMONARY TISSUES

Within the lung itself, there are a variety of tissues that possess unique radiation tolerance characteristics, namely, the airways (both large and small functioning as serial structures), the alveoli/capillary complexes (functioning as parallel structures), and the arterial and venous network (likely functioning as serial structures).

The classic tolerance-defining toxicity for conventional radiation delivery in most prospective trials has been pneumonitis. Radiation pneumonitis is a subacute (weeks to months from treatment) inflammation of the end bronchioles and alveoli. The clinical picture may be very similar to acute bacterial pneumonia with fatigue, fever, shortness of breath, nonproductive cough, and a pulmonary infiltrate on chest X-ray. The infiltrate on chest X-ray should include the area treated to a high dose, but may extend outside of these regions. The infiltrates may be characteristically "geometric" corresponding to the radiation portal, but may also be ill-defined. Pneumonitis is generally treated with corticosteroids. It may resolve over time, but many progress into fibrosis with linear opacities appearing on imaging studies. Based on the pattern of infiltration during the initial presentation of pneumonitis, it is most likely that pneumonitis is a toxicity related to damage to end bronchioles and alveolar/capillary complexes. As such, this damage is to parallel functioning tissue and is most likely more volume dependent than dose dependent. Furthermore, the incidence of pneumonitis likely occurs at a relatively low threshold dose, in the range of the equivalent of 15–20 Gy in conventional fractionation. As such, high

dose per fraction stereotactic body radiation therapy likely causes pneumonitis within the high dose rim surrounding the tumor target in most cases.
Whether pneumonitis becomes symptomatic depends on the volume of
tissue that exceeds this threshold dose. Because normal lung volume is
relatively small in stereotactic treatments with little or no prophylactic irradiation, it would be potentially a less likely outcome as compared to conventional radiation therapy. Indeed, in the Indiana University phase I dose
escalation trial, symptomatic radiation pneumonitis occurred relatively
infrequently despite very potent effective dose delivery (23).

Conventional radiotherapy commonly causes large serially functioning
airway irritation, such as cough, but rarely dose limiting toxicity. In contrast, high dose stereotactic body radiation therapy treatment schemes
may cause significant large airway damage by both mucosal injury and ultimate collapse of the airway. This loss of functional capacity results from
both mucosal sloughing, cartilage damage, and peribronchial fibrosis; all
effectively causing bronchial stenosis. In turn, bronchial stenosis will in
many cases lead to distal atelectasis of lung parenchyma downstream from
the obstruction. This loss of lung function appears to mostly affect oxygenation parameters including diffusing capacity for carbon monoxide (DLCO),
arterial oxygen tension (pressure) on room air (PO_2), and supplemental
oxygen requirements (FIO_2) (23). Because the degree of this airway injury
toxicity is related to the proximity of the target to proximal trunks of the
branching tubular lung structure, great care should be taken when considering treatment to tumors near the hilum or central chest. More protracted
fractionation schedules for central tumors may facilitate treatments in these
locations at the expense of potentially less effective tumor control.

Unexpected toxicity may also occur when treating central chest target
relating to toxicity to mediastinal structures, including esophagus and heart.
While acute and sometimes severe esophageal toxicity is commonly seen
after conventionally fractionated radiation for lung cancer, most of the
injury is self-limiting and resolves after treatment. After high dose stereotactic body radiation therapy, esophageal strictures may form as a late effect.
Another more unique toxicity from stereotactic body radiation therapy
relates to pericardial injury. In the Indiana University phase I study, several
patients with tumors adjacent to the heart had asymptomatic pericardial
effusions, while one patient treated at the highest dose level had a large
and symptomatic pericardial effusion that required surgical intervention
to resolve (unpublished data).

Most reports of stereotactic body radiation therapy do not include
long-term follow-up data. As such, there may be unexpected toxicities that
need to be recognized, monitored, and evaluated. Particularly with large
doses per fraction there may be unexpected injury related to nerve tissue
and vascular tissue. Ideally, the dose to brachial plexus, spinal cord,
phrenic nerves, and intercostal nerves will be kept low via prudent

treatment planning. Furthermore, avoiding large blood vessels in the central chest may be reasonable as well. While there have not been reports of vascular wall damage including aneurysms and fistulas with hemoptysis or internal bleeding, these events may only manifest after many years of follow-up.

With a paucity of long-term data relating tissue effects after large dose per fraction radiation, it is difficult and somewhat dangerous to identify specific normal tissue tolerances. Nonetheless, in order for thoughtful investigation to proceed, a starting point must be established. The Radiation Therapy Oncology Group in the United States has developed a protocol for using stereotactic radiation to treat early stage lung cancer. The prescription dose to the margin of the planning target volume (PTV) for this protocol that treats tumors up to 5 cm in dimension is 60 Gy total over three fractions (20 Gy per fraction). A committee of experienced radiation oncologists, physicists, and biologists has established organ dose limits for this protocol based on limited institutional follow-up and linear–quadratic conversions of known dose tolerance parameters from conventional radiation fractionation schemes. The tolerances for this protocol are shown in Table 2 for several critical organs. These are absolute limits relating to a point rather than a volume. Obviously, a goal of radiation dosimetry for planning stereotactic lung radiation therapy should be to minimize the volume of normal tissue, even getting lower doses than those listed in Table 2. It must be emphasized that these tolerances figures have not been validated with long-term follow-up.

A proposed tolerance of the lung itself is not identified in Table 2. Based on the critical volume model of Yeas described above, it is assumed that the lung within the PTV exceeds tolerance and is no longer functional after high dose per fraction stereotactic radiation therapy. A dose fall-off region exists outside of the PTV, the volume of which depends on the size of the PTV, the location of the PTV within the chest, the quality of the radiation dosimetry (e.g., number of beams, beam arrangements, radiation energy, etc.), and the type of radiation (e.g., photon vs. proton, etc.). This

Table 2 RTOG Proposed Radiation Tolerances of Thoracic Normal Tissue

Organ	Volume	Dose
Spinal cord	Any point	18 Gy total over three fractions
Esophagus	Any point	27 Gy total over three fractions
Ipsilateral brachial plexus	Any point	24 Gy total over three fractions
Heart	Any point	30 Gy total over three fractions
Trachea and ipsilateral bronchus	Any point	30 Gy total over three fractions

dose fall-off region, also called the gradient region, constitutes unintended radiation exposure and should be kept as small as possible. The lung tolerance criteria used in conventionally fractionated radiotherapy, such as the percentage volume receiving 20 Gy (V_{20}), do not lend themselves to stereotactic body radiation therapy since these volumes are already relatively small. For the RTOG study, it is required that the ratio of the prescription isodose to 50% of the prescription isodose (which occurs in normal tissue) be no greater than 3.2. Considering then the maximum lesion size treated (5 cm), these constraints would allow no more than 320 cc of normal lung (excluding PTV) to exceed 30 Gy total over three fractions (10 Gy per fraction). It should be possible to keep this volume of normal lung considerably less for smaller lesions.

Treatment Delivery

Patient Immobilization and Target Reproducibility

The purpose of stereotactic radiotherapy of pulmonary targets is improved local tumor control achieved by dose escalation and volume restriction. Therefore setup inaccuracy and target mobility have to be minimized as much as possible.

Several immobilization devices have been developed during the last decade. All of them rely on a vacuum pillow, which is individually molded to the patient's body and fixed to a stereotactic frame. The frame itself is not only an immobilization device but also an external reference system, which allows identification of the isocenter by 3D-stereotactic coordinates. Although a stereotactic treatment might be performed without a dedicated immobilization device (24–28) the time for verification of the correct target position and irradiation itself of fraction doses up to 30 Gy often lasts for 30–60 min. During that time sufficient immobilization has to be ensured if the efforts for treatment precision should not be diminished by (uncontrolled) patient motion during treatment.

The other important factor which has to be addressed is breathing mobility. Uncontrolled breathing mobility of pulmonary tumors ranges up to more than 20 mm (29,30). The amount of mobility is related to the target location in the lung with larger mobility in the lower lobes. Breathing mobility can be evaluated by fluoroscopy or by CT scans. The CT-evaluation relies on dynamic examination of the tumor at the same couch position during some breathing cycles. The change of the axial tumor shape represents the amount of mobility and can be measured directly by comparing the different slices during the breathing phases. The longitudinal mobility can be measured by multi-slice technique or estimated by comparison of the evaluated slice level to slices cranio-caudal of that level. The CT evaluation has the advantage that even small targets and targets covered by other structures such as heart or diaphragm in fluoroscopy are clearly visible.

If breathing mobility of the target exceeds 5 mm in any direction attempts to reduce these motions are performed. While some groups irradiate patients just by shallow breathing with oxygen support (25,26), most authors use a mechanical breathing control device. It is attached to the immobilization frame and consists of a template pushed into the patient's epigastrium to a reproducible amount. By the use of this very easy-to-handle system, abdominal pressure is increased leading to decreased mobility of the diaphragm and secondary reduced target mobility. This technique allows reduction of breathing mobility down to 5 mm (31–36). Although most patients tolerate this technique very well, in cases such as patients with very poor lung function (e.g., after pneumonectomy), the effect is limited. In these patients breathing mobility has to be evaluated carefully and taken into account for PTV definition with enlarged margins.

Because increasing volume due to increased security margins is clearly not desirable, especially in patients with poor lung function, more advanced techniques have been developed. While jet ventilation under general anesthesia (37) needs high logistical efforts and to some extent contradicts the non-invasive character of the stereotactic approach, other authors have inaugurated active breathing control systems or breathing-triggered radiotherapy. If performed properly, breathing mobility intrafractionally can be reduced to almost zero (38,39). A still unresolved problem is inter-fractional reproducibility, which can be again up to 5 mm (39). To resolve this problem further evaluation supported by technical improvements, such as CT verification in the treatment room prior to irradiation or cone-beam CT, has to be performed. Another disadvantage is prolongation of treatment time due to restriction of irradiation to defined phases of the breathing cycle. An extreme of this approach is irradiation of lung tumors by the CyberKnife. The tumor is marked by intralesional gold seeds and irradiated by a robot-like accelerator, which calculates the actual target position from real-time flat-panel fluoroscopy. Nevertheless the pneumothorax-rate from gold seed implantation was 15% (3/21 patients) and an irradiation session of a single fraction treatment lasted for four hours at mean (2–6 hr) (40).

The accuracy of target reproducibility in a stereotactic body frame using oxygen supported shallow breathing (26,28) or mechanical breathing control (33,35) ranges from 3.1 to <5 mm in axial and 4.4–5.5 mm in longitudinal direction (median, for both 1 SD) evaluated by comparison of CT data from treatment planning and CT verification prior to treatment. According to these results most groups use security margins for PTV definition of 5 mm in axial and 5–10 mm in the longitudinal direction added to the CTV.

For definition of security margins the absolute target reproducibility independent on its origin from setup-inaccuracy or breathing mobility is the relevant parameter. Nevertheless for the process of minimizing setup-inaccuracy and for improvement of skills, information on the contribution of both factors separately is necessary. Setup accuracy can be measured by comparison of non-mobile bony structures relative to an external reference system, such as the stereotactic frame. This can be evaluated from the two different CT scans performed for treatment planning and for CT verification prior to irradiation. According to our own analysis this setup inaccuracy is about 2 mm: SD in lateral direction was 1.9 mm, AP 1.8 mm, and longitudinal 2.0 mm leading to a 3D-vector of 2.6 mm (35). These data were confirmed by Yenice et al. (41), who evaluated a self-constructed, non-invasive frame for stereotactic irradiation of paraspinal tumors.

Isocenter and Target Verification

The described data on target reproducibility are numbers representing the median or 1 SD; therefore it will be representative for the majority of cases. Nevertheless there will also be extremes of deviation, which will not be covered by the usual security margins of 5 mm in axial and 5–10 mm in longitudinal direction. In our own analysis target deviation (including setup inaccuracy and target mobility) exceeded 5 mm in 16% (AP), 12% (lateral), and 9% (longitudinal) of targets. A deviation of more than 10 mm was observed in 2% in the anteroposterior and lateral, respectively, and of 6% in longitudinal direction (35). Target miss due to deviations of >5 mm might not only lead to significant underdose of the tumor but also to eventually dangerous overdose to organs at risk due to the very high fraction doses used in stereotactic radiotherapy. Therefore major target deviations should be recognized and corrected prior to irradiation.

For that purpose three different approaches are used:

1. isocenter verification relative to bony structures by comparison of DRRs to beam views or portal images,
2. CT simulation prior to irradiation at the CT unit with subsequent transport of the patient to the linac,
3. CT verification on the treatment couch at the linac.

Isocenter verification relative to bony landmarks is the easiest and most widespread method to control accuracy of radiotherapy. Nevertheless by using this method it is assumed that the deviation of the (often invisible target) is represented by deviation of bony reference structures. To analyze this assumption we evaluated the congruence of deviation of bony reference structures to different types of targets, such as soft tissue targets fixed to other structures or mobile soft tissue targets, with or without use of the breathing control achieved by abdominal pressure. Because the security margins used for PTV definition were 5 mm at least in axial direction, congruence of the target to bony structures was assumed if the difference of deviation of both structures was less than 5 mm. This was the case in 80% of fixed soft tissue targets but only in 33% of mobile soft tissue targets (37.5% without breathing control and only 28.5%

with breathing control) (35). From these results it was concluded that bony reference structures are not reliable to control correct target reproducibility within the security margins of 5 mm. Therefore, many centers use CT verification prior to irradiation to control the correct isocenter position in the target as is common practice in intracranial stereotactic radiotherapy.

While CT verification would be most appropriate directly at the treatment couch without subsequent transport of the patient from the CT unit to the linac, this opportunity is not available at most institutions at this time. Nevertheless even if it is performed outside the treatment room CT-verification should allow for evaluation of target reproducibility.

To confirm target reproducibility after CT-simulation over the complete target volume and the complete course of three treatment fractions we analyzed the data of 60 CT-verifications in 22 pulmonary targets (42). For that purpose the anatomically corresponding isocenter slices of the planning-CT and the three verification-CTs of each patient were matched to each other using a digital matching tool of the 3D-treatment planning system. The CTV segmented in each verification CT was matched into the planning study and a DVH for this volume was calculated using the original treatment plan. Major deviations at any position of the CTV from the verification study should result in a decrease of dose coverage of the simulated CTV, if the deviation exceeds beyond the PTV-related reference isodose. As a result, in only three of 60 CT verifications (5%), the proportion to the CTV beyond the reference isodose exceeded 5%. Two of these major deviations were noticed in one patient treated for a lung metastasis in the left lower lobe after pneumonectomy. It is concluded that target reproducibility confirmed and eventually corrected due to CT-verification is accurate. Nevertheless for single patients treated under difficult conditions eventually increased security margins or more advanced techniques for breathing control have to be used.

Target Definition

Most reports on clinical results of stereotactically irradiated lung tumors do not focus on target definition in detail but give only information on security margins for PTV definition added to either the GTV or CTV. Therefore the practice of target definition might be potentially inhomogeneous among the different groups working on stereotactic irradiation of lung tumors. From surgical data on limited wedge or segmental resection it can be derived that not only the macroscopic tumor should be treated to achieve high local control rates. Therefore the GTV should include the small spiculae often seen in the periphery of the tumor and eventually the parts of infiltrated pleura. For this purpose target definition in the lung window (e.g., 1600, −400 HU) is preferred. In targets close to mediastinal or hilar structures, i.v. contrast eases the differentiation of tumor to blood vessels. To this GTV 2–3 mm of potential microscopic disease may be added to achieve the CTV. Another

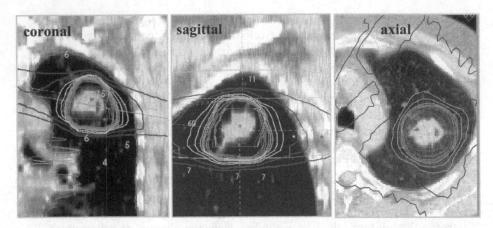

Figure 1 CTV-definition and conformal dose distribution in a 43-year-old male with primary lung cancer cT2 cN0 cM0 (adenocarcinoma grade II) in the left upper lobe medically inoperable due to severe heart disease. The CTV was 45 cm^3, the PTV was 100 cm^3. The tumor was treated by 3×10 Gy to the PTV-enclosing 100%-isodose (the inner orange isodose) with normalization to 150% at the isocenter. For CTV definition not only the macroscopic tumor but also the small tumor extensions into the periphery have to be included into the target volume (the numbers in the coronal and sagittal reconstruction show the point dose in percent to the prescribed fraction dose of 10 Gy). (*See color insert.*)

5 mm in axial and 5–10 mm in longitudinal direction are added for PTV definition, depending on the results of individual evaluation, e.g., of breathing mobility. An example for target definition with the consecutive 3D-dose distribution is shown in Figure 1.

Treatment Planning

For treatment planning usually CT slices of 3–5-mm thickness with or without i.v. contrast medium are sufficient. In general and especially in patients with impaired lung function the planning study should cover the complete lung to allow for assessment of the amount of lung irradiated. The planning study can be performed as an incremental or spiral scan, but it must be ensured that the target is not randomly scanned in an extreme phase of the breathing cycle. Therefore evaluation of breathing mobility and eventual use of breathing control techniques should be evaluated prior to the definite planning study.

The 3D-conformal treatment planning depends on dose prescription, which differs considerably among the published results. Some groups prescribe their dose to the isocenter (24,43–45), others to the PTV-enclosing isodose (23,25,27,31,32,36,37,40,46). Some groups use homogeneous dose distributions (44), some allow slight inhomogeneity with the 80%-isodose encompassing the PTV (23,25,26,37,40,46), and others prefer increased inhomogeneity such as prescribing the dose to the PTV-enclosing 65%-isodose (which is equivalent to dose prescription to the PTV-enclosing 100%-isodose with normalizing 150% at the isocenter) (31–36).

There are no detailed publications on treatment techniques and beam arrangement. Most groups use 5–9 coplanar static fields to achieve a conformal dose distribution encompassing the PTV. Especially in larger volumes rotational beams with leaf adaptation every 20–40° are useful to avoid triangulated high dose spikes from overlapping parts of static fields. Under some circumstances non-coplanar beams or the use of wedges have to be considered, but the benefit of optimized dose distribution has to be balanced against prolongation of irradiation time.

The quality of a dose distribution can be evaluated by comparison of the volume of the reference isodose to the volume of the PTV (conformity index = 1, if these volumes are identical). Because the volume of the reference isodose does not necessarily cover the PTV but also potentially normal tissue outside the PTV, the conformity index has to be related to the target coverage (TC) of the PTV. The TC represents the amount of the PTV covered by the reference isodose. According to Van't Riet et al. (47), the product of TC and conformity index results in a conformation number (CN), which optimally is one if both parameters are one. The evaluation of our own treatment plans for 22 lung tumors achieved by static or rotational beams revealed a TC of the PTV by the reference isodose of at mean 96% ± 2.3% (SD) and a conformity index of at mean 0.51 ± 0.13 (SD). The resulting CN was at mean 0.73 ± 0.09 (SD) (48).

Tissue Heterogeneity Issues

Important for the quality and reliability of treatment plans is the dose calculation algorithm. Recent studies revealed an energy dependent potential dose decrease at the tumor margin of up to 10–20% if simple dose calculation algorithms such as the widespread pencil-beam algorithm are used instead of more sophisticated models such as the point kernel-based collapsed cone algorithm (49,50,55).

The most obviously unique aspect of lung tissues vs. tissues elsewhere in the body in regard to photon dosimetry is the spectrum of densities across the organ. Within the lung and chest are areas of air density (large airways), water density (mediastinum and tumor bearing tissue), bone density (chest wall), and intermediate density (lung parenchyma). The density of the lung parenchyma may vary between patients from 0.15 to 0.35 g/cm^3, depending on host factors like history of emphysema, etc. This heterogeneity of density has significant implications toward dose deposition, especially in areas of inherent electronic dysequilibrium like the edge of a tumor.

As a beam of photon radiation passes through a patient toward a tumor target, it first is attenuated by the chest wall or perhaps mediastinum.

The physics of this interaction are well described. However, once the beam passes into lung parenchyma, there is considerably less energy loss through attenuation. Effectively, more photon fluence will be delivered to the edge of the tumor resulting in higher central tumor doses than predicted by algorithms considering all tissues to have water density ($1.0\,\text{g/cm}^3$). At the edge of the tumor, a secondary buildup will occur resulting in relative under-dosing as compared to what would be predicted by algorithms considering all tissues to have water density. These effects have implications both to tumor control and toxicity.

Beam energy also dramatically influences the dose buildup characteristics at the edge of a tumor. While higher energy beams will deliver more radiation fluence to the core of a tumor target relative to the skin dose compared to low energy beams, the deeper location of achieving equilibrium (D_{max}) may result in significant underdosing of the tumor margin. Rather than use high energy beams to overcome problems with skin toxicity, it is probably more prudent to add additional lower energy beams, thereby spreading out the entrance dose among all beams.

Stereotactic body radiation therapy typically involves the use of many beams with relatively small apertures. Heterogeneity effects are magnified by such arrangements in that field edges are very close to target edges. Strikingly steep dose gradients result in the region, where accurate prescription dose must be appreciated. The edge of a tumor can be effectively "missed" or underdosed if these effects are improperly characterized. With stereotactic radiation, greater care must be taken to commission beams with small apertures, especially toward the edge of the fields. Otherwise the minimum tumor dose, which will nearly always occur at the edge of the tumor, will be mischaracterized.

Historically, treatment planning software systems did not account for these heterogeneity effects. As such, knowledge of radiation response reflects an inaccurate characterization of dose both in terms of tumor control and toxicity. Newer generation planning software makes approximations for both attenuation and scatter effects in heterogeneous tissues. The attenuation algorithms from vendor to vendor consistently account for this effect. However, the scattering corrections are not consistent and may lead again to significant differences in reported tumor doses from center to center, especially at the edge of the target. Monte Carlo dosimetry will likely overcome these difficulties, but is generally not available for treatment planning. Until these obstacles are overcome, it is important that investigators report the nature of their institution's calculation, including algorithms used for calculating dose to the target margin.

TREATMENT OUTCOME

More published outcomes have been available for treating lung tumors with stereotactic body radiation therapy than any other site. To the credit of the investigators, much of this work describes prospective trials. The first authors inaugurating the stereotactic method for irradiation of extracranial targets were Blomgren and Lax from Karolinska Hospital, Stockholm, Sweden. They started with a hypofractionated treatment approach in the early 1990s irradiating pulmonary, liver, and abdominal targets with 2×15 Gy or 3×10 Gy, prescribed to the PTV-enclosing 65%-isodose and normalizing the 100% dose to the isocenter (31–34). While almost all groups treat NSCLC of stage I/II and lung metastases, up to now no homogeneous treatment concept has been established. The published data show a wide variety of doses, fractionation, dose prescription, and normalization. In general there are three groups of fractionation: single dose treatment (37,40,43,46), hypofractionated treatment with 3–4 fractions (23,31,32,36, 44,51), and hypofractionated treatment in 5–15 fractions (24,25,27,45). An overview on treatment concepts, tumor volumes and diameter, follow-up, and local control rates is given in Table 3.

Single Dose Irradiation

The prescribed dose ranges from 15 to 30 Gy. Some groups started with lower doses and increased the dose over time in a dose escalation study and some groups adapted to the tumor size and location. Dose prescription varies from "peripheral" dose $\pm$ conventional fractionated irradiation (46), prescription to the PTV-enclosing 80%-isodose (40) or the isocenter with having the 80%-isodose enclosing the PTV (37), or as "minimal dose to the GTV" (43).

Hypofractionation with 3–4 Fractions

In this group the Swedish concept of an inhomaogeneous dose distribution was mainly used with 2×15 Gy or 3×10 Gy, prescribed to the PTV-enclosing 65%-isodose and normalization to 100% at the isocenter (31–36). This prescription results in a peripheral fraction dose at the PTV of 15 Gy, respectively, 10 Gy and isocenter doses of 22.5 Gy/15 Gy. (In terms of doses the prescription to the PTV-enclosing 65%-isodose is identical to the otherwise used nomenclature of prescribing the dose to the PTV-enclosing 100%-isodose with normalization to 150% at the isocenter.) Nagata et al. (44) reported on 4×10–12 Gy, prescribed to the isocenter. Lee et al. (51) prescribed 3–4×10 Gy to the 90%-isodose. Timmerman et al. (23) performed a phase I dose escalation study in patients with medically inoperable NSCLC with three fractions using dose per fraction ranging from 8 up to 20 Gy to generally the 80% isodose.

Hypofractionation with 5–15 Fractions

Uematsu et al. (25) treated their patients with more fractions ranging from 5 to 15 and doses ranging from 30 to 76 Gy prescribed to the 80%-isodose,

Table 3 Published Treatment Concepts and Results of Stereotactic Radiotherapy of Targets in the Lung

Study	Tumor type	Targets (n)	n/Normalization	Median (cm³)[a]	Min-max (Month)	Local control (All targets)	Local control prim. LC	Local control metastases
Blomgren et al. (31) J Radiosurg 1998	Prim. tumors/ metastases	17	3×10 to 2×15 Gy/65%-isodose	3-198 (15)[a]	8 (mean) (3.5-25)	16/17 (94%)	3/3 (100%)	13/14 (93%)
Uematsu et al. (25) Cancer 1998	Prim. tumors/ metastases	66	5-15 fractions 30-76 Gy/80%-isodose	1-4.8 cm tumor diameter 0.5-55 cm³ [3a]	11 (3-31)	64/66 (97%)	22/23 (96%)	42/43 (98%)
Nakagawa et al. (46) IJROBP 2000	Metastases	22	1×15-1×24 Gy "peripheral dose" ± conv. fract. RT	Chest wall 5-126 (40) Central lung 0.8-13 (4.5)	10 (2-82)	20/21 (95%)	1/1 (100%)	20/21 (95%)
Uematsu et al. (27) IJROBP 2001	Prim. tumors	50	5-10 fract. 50-60 Gy Tu encl. 80%-isodose (18 pts boost after CFRT)	0.8-5.0 cm tumor diam. (median 3.2 cm)	36 (22-66)	—	47/50 (96%)	—
Wulf et al. (36) Strahlenther Onkol 2001	Prim. tumors/ metastases	27	3×10 Gy/100%-isodose, norm. 150%	5-277 (57)	8 (2-33)	23/27 (85%)	11/12 (92%)	8/11 (73%)
Nagata et al. (44) IJROBP 2002	Prim. tumors/ metastases	40	4×10 Gy to 4×12 Gy isocenter	<4cm diameter	19 (4-39)	31/33 (94%)	16/31 evaluated 16/16 (100%)	6/9 (66%)

Study	Type	n	Dose/technique	Tumor size	Follow-up			
Hara et al. (43) Radiother Oncol 2002	Prim. tumors/ metastases	23	1×20-30 Gy to minimal dose to the GTV	<4cm diameter CTV: 1-16 (4)	13 (3-24)	19/23 (83%)	5/5 (100%)	14/18 (78%)
Whyte et al. (40) Ann Thorac Surg 2003	Prim. tumors/ metastases	23	1×15 Gy/80%-isodose (?) Cyberknife	1-5cm tumor diameter	7 (mean) (1-26)	21/23 (91%)	n = 15 (no detailed report on local control)	n = 8
Onimaru et al. (24) IJROBP 2003	Prim. tumors/ metastases	57	48-60 Gy/8fx isocenter or PTV- encl. 80%-isodose	0.6-6cm (2.6cm)	18 (2-44)	50/57 (88%)	20/25 (80%)	18/20 (90%)
Hof et al. (37) IJROBP 2003	Prim. NSCLC stage I	10	1×19-26 Gy/ isocenter, 80%-isod. encl. PTV	5-19 (12)	15 (8-30)	—	8/10 (80%)	—
Lee et al. (51) Lung Cancer 2003	Prim. tumors/ metastases	34	3-4×10 Gy/90%-isodose	4.4-230 (41) (PTV)	18 (7-35)	31/34 (91%)	8/9 (89%)	23/25 (92%)
Timmerman et al. (23) Chest 2003	Prim. tumors	37	Dose escalation from 3×8 Gy/80% to 3×20 Gy/80% isodose	1.5-157 (22.5)	15 (2-30)	—	31/37 (84%)	—

[a]Data have been recalculated from that given in the original publications.

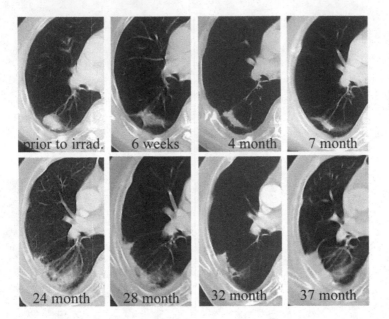

Figure 2 (*Caption on facing page*)

respectively, 50–60 Gy in 5–10 fractions with the 80%-isodose enclosing the tumor. Within the latter concept stereotactic irradiation was given as boost after conventional fractionated radiotherapy (CFRT; $n = 18$) (27). Fukumoto et al. (45) and Onimaru et al. (24) reported on eight fractions of 6 Gy with dose prescription to the 80%-isodose in peripheral and 6 Gy to the isocenter in targets close to the mediastinum.

Target Volume

The reported target volumes again show a large variety. Some authors report the tumor diameter; others the GTV, CTV, or the PTV. The tumor diameters range from 0.6 to 6 cm. The CTV ranges from a minimum of $0.5 \, \text{cm}^3$ to a maximum of $277 \, \text{cm}^3$ (median 4–$40 \, \text{cm}^3$) (Table 3).

LOCAL CONTROL AND SURVIVAL

Unfortunately, as expected for an emerging technology, follow-up on most of these reports is relatively short. Median follow-up ranged from 7 to 19 months [36 months of surviving patients by Uematsu et al. (27)] the reported maximum follow-up was 82 months (46). An overview on treatment parameter and results is given in Table 3, which encompasses 12 studies (23–25,27,31,36,37,43,44,46,51). (The treatment results of two additional studies—Blomgren et al. (32) and Fukumoto et al. (45)—were

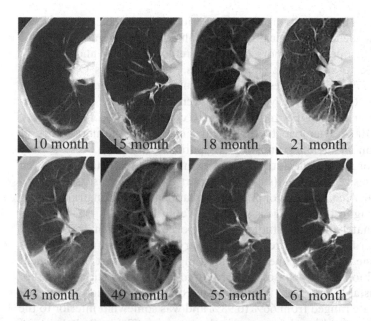

Figure 2 CT follow-up over 61 months in a 62-year-old male with a medically inoperable squamous cell lung cancer cT3 cN0 cM0 in the right lower lobe treated by stereotactic irradiation of 3×10 Gy/PTV-enclosing 100%-isodose, normalization to 150% with a CTV of 91 cm^3 and a PTV of 174 cm^3. After initial tumor regression progressive fibrosis occurred with continuous changes of CT morphology during follow-up. At 15 months a CT-assisted biopsy of the suspicious mass at the thoracic wall revealed fibrous tissue and no evidence of malignant tumor. Typically the appearance of the irradiated lung tissue changes rapidly over time without tumor recurrence or clinical symptoms reported by the patient.

included in later publications by Blomgren et al. (31) and Onimaru et al. (24). Only the data from the most recent papers appear in this overview.) Most authors define local control as complete or partial remission or stable disease. Local failure is defined as progressive disease or regrowth after initial response. A clinical example of a locally controlled tumor and changes during follow-up is shown in Figure 2.

Summarizing the published data from the 12 studies, a total of 206 patients (ranging from 1 to 50 per study) with primary lung cancer have been treated by stereotactic irradiation. Crude local control rates ranged from 80% to 100%.

The largest cohort consisting of 50 patients with NSCLC stage I has been published by Uematsu et al. (27). They reached a crude local control rate of 96% with only three local failures. The actuarial cause specific survival (overall survival) was 98% (98%) after six months, 96% (90%) after one year, 91% (77%) after two years, 88% (66%) after three years, and 81% (55%)

after four years. These results are clearly superior to these achieved by CFRT and reach equivalency to surgical results. Evaluating the overall survival of 29 patients with operable tumors, who had refused surgery and therefore are comparable to surgically treated patients, the four-years OS of these patients was 77%. Similar results with actuarial local control rates of 90–100% after two to three years have been achieved by other groups (36,44,51). Nevertheless DFS and OS differed considerably from only 11%/27% to 73%/100% after two to three years, indicating the importance of patient selection. While the groups treating patients with stage I disease only achieve superior results, the authors also treating patients of stage II or even initially metastasized patients (stage IV) report on inferior disease-free and overall survival. A comparison of published treatment results on primary lung cancer according to tumor stage is shown in Table 4.

Unfortunately, in most studies, no time-event analyses have been performed to describe treatment results of primary lung cancer and metastases separately. Nine of the 12 papers presented in Table 3 report on treatment results for pulmonary metastases. According to these publications a total of 169 lung metastases have been treated by stereotactic irradiation. The crude local control rate ranged from 66% to 98% and was somewhat inferior to the local control rates achieved for primary lung cancer (Table 4). Because of the small number of local failures (a total of 30, ranging from 1 to 7 local failures for the individual studies) no reliable evaluation of factors associated with locally uncontrolled failure could be performed up to now. Additionally the treated patient groups, especially for metastases from different primaries, are inhomogeneous and therefore the role of tumor size or histology on treatment results could not be evaluated sufficiently.

Nevertheless some authors observed a dose dependence of local tumor control without respect to differentiation in primary lung cancer or metastases. Hara et al. (43) reported an actuarial local control rate after 13 months of 88% for tumors receiving a single dose ≥ 30 Gy, but only of 63% for dose < 30 Gy ($p = 0.102$). Onimaru et al. (24) evaluated a three years' local control rate for pulmonary tumors (NSCLC and metastases) of 100% for doses of 60 Gy compared to 70% for 48 Gy, both given in eight fractions ($p = 0.0435$). In our own data from Wuerzburg 65 lung tumors (24 primary lung cancer and 41 metastases) were treated either by 3×10 Gy/PTV-enclosing 100%-isodose, normalization 150% at the isocenter ($n = 27$) or 3×12–12.5 Gy (same dose prescription, $n = 19$) and single dose irradiation of 26 Gy/PTV-enclosing 80%-isodose ($n = 19$). After a median follow-up of 10 months (2–61 months) the actuarial local control after one year and later was 72% for the patients treated with 3×10 Gy compared to 100% for those treated by 3×12–12.5 Gy or single dose irradiation (log-rank test: 0.026; 56). Evidence of a dose response relationship for primary lung cancer was also observed in the Indiana University phase I dose escalation study. Although this study was primarily a toxicity evaluation, six patients had local failure

Table 4 Actuarial Local Control Rates, Disease Free Survival (DFS) and Overall Survival (OS) for Primary Lung Cancer

Study	Tumor stage	Crude local control	Actuarial data available	Local control/DFS/OS (%)				
				6 months	1 year	2 years	3 years
Blomgren et al. (31) J Radiosurg 1998	cT1-2 cN0 cM0	3/3 (100%)	No	100/x/x	100/x/x	100/x/x	—
Nakagawa et al. (46) IJROBP 2000	cTx cN0 cM1 (GTV 6 cm³)	1/1 (100%)	No	—	—	—	—
Uematsu et al. (27) IJROBP 2001	cT1 cN0 cM0 (n = 24) cT2 cN0 cM0 (n = 26)	47/50 (96%)	Yes	x/98*/98 (*cause specific survival)	x/96*/90	x/91*/77	x/88*/66 [4 years: x/ 81*/55]
Wulf et al. (36) Strahlenther Onkol 2001	cT2 cN0 cM0 (n = 3) cT3 cN0 cM0 (n = 5) cT2-3 cN0 cM1 (n = 4)	11/12 (92%)	Yes (recalculated from original data)	91/82/92	91/42/52	91/11/27	91/11/27
Nagata et al. (44) IJROBP 2002	cT1 cN0 cM0	16/31 evaluated 16/16 (100%)	Yes	100/100/93	100/81/87	100/73/79	100/73/79
Hara et al. (43) Radiother Oncol 2002	GTV 3,4,6,8 cm³	5/5 (100%)	No	—	—	—	—

(*Continued*)

Table 4 Actuarial Local Control Rates, Disease Free Survival (DFS) and Overall Survival (OS) for Primary Lung Cancer (*Continued*)

Study	Tumor stage	Crude local control	Actuarial data available	Local control/DFS/OS (%)			
				6 months	1 year	2 years	3 years
Whyte et al. (40) Ann Thorac Surg 2003	n.a.	n = 15 (no detailed report on local control of primary lung cancer)	No	—	—	—	—
Onimaru et al. (24) IJROBP 2003	I (n = 19), II (n = 1), III (n = 1), IV (n = 4)	20/25 (80%)	Yes	x/x/x	x/x/x	x/47/60	55/x/x
Hof et al. (37) IJROBP 2003	cT1 cN0 cM0 (n = 2) cT2 cN0 cM0 (n = 8)	8/10 (80%)	Yes	100/x/100	89/x/80	71/x/64	—
Lee et al. (51) Lung Cancer 2003	n.a. (7 medically inop., 2 refused surgery)	8/9 (89%)	Yes	90/x/100	90/x/100	90/x/100	—
Timmerman et al. (23) Chest (in press)	cT1 cN0 cM0 (n = 19) cT2cN0 cM0 (n = 18) max tumor 7 cm	31/37 (84%)	Yes (only at 15.2 months)	—	x/50/64 at 15.2 mo.	—	—

Some authors did not perform time–event analyses or did not differentiate results of primary lung cancer to pulmonary metastases.

at dose of 3 × 16 Gy or below while no patient had local failure at 3 × 18 Gy or higher (23).

Toxicity

Published reports of stereotactic irradiation of pulmonary targets describe a very low acute and late toxicity rate compared to conventional radiation techniques to high dose used in medically impaired patients. Acutely, some hours after irradiation, about 10–22% of patients will exhibit pain, fever, chills, nausea, or vomiting, which lasts for a few hours with spontaneous remission and only rarely requires treatment by antipyretic pain killers (31,32,36). The reported rate of radiation pneumonitis is low. It is diagnosed without clinical symptoms by CT-scans during follow-up in 5–9% (27,36,46). Symptomatic pneumonitis requiring steroid treatment is observed with a rate of about 4% (24,43). Only two cases have been reported with impairment of lung function due to stereotactic irradiation (40,43). Three cases of pneumothorax occurred due to seed insertion into the tumor for preparation of CyberKnife-treatment, two of them requiring a chest tube (40).

The most obvious late toxicity is fibrosis of the lung in the high dose area, potentially associated with atelectasis distantly. This fibrosis occurs in almost every patient after stereotactic irradiation. Severe late complications are very rare. Two cases of esophageal ulceration have been reported, one of these with consecutive fatal bleeding (24,36). Another patient suffered from grade 3 chronic cough after irradiation of a target close to the trachea by 2×10 Gy (31,32). At this time there are no data on radiosensitivity of the wall of large vessels. One fatal bleeding from the pulmonary artery was reported nine months after stereotactic treatment with 3×10 Gy to a tumor recurrence progressively compressing the artery after preirradiation with 66 Gy a year before (36). Uematsu et al. (27) reported on two patients with bones within the 80%-isodose, who suffered from a rib fracture or a vertebral compression fracture after irradiation.

The potential for dose escalation by stereotactic irradiation related to toxicity has been evaluated in a phase I dose escalation toxicity study from Timmerman et al. (23) in patients with medically inoperable early stage lung cancer. The treatment population generally had very poor pulmonary function at the outset with mean FEV1 1.24 (46% predicted) and range 0.4–2.5 (19–94% predicted). Despite their general frailty, dose escalation to dramatically high doses was accomplished from 3 × 8 Gy to 3 × 20 Gy prescribed to the PTV-enclosing 80%-isodose in steps of 2 Gy per fraction. Sporadic pneumonitis and hypoxia was observed irrespective of dose level. At the higher doses, fibrosis in the treatment area with distal collapse of airway was observed in all patients although rarely symptomatic. Pulmonary function testing after treatment showed trends toward worsening of diffusing capacity and arterial oxygen tension. Spirometry indices showed no significant decline after treatment; indeed, in many patients FEV_1 and FVC improved for unknown reasons. Overall, this study demonstrated that very high biologically potent dose levels could be reached in a frail population using stereotactic techniques likely owing to the care taken to exclude uninvolved lung volume.

Summarizing these data, no relevant toxicity has been reported due to stereotactic irradiation of peripheral lung tumors. Only targets close or adjacent to the mediastinum with high dose spots to the organs at risk, such as trachea, major bronchi, or esophagus, are associated with increased risk toxicity.

CONCLUSION AND FUTURE DIRECTIONS

Summarizing the clinical data achieved by stereotactic irradiation of lung tumors it can be concluded that high actuarial local control rates of 80–100% after three years can be achieved for primary lung cancer and somewhat lower for pulmonary metastases. At the same time the treatment is associated with very low acute and late toxicity if high doses to organs at risk at the mediastinum are avoided. The results of disease-free survival and overall survival may reflect the practice of patient selection for a new treatment approach. Most authors report on case numbers of less than 30 targets, indicating publication of the treatment results of the very first patients. Nevertheless the published results support the concept of dose escalation and volume restriction due to the stereotactic approach with minimizing setup-inaccuracy and target (breathing) mobility to achieve local tumor control. Therefore, from the published data it seems justified to consider stereotactic irradiation of lung tumors even for curative treatment. Despite the heterogeneity of treatment concepts all approaches seem to lead to very promising treatment results. Nevertheless there is evidence on dose dependency of local control rates so that doses that have been reported with inferior results should be avoided.

Stereotactic body radiotherapy will likely play an increasing role in lung cancer treatment, particularly early stage NSCLC. Treatment toxicity is related to the volume of normal tissue treated at or near the target dose. The main challenge will be to better account for target motion and other uncertainties allowing further field reductions without missing the targets. This will be of particular importance when treating larger tumors and tumors closer to the central chest.

The Radiation Therapy Oncology Group in the United States is about to embark on a phase II trial of stereotactic body radiation therapy in early stage NSCLC using the Indiana University phase I study as the basis for dose selection. This will be a multi-institutional trial assessing not only patient outcome, but also feasibility of these treatments on a wider scale. Comprehensive central review and quality assurance are incorporated into this pilot trial. Eventually, it is envisioned that this therapy will be tested against other therapies, including surgical resection, in a phase III trial. Several institutions are studying the implementation of stereotactic body radiation therapy as a boost only with more conventionally fractionated radiation in locally advanced lung cancer. This approach is being used in both initial treatment regimens as well as for patients with recurrent tumors. Many of these types of patients also get chemotherapy as part of their treatment. Whether higher than conventional dose per fractions will alter the chemotherapy response in tumor or normal tissues remains to be evaluated.

In future efforts to reduce the irradiated volume by further decrease of security margins to compensate for target mobility and setup-inaccuracy will be undertaken. In this direction "4D"-image-guided radiotherapy, e.g., by implementation of CT verification in the treatment room ("cone beam CT") or chased beam irradiation with the beam or treatment couch following a moving target will be introduced (45). Other approaches will focus on further reduction of breathing mobility by, e.g., breathing-triggered irradiation (52–54).

REFERENCES

1. Becker N, Wahrendorf J. Atlas of Cancer Mortality in the Federal Republic of Germany 1981–1990. 3rd. Berlin, Heidelberg, New York: Springer-Verlag, 1997.
2. Janssen-Heijnen MLG, Coebergh JWW. The changing epidemiology of lung cancer in Europe. Lung Cancer 2003; 41:245–258.
3. Hoelzel D, Klamert A, Schmidt M. Krebs: Häufigkeiten, Befunde und Behandlungsergebnisse. W. Zuckschwerdt Verlag 1996:247–261.
4. Nesbitt JC, Putnam JB Jr, Walsh GL, et al. Survival in early-stage non-small cell lung cancer. Ann Thorac Surg 1995; 114:535–543.
5. Mountain CF. Revisions in the international system for staging lung cancer. Chest 1997; 111:1710–1717.
6. Adebonojo SA, Bowser AN, Moritz DM, et al. Impact of revised stage classification of lung cancer on survival: a military experience. Chest 1999; 115(6):1507–1513.
7. Kaseda S, Aoki T, Hangai N, et al. Better pulmonary function and prognosis with video- assisted thorascopic surgery than with thoractomy. Ann Thorac Surg 2000; 70:1644–1646.
8. Martini N, Bains MS, Burt ME, et al. Incidence of local recurrence and second primary tumors in resected stage I lung cancer. J Thorac Cardiovasc Surg 1995; 109:120–129.
9. Ginsberg RJ, Rubinstein LV. Lung Cancer Study Group: Randomized trial of lobectomy versus limited resection for T1 N0 non-small cell lung cancer. Ann Thorac Surg 1995; 60:615–623.
10. Jeremic B, Classen J, Bamberg M. Radiotherapy alone in technically operable, medically inoperable, early-stage (I/II) non-small cell lung cancer. Int J Radiat Oncol Biol Phys 2002; 54:119–130.

11. Sibley GS. Radiotherapy for patients with medically inoperable stage I non-small cell lung carcinoma. Smaller doses and higher doses. A review. Cancer 1998; 82:433–438.

12. Sibley GS, Jamieson TA, Marks LB, et al. Radiotherapy alone for medically inoperable stage I non-small cell lung cancer: the Duke experience. Int J Radiat Oncol Biol Phys 1998; 40:149–154.

13. Belderbos JSA, De Jaeger K, Heemsbergen WD, et al. First results of a phase I/II dose escalation trial in non-small cell lung cancer using three-dimensional conformal radiotherapy. Radiother Oncol 2003; 66:119–126.

14. Slotman BJ, Antonisse IE, Njo KH. Limited field irradiation in early stage (T1-2N0) non-small cell lung cancer. Radiother Oncol 1996; 41:41–44.

15. Krol ADG, Aussems P, Noordijk EM, Hermans J, Leer JWH. Local radiation alone for peripheral stage I lung cancer: could we omit the elective regional nodal irradiation? Int J Radiat Oncol Biol Phys 1996; 34(2):297–302.

16. Bradley JD, Wahab S, Lockett MA, et al. Elective nodal failures are uncommon in medically inoperable patients with stage I non-small cell lung carcinoma treated with limited radiotherapy fields. Int J Radiat Oncol Biol Phys 2003; 56:342–347.

17. Pastorino U, Buyse M, Friedel G, et al. Long-term results of lung metastasectomy: prognostic analyses based on 5206 cases. J Thorac Cardiovasc Surg 1997; 113:37–49.

18. Davidson RS, Nwogu CE, Brentjens MJ, Anderson TM. The surgical management of pulmonary metastasis: current concepts. Surg Oncol 2001; 10:35–42.

19. Wolbarst AB, Chin LM, Svensson GK. Optimization of radiation therapy: integral-response of a model biological system. Int J Radiat Oncol Biol Phys 1982; 8:1761–1769.

20. Yeas RJ, Kalend A. Local stem cell depletion model for radiation myelitis. Int J Radiat Oncol Biol Phys 1988; 14:1247–1259.

21. Douglas BG, Fowler JF. The effects of multiple small doses of x-rays on skin reactions in the mouse and a basic interpretation. Radiat Res 1976; 66:401–426.

22. De Jaeger K, Merlo FM, Kavanagh MC, et al. Heterogeneity of tumor oxygenation: relationship to tumor necrosis, tumor size, and metastasis. Int J Radiat Oncol Biol Phys 1998; 42(4):717–721.

23. Timmerman RD, Papiez L, McGarry R, Likes L, DesRosiers C, Bank M, Frost S, Randall M, Williams M. Extracranial stereotactic radioablation: results of a phase I study in medically inoperable stage I non-small cell lung cancer. Chest 2003; 124(5):1946–1955.

24. Onimaru R, Shirato H, Shimizu S, Kitamura K, et al. Tolerance of organs at risk in small-volume, hypofractionated, image-guided radiotherapy for primary and metastatic lung cancers. Int J Radiat Oncol Biol Phys 2003; 56:126–135.

25. Uematsu M, Shioda A, Tahara K, Fukui T, Yamamoto F, Tsumatori G, Ozeki Y, Aoki T, Watanabe M, Kusano S. Focal, high dose, and fractionated modified stereotactic radiation therapy for lung carcinoma patients. Cancer 1998; 82: 1062–1070.

26. Uematsu M, Shioda M, Suda A, Tahara K, Kojima T, Hama Y, Kojima T, Kono M, Wong JR, Fukui T, Kusano S. Intrafractional tumor position stability during computed tomography (CT)-guided frameless stereotactic radiation therapy for lung or liver cancers with a fusion of CT and linear accelerator (focal) unit. Int J Radiat Oncol Biol Phys 2000; 48(2):443–448.

27. Uematsu M, Shioda M, Suda A, et al. Computed tomography-guided frameless stereotactic radiotherapy for stage I non-small cell lung cancer: a 5-year experience. Int J Radiat Oncol Biol Phys 2001; 51(3):666–670.
28. Uematsu M, Sonderegger M, Shioda A, Tahara K, Fukui T, Hama Y, Kojima T, Wong J, Kusano S. Daily positioning accuracy of frameless stereotactic radiation therapy with a fusion of computed tomography and linear accelerator (focal) unit: evaluation of z-axis with a z-marker. Radiother Oncol 1999; 50:337–339.
29. Shimizu S, Shirato H, Ogura S, Akita-Dosaka H, et al. Detection of lung tumor movement in real-time tumor-tracking radiotherapy. Int J Radiat Oncol Biol Phys 2001; 51(2):304–310.
30. Erridge SC, Seppenwoolde Y, Muller SH, van Herk M, et al. Portal imaging to assess set-up errors, tumor motion and tumor shrinkage during conformal radiotherapy of non-small cell lung cancer. Radiother Oncol 2003; 66:75–85.
31. Blomgren H, Lax I, Göranson H, Kräpelien T, Nilsson B, Näslund I, Svanström R, Tilikidis A. Radiosurgery for tumors in the body: clinical experience using a new method. J Radiosurg 1998; 1(1):63–74.
32. Blomgren H, Lax I, Näslund I, Svanström R. Stereotactic high dose fractionation radiation therapy of extracranial tumors using an accelerator. Acta Oncol 1995; 34:861–870.
33. Lax I, Blomgren H, Larson D, Näslund D. Extracranial stereotactic radiosurgery of localized targets. J Radiosurg 1998; 1(2):135–148.
34. Lax I, Blomgren H, Näslund I, Svanström R. Stereotactic radiotherapy of malignancies in the abdomen. Methodological aspects. Acta Oncol 1994; 33:677–683.
35. Wulf J, Haedinger U, Oppitz U, Olshausen B, Flentje M. Stereotactic radiotherapy of extracranial targets: CT-simulation and accuracy of treatment in the stereotactic body frame. Radiother Oncol 2000; 57:225–236.
36. Wulf J, Haedinger U, Oppitz U, Thiele W, Ness-Dourdoumas R, Flentje M. Stereotactic radiotherapy of targets in the lung and liver. Strahlenther Onkol 2001; 177:645–655.
37. Hof H, Herfarth KK, Munter M, Hoess A, Motsch J, Wannenmacher M, Debus J. Stereotactic single-dose radiotherapy of stage I non-small-cell lung cancer (NSCLC). Int J Radiat Oncol Biol Phys 2003; 56(2):335–341.
38. Wong JW, Sharpe MB, Jaffray DA, Kini VR, Robertson JM, Stromberg JS, Martinez AA. The use of active breathing control (ABC) to reduce margin for breathing motion. Int J Radiat Oncol Biol Phys 1999; 44(4):911–919.
39. Dawson LA, Brock KK, Kazanjian S, Fitch D, et al. The reproducibility of organ position using active breathing control (ABC) during liver radiotherapy. Int J Radiat Oncol Biol Phys 2001; 51:1410–1421.
40. Whyte RI, Crownover R, Murphy MJ, Martin DP, et al. Stereotactic radiosurgery for lung tumors: preliminary report of a phase I trial. Ann Thorac Surg 2003; 75:1097–1101.
41. Yenice KM, Lovelock DM, Hunt MA, et al. CT image-guided intensity-modulated therapy for paraspinal tumors using stereotactic immobilization. Int J Radiat Oncol Biol Phys 2003; 55:583–593.
42. Wulf J, Haedinger U, Oppitz U, Thiele W, Flentje M. Impact of target reproducibility on tumor dose in stereotactic radiotherapy of targets in the lung and liver. Radiother Oncol 2003; 66:141–150.

43. Hara R, Itami J, Kondo T, Aruga T, Abe Y, et al. Stereotactic single high dose irradiation of lung tumors under respiratory gating. Radiother Oncol 2002; 63:159–163.
44. Nagata Y, Negoro Y, Aoki T, et al. Clinical outcomes of 3D conformal hypo-fractionated single high dose radiotherapy for one or two lung tumors using a stereotactic body frame. Int J Radiat Oncol Biol Phys 2002; 52(4):1041–1046.
45. Fukumoto S, Shirato H, Shimizu S, Ogura S, Onimaru R, et al. Small volume image-guided radiotherapy using hypofractionated, coplanar and noncoplanar multiple fields for patients with inoperable stage I nonsmall cell lung carcinomas. Cancer 2002; 95:1546–1553.
46. Nakagawa K, Aoki Y, Tago M, Terahara A, Ohtomo K. Megavoltage CT-assisted stereotactic radiosurgery for thoracic tumors: original research in the treatment of thoracic neoplasms. Int J Radiat Oncol Biol Phys 2000; 48(2):449–457.
47. Van't Riet A, Mak ACA, Moerland MA, Elders LH, Van der Zee W. A conformation number to quantify the degree of conformality in brachytherapy and external beam irradiation: application to the prostate. Int J Radiat Oncol Biol Phys 1997; 37(3):731–736.
48. Haedinger U, Thiele W, Wulf J. Extracranial stereotactic radiotherapy: evaluation of PTV coverage and dose conformity. Z Med Phys 2002; 12:221–229.
49. Engelsman M, Damen EMF, Koken PW, van't Veld AA, van Ingen KM, Mijnheer BJ. Impact of simple tissue inhomogeneity correction algorithms on conformal radiotherapy of lung tumors. Radiother Oncol 2001; 60:299–309.
50. Engelsman M, Remeijer P, van Herk M, Lebesque JV, et al. Field size reduction enable Iso-NTCP escalation of tumor control probability for irradiation of lung tumors. Int J Radiat Oncol Biol Phys 2001; 51(5):1290–1298.
51. Lee S, Choi EK, Park HJ, et al. Stereotactic body frame based fractionated radiosurgery on consecutive days for primary or metastatic tumors in the lung. Lung Cancer 2003; 40:309–315.
52. Kuriyama K, Onishi H, Sano N, et al. A new irradiation unit constructed of self-moving gantry-CT and linac. Int J Radiat Oncol Biol Phys 2003; 55:428–435.
53. Onishi H, Kuriyama K, Komiyama T, et al. CT evaluation of patient deep inspiration self-breath-holding: how precisely can patients reproduce the tumor position in the absence of respiratory monitoring devices? Med Phys 2003; 30(6):1183–1187.
54. Onishi H, Kuriyama K, Komiyama T, Tanaka S, et al. A new irradiation system for lung cancer combining linear accelerator, computed tomography, patient self-breath-holding and patient directed beam control without respiratory monitoring devices. Int J Radiat Oncol Biol Phys 2003; 56:14–20.
55. Haedinger U, Krieger T, Flentje M, Wulf J. Influence of calculation model on dose distribution in stereotactic radiotherapy for pulmonary targets. Int J Radiat Oncol Biol Phys 2005; 61(1):239–249.
56. Wulf J, Haedinger U, Oppitz U, Thiele W, Mueller G, Flentje M. Stereotactic radiotherapy for primary lung cancer and pulmonary metastases: a noninvasive treatment approach in medically inoperable patients. Int J Radiat Oncol Biol Phys 2004; 60(1):186–196.

10

Prostate Tumors

Raymond Miralbell

Servei de Radio-oncologia, Instituto Oncológico Teknon, Barcelona, Spain and Service de Radio-oncologie, Hôpitaux Universitaires, Geneva, Switzerland

Meritxell Mollà and Lluis Escudé

Servei de Radio-oncologia, Instituto Oncológico Teknon, Barcelona, Spain

Dirk Verellen, Guy Soete, and Guy Storme

Department of Radiotherapy, AZV-UB, Brussels, Belgium

THE TEKNON EXPERIENCE

INTRODUCTION AND RATIONALE

Rationale for Dose Escalation in Curative Treatment of Localized Prostate Cancer

Dose escalation above 70 Gy may prove beneficial in prostate cancer radiotherapy (RT) (1–3). The results of curative RT performed in the 1970s and 1980s, assessed with sequential PSA tests, have shown a higher than previously expected treatment failure rate (40–50%) when delivering a dose below 70 Gy (the recommended dose at that time) (1). Dose escalation studies performed at Memorial Sloan Kettering Cancer Center (2) and at M.D. Anderson Hospital (3) have shown an improved outcome with doses 78 Gy and above. Patients with poorly differentiated tumors (i.e., Gleason scores 7–10) and/or perineural invasion in the biopsy specimen are at higher than average risk for local failure and may benefit most from the administration of a high dose to the tumor (4–6).

Optimization of Target Repositioning Reproducibility May Lead to Treatment Volume Reduction

In order to deliver high doses to the prostate, tight margins around the target are necessary to spare critical organs such as the rectum and the bladder. The urethra, though contained within the target volume, may also be a dose-limiting organ if postirradiation stricture is to be considered (7). A significant reduction of the irradiated target volume may facilitate delivery of a higher, more effective dose, while at the same time reducing treatment side effects. However, suboptimal reproducibility of daily treatment setup and random internal organ motion (8–11) may defeat any attempt to reduce the usually generous safety margins around the clinical target volume (CTV) (12). Improving patient repositioning and reducing random prostate shifts, largely due to rectal volume changes, may help to tighten the margins around the CTV enough to allow further dose reduction to critical structures.

Non-Uniform Tumor Cell Distribution Within the Prostate

Largest tumor clonogen clusters are preferentially located in the peripheral zone or in the central zone (base) of the prostate, especially in more advanced local tumor stages and/or in high (i.e., 7–10) Gleason scores (13). Thus, a heterogeneous density distribution of tumor cells within the prostate supports the notion of an intentionally inhomogeneous dose distribution to deliver a relatively higher dose to the high-density tumor bearing areas and relatively lower doses to areas with smaller tumor foci (e.g., transitional zone). Progress in imaging (e.g., endorectal spectroscopic magnetic resonance, ^{11}C-choline or -acetate positron emission tomography) may help to further improve definition of local tumor extent within the prostate (14–16).

Radiobiology of Prostate Cancer: Hypofractionation

In RT, one of the main arguments for delivering a treatment in many fractions is that late sequelae are generally more sensitive than tumor control to changes in fractionation. Thus, delivering the treatment in a large number of small daily fractions (e.g., 1.8–2 Gy/fraction) generally spares late-responding tissue (able to repair sublethal damage between fractions) more than the tumor (unable to repair sublethal damage between fractions). The α/β ratio is a parameter that purportedly defines the sensitivity of each tissue (normal or tumoral) to changes in treatment fractionation (17). A low α/β ratio (2–4 Gy) implies a high sensitivity to changes in fractionation. In general, tumors are characterized by large α/β ratios (>8 Gy).

Prostate tumors, however, can be considered relatively exceptional with regard to their fractionation sensitivity. Prostate cancer cells have a long doubling time (42 days median potential doubling time, range 15–170 days) and an effective repair of sublethal radiation damage at low dose per fraction (18). Indeed, combined analysis of patient outcome after external beam radiotherapy or brachytherapy has recently led to the conclusion that prostate cancer is characterized by a low α/β ratio (i.e., 1.5 Gy and 0.8–2.2 Gy confidence interval), lower than that of most tumors or even of the late-responding normal tissues surrounding the tumor: the rectum and the bladder (i.e., α/β ratio $= 4$ Gy) (18–20). Thus, large treatment fractions (hypofractionation) may increase the tumor cell killing effect. Several authors have reported their respective experiences with doses per fraction above 2 Gy (2.5, 2.75, and 3.13 Gy) in prostate cancer. They all found the treatment to be efficient and well tolerated (21–23).

In summary, if the above observations are substantiated, hypofractionated treatments may have the potential to either increase tumor control for a given level of late complications or decrease normal tissue complications for a given level of tumor control. Hypofractionation in radiotherapy may not only be biologically sound, but also economically advantageous (by increasing availability of treatment slots in each department) and may also improve patient convenience (by reducing the number of treatment sessions).

HYPOFRACTIONATED BOOST WITH INTENSITY MODULATED X-RAY BEAMS UNDER STEREOTACTIC CONDITIONS: A PILOT STUDY

Preliminary Considerations

Clinical data suggest that 64 Gy in 32 daily "standard" 2 Gy fractions can cure residual or relapsing microscopic local disease after postprostatectomy biochemical failure (24). This notion can be extrapolated to the curative treatment of gross disease, by prescribing a similar dose level (i.e., 64 Gy) to areas of potentially microscopic foci in the transitional zone (near the urethra), while reserving higher dose levels to boost gross tumor-bearing regions (peripheral and/or central zones, and/or seminal vesicles) with >80 Gy total dose to reach the desired local cure. Indeed, two fractions of 5, 6, 7, or 8 Gy to the tumor-bearing region in addition to 64 Gy in 2 Gy daily fractions of standard RT to the whole prostate and seminal vesicles are equivalent to 82, 88, 96, and 104 Gy of standard fractionated RT, respectively (α/β for prostate cancer $= 2$ Gy). Thus, a local control probability well above 80% might be expected (18).

Such a hypofractionated treatment approach has been applied since June 2000 at the University Hospital of Geneva to treat patients with non-metastatic, high-risk (e.g., perineural invasion and/or Gleason 8–10) tumors. High dose rate (HDR) brachytherapy with temporary open MRI-guided iridium implants have been used to escalate the dose in the boost region. Through March 2004, 64 such patients have been implanted with a low incidence of moderate acute toxicity and no significant severe late side effects (25). About 19, 21, and 24 patients were treated with two fractions of 6, 7, and 8 Gy, respectively, to the boost volume. Unfortunately, the coverage of the prostatic primary tumor volume with brachytherapy needles has not been always optimal in the Geneva series, especially in very large prostates or when the tumor infiltrated the base of the gland or the seminal vesicles.

Intensity modulated radiotherapy (IMRT) under stereotactic conditions to boost exclusively the tumor-bearing region, as defined by endorectal MRI, may be an interesting alternative to the above brachytherapy technique. Hypofractionated IMRT has the additional advantage of improving tumor coverage and reducing costs, pain, and time compared with HDR brachytherapy. Indeed, neither anesthesia, hospitalization, nor major pain relievers (morphine) are necessary with IMRT.

We performed a study aiming to assess feasibility, tolerance, and outcome of patients (with non-metastatic prostate cancer) treated according to a dose escalation protocol to the boost region with IMRT under stereotactic conditions. The preliminary results of this study are presented below.

Clinical Material

From June 2001 through May 2003, a dose escalation pilot study for prostate cancer with high-precision RT was undertaken at Centro Médico Teknon (CMT), Barcelona. Treatment was delivered with a commercially available extracranial stereotactic repositioning system (ExacTrac, Brain-LAB A.G., Heimstetten, Germany) and 6 MV X-ray beams IMRT with a micromultileaf collimator-based linear accelerator (Novalis, BrainLAB A.G., Heimstetten, Germany). Forty-three patients were included in the study. The distribution of patients according to clinical stage, Gleason score, and blood PSA level at diagnosis are presented in Table 1. The patients have been followed for a median time of 19 months (range, 9–34 months).

Table 1 Patient Distribution According to Clinical Stage, Gleason Score, and PSA at Diagnosis

Stage	$T1_c$	15 pts
	$T2_{a-c}$	11 pts
	$T3_{a,b}$	17 pts
Gleason	4–6	21 pts
	7–10	22 pts
PSA at diagnosis	<10 ng/mL	22 pts
	10–20 ng/mL	14 pts
	>20 ng/mL	07 pts

Treatment Description

Neoadjuvant full androgen deprivation with leuprolide and bicalutamide was given to 26 patients (those with a PSA at diagnosis >15 ng/mL and/or those with a total Gleason score >7) for a duration of 6–24 months, with radiotherapy starting one to three months after the first day of hormonal blockade. Three patients were referred for RT after orchidectomy.

The first part of the radiation treatment included conventional fractionated 3D conformal external RT or IMRT (Fig. 1). The prostate and seminal vesicles (CTV1) were to receive 64 Gy in 2 Gy daily fractions if the risk of nodal involvement (according to Ref. 26) was <15% (22 patients). If nodal risk was >15%, pelvic nodes, in addition to the prostate and seminal vesicles, were treated with 50.4 Gy (in 1.8 Gy daily fractions) followed by a volume reduction up to a total tumor dose of 64.4 Gy to CTV1 (21 patients). Thirty-two patients were treated with 15 MV X-rays from a Clinac 23-EX (Varian, Associates, Palo Alto, California, U.S.A.) in the supine position without special immobilization devices. Eleven patients, all presenting with low-risk disease, were treated to CTV1 with 6 MV X-rays from the Novalis linear accelerator using IMRT or dynamic arc techniques. These patients were immobilized in a customized vacuum body cast and repositioned with ExacTrac as described below.

All patients received a final boost to a reduced prostate volume using IMRT under stereotactic conditions (Fig. 1). The reduced prostate boost

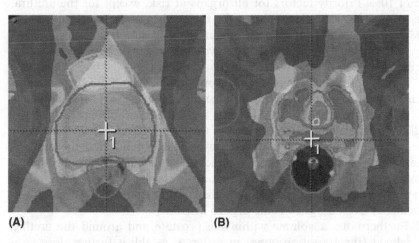

(A) **(B)**

Figure 1 Dose distribution of an intensity modulation radiotherapy plan in the axial central plane of the planning target volume (PTV). (**A**) 64–64.4 Gy delivered to the prostate and seminal vesicles (PTV1); (**B**) 10–16 Gy boost delivered to a reduced horseshoe-shaped volume (the prostate peripheral zone) (PTV2). Dose distribution is given in percent values and is displayed in color bands. The yellow crosses in the figures represent the treatment isocenters for PTV1 and PTV2, respectively. (*See color insert.*)

volume (CTV2) included the peripheral and central zone tumor-bearing regions, together with the seminal vesicles if involved (or the prostate excluding the urethra if massive involvement of the gland). The CTV2 was expanded with a surrounding margin of 3 mm in order to define a PTV2. Two fractions of 5, 6, 7, and 8 Gy each were delivered with a time interval of 3 to 7 days between fractions to 6, 7, 7, and 23 patients, respectively. This represents a biological equivalent tumor dose (in 2 Gy fractions and α/β ratio $= 2$ Gy) of 82, 88, 96, and 104 Gy, respectively.

Boost (PTV2) Treatment Planning

A standard single-isocenter seven-field coplanar technique was most frequently selected. This was the optimal technique for achieving the "doughnut" or "horseshoe" shaped dose distributions around the urethra (localized with a urinary catheter at simulation) needed to correctly treat the relatively complex PTV2 (Fig. 1). In order to reduce the overall treatment time a dynamic MLC IMRT technique was preferred, rather than a static "step and shoot" IMRT technique.

Dose constraints were established to optimize the dose distribution for the PTV2 and the organs at risk (i.e., bladder, rectum, femoral heads, periprostatic neurovascular bundles, and, most of all, the urethra). The rectum was set to receive a maximum dose of 80% of the prescribed dose but to no more than 20–50% of the volume. The urethra was set to receive a maximum dose of 10%. Priority factors for all organs at risk, except for the urethra, were set to 50%. The priority factor for the urethra was set to 100%. These values were used as a starting point but often had to be modified according to the results of the calculation cycles in order to optimize the dose distribution.

The femoral heads were distant from the PTV2 and did not present a major dosimetric problem. Dose–volume histograms (DVHs) requirements were thus easily met. Nor were bladder and rectum problematical, as only small portions of their volumes received the highest doses (those lying close to the PTV2). Both periprostatic neurovascular bundles and the urethra, however, are so small that their volumes were included in the penumbra surrounding PTV2. Hence, uncertainties in target repositioning might have strongly influenced overall dose distribution, potentially resulting in a significant overdosage to some organs at risk.

Furthermore, a volume within the prostate and around the urethra was defined (the transition zone) in order to establish further dose constraints that could help to improve the dose gradient between the PTV2 and the urethra. Frequently, the size of the transition zone was so reduced that such an optimal dose gradient was not obtained. In these cases a trade-off between PTV2 dose distribution homogeneity and the dose to the urethra had to be found.

Treatment Planning Quality Assurance Procedure

After physician approval, treatment plans were transferred to the treatment network in order to test the procedure on a plastic stacked slab phantom (PMMA) with the selected beam fluences, gantry angles, collimator angles, and monitor units. Only the position of the isocenter and the monitor unit scaling were modified. The aim was to compare dosimetric measurements with calculations obtained by the treatment planning with the same phantom system. The agreement between in-phantom measurement and calculation was assumed to be applicable to patient treatment.

Two types of measurements were performed: a film (Kodak EDR) dose distribution on a coronal plane and a point dose measurement with a small volume (0.125 cc) ionization chamber at a defined depth in the beam central axis. In both scenarios, only the composite plan corresponding to the sum of all the fields was checked.

The film dose distribution was compared with the corresponding dose distribution obtained with the treatment planning system and analyzed with an in-house computer program. After automatic registration of both dose distributions, isodose curves and dose profiles were plotted and compared. A "gamma index" was calculated according to Low et al. (27) and Depuydt et al. (28) helping to standardize comparison criteria based on "dose differences" in low-dose gradient areas and "distance to agreement" (DTA) in high-dose gradient regions. Tolerance values were established to 3% for the dose difference and 2 mm for the DTA. For the point dose measurements the tolerance was set to ±4%.

In an earlier phase of our prostate treatment program, the individual fields at 0° incidence angle were also checked and measured. This helped us to gain an insight into the dynamic behavior of the MLC measurements of individual beams impinging perpendicularly on a flat surface of an homogeneous medium (less dependent on the patient or phantom-geometry).

Patient Immobilization

ExacTrac was used to reposition all patients for the final high-dose boost (CTV2) and 11 low-risk patients treated with Novalis to CTV1. The repositioning procedure with ExacTrac starts with immobilizing the patient in a customized vacuum body cast. Five to seven metallic infrared (IR) reflecting markers are asymmetrically taped to the skin of the abdomen (Fig. 2). Starting from the planning CT, the position of the isocenter with regard to the IR markers is calculated by the planning system. Before each treatment session the markers are placed back on the patient. Their spatial arrangement is detected by a pair of IR cameras mounted to the treatment room's ceiling to reproduce the same coordinates when repositioning the patients for daily treatment.

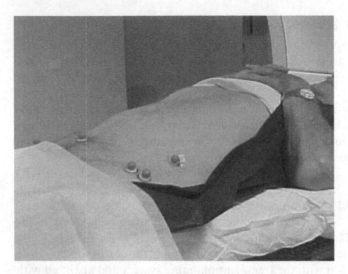

Figure 2 Immobilization and stereotactic repositioning system (ExacTrac). The patient is immobilized with a customized vacuum body cast and is repositioned with several infrared reflecting metallic markers taped to the skin of the abdomen.

In our study, patients were requested to void their bladders immediately before simulation and before each treatment fraction. To further limit target motion and to help to improve file target defining process in the simulation CT, a magnetic resonance (MR)-based endorectal probe was used for the CTV2 simulation and treatment (Figs. 3 and 4). Sodium phosphate enemas were used to evacuate the rectum the night before and again one to two hours before each procedure. In order to reduce anxiety and prevent or alleviate potential painful rectal spasms during the simulation or treatment intervals, alprazolam 0.5 mg per os was prescribed in later patients. After introducing the probe in the rectum, 60 cc were introduced with a syringe. The inflated probe was then gently pulled toward the anus. Patients were then fitted in their immobilization casts, skin metallic markers were fixed on their respective spots, and the IR guided setup was undertaken.

Preliminary Results: Feasibility, Treatment Tolerance, and Outcome

Patient compliance with treatment was optimal. All 43 patients completed treatment as planned. Few patients complained of anal–rectal pain or spasms while on treatment with the inflated rectal balloon.

   Urinary and lower gastro-intestinal (GI) acute effects were scored according to the RTOG/EORTC scoring system (Table 2) (29). Tables 3 and 4 show the observed urinary and lower GI acute toxicity scores for

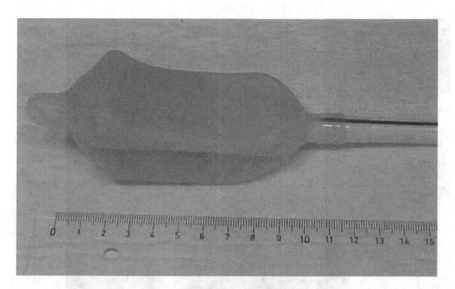

Figure 3 MR endorectal probe used to reduce the internal organ motion of the prostate during extracranial stereotactic radiotherapy and to help to optimize image registration between the endorectal MR at diagnosis and the simulation CT.

all patients according to the delivered boost dose. Acute toxicity was scored every week during treatment and five to six weeks and again three months after treatment completion.

Acute urinary toxicity was minimal (grade 1) to moderate (grade 2) for most patients. A correlation between acute urinary toxicity score and dose escalation was not observed. Acute lower GI toxicity was minimal (grade 1) or moderate (grade 2) in more than one-third of patients with no relation to dose escalation. It is noteworthy that no acute lower GI toxicity was observed among the 11 patients treated with Novalis-IMRT to CTV1 and receiving the highest boost dose (2×8 Gy) to CTV2. This compared favorably with patients receiving the same 2×8 Gy-boost after being treated to CTV1 with a non-IMRT technique. Almost half of them presented grade 1 or 2 acute lower GI toxicity.

Late urinary and lower GI toxicities were scored after a minimum six-month post-treatment follow-up interval. Scoring was done according to the SOMA and to the EORTC/RTOG systems (Table 5) in order to grade urinary and lower GI toxicities, respectively (29,30). So far only moderate late toxicity scores have been obtained for both urinary and lower GI morbidities. Five patients (12%) presented with late urinary grades 1–2 toxicity (Table 6) while 13 (30%) presented with late lower GI grades 1–2 toxicity (Table 7).

A systematic assessment of lower GI toxicity was designed as part of the study protocol. At 18–24 months postradiotherapy (the peak risk for late

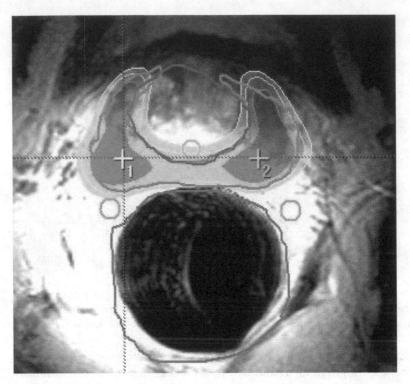

Figure 4 Dose distribution overlying the axial central plane of an endorectal MR image of the prostate containing the PTV2 (bilateral prostatic peripheral zone). Isodose bands of 100% or above (*red*), 90–100% (*yellow*), and 80–90% (*green*) are displayed. (*See color insert.*)

rectal toxicity), patients are requested to undergo recto-sigmoidoscopy with an assessment of the rectal mucosa and scoring of erythema and/or of telangiectasia. In addition, random biopsies of the normal rectal mucosa, or of suspected areas of proctitis are undertaken. Functional testing with an endorectal barostat is also performed in order to assess for potential passive mechanical changes due to fibrosis and to evaluate changes in sensitivity to rectal wall distension.

So far, 16 patients have undergone a rectosygmoidoscopy with 10 grade 0, three grade 1, and three grade 2 RTOG clinical toxicity scores (see above). Rectal mucosa was normal in five patients without late rectal toxicity (grade 0). Erythema was observed in three and two patients with grade 1 and grade 2 late rectal RTOG toxicity, respectively. Grade 1 telangiectasia (focal and isolated) was observed in five patients with no clinical late rectal toxicity. Grade 2 telangiectasia was observed in one patient suffering from grade 2 (2×8 Gy boost) late rectal RTOG toxicity.

Table 2 RTOG/EORTC Acute Radiation Morbidity Scoring System

Urinary	
Grade 1	– Frequency of urination twice pretreatment habit
	– Dysuria, urgency not requiring medication
	– Incontinence not requiring sanitary pads
Grade 2	– Frequency of urination less frequent than every hour
	– Dysuria, urgency, bladder spasms requiring non-narcotic medication
	– Incontinence requiring medication or pads
Grade 3	– Frequency of urination hourly or more frequently
	– Dysuria, pain or spasms requiring narcotics
	– Gross hematuria
Lower GI	
Grade 1	– Increased frequency or change in quality of bowel habits not requiring medication
	– Rectal or anal discomfort not requiring medication
	– Urgency not requiring medication
Grade 2	– Diarrhea requiring medication
	– Mucous or blood discharge or soiling not necessitating sanitary pads
	– Rectal or anal pain, urgency, requiring medication

Source: From Ref. 29.

Although biochemical relapse has not yet been observed in any of our patients, much longer follow-up will be required before conclusions can be drawn regarding the potential value of IMRT dose escalation in the curative treatment for prostate cancer.

Quality Assessment on Patient and Target Repositioning Reproducibility

In order to simulate repositioning reproducibility a second pelvic CT, under simulation conditions, was performed before the last boost fraction (usually 10–15 days after the first CT used for boost simulation). Prostate repositioning

Table 3 Acute Urinary Toxicity According to Boost Dose (EORTC Score)

Dose (Gy)	G-0	G-1	G-2	G-3
5	0	4	2	0
6	2	2	3	0
7	1	2	4	0
8[a]	5(3)	7(3)	10(4)	1(1)

[a]11/22 patients, in brackets, treated with IMRT.

Table 4 Acute Rectal Toxicity According to Boost Dose (EORTC Score)

Dose (Gy)	G-0	G-1	G-2
5	2	2	2
6	4	2	1
7	3	2	2
8[a]	17(11)	4(0)	2(0)

[a]11/22 patients, in brackets, treated with IMRT to CTV1.

was assessed, first, after CT-to-CT registration of the stereotaxic IR reflecting metallic body markers (to simulate the setup reproducibility with ExacTrac) (Fig. 5) and, second, after CT-to-CT registration of the pelvic bony structures (to simulate for potential further improvement of patient repositioning with pelvic bone registration as it is performed by the Novalis Body system from BrainLAB, not used for patient treatment in our study). A study has been recently reported assessing prostate and rectal probe repositioning in 22

Table 5 Late Radiation Morbidity Scoring System

Urinary (SOMA):	
Grade 1	– Occasional dysuria
	– Occasional hematuria
	– Microscopic hematuria
	– Occasional use of incontinence pads
	– Occasional medication for dysuria
Grade 2	– Intermittent dysuria
	– Intermittent macroscopic hematuria
	– Intermittent use of incontinence pads
	– Regular non-narcotic medication for dysuria
Grade 3	– Persistent or intense dysuria
	– Incomplete obstruction
	– Persistent macroscopic hematuria with clots
	– Regular use of incontinence pads
	– Regular narcotic medication for dysuria
Lower GI (RTOG/EORTC):	
Grade 1	– Slight rectal discharge or bleeding
	– Urgency, anal pain, soiling
Grade 2	– Excessive rectal mucus or bleeding requiring medical treatment
	– Urgency, anal pain, or soiling requiring medication
Grade 3	– Bleeding requiring surgery or formolinization
	– Obstruction

Source: From Refs. 29, 30.

Table 6 Late Urinary Toxicity According to Boost Dose (SOMA)

Dose (Gy)	G-0	G-1	G-2
5	6	0	0
6	7	0	0
7	6	1	0
8	19	2	2

patients treated under optimal immobilization conditions according to the present protocol (31).

The shifts between the center of mass of the prostate in the first CT and the center of mass of the prostate in the second CT were measured in the three axes: latero-lateral (X), antero-posterior (Y), and cranio-caudal (Z). The mean and standard deviation (SD) of the displacements in the three axes of the prostate's center of mass were calculated for all patients. This measurements helped to estimate margins around the CTV2 to define an ideal PTV using the model described by McKenzie et al. (32) with the following formula:

$$\text{CTV} \rightarrow \text{PTV margin width} = 2.5 \sum + \beta \left(\sigma - \sigma_p \right)$$

in which "Σ" is the SD of the individual displacements of the prostate center of mass; "σ" the random error (takes in account organ motion and penumbra) and "σ_p" the SD describing the width of the beam penumbra (3.2 mm); "β" is the penumbra correction coefficient that depends on the number of beams used to treat a spherical volume in order to deliver at least 95% of the dose to the CTV (0.52 for the transverse plane, and 1.64 in the cranio-caudal direction for a six non-parallel and opposed field arrangement).

As mentioned above, 11 patients were also treated with Novalis for the first part of the treatment (64 Gy in 2 Gy daily fractions to CTV1). They underwent weekly resimulation CT scans on treatment position (average, six CTs for each patient). All of these patients were treated without an endorectal balloon during the first treatment phase. Assessing the displacements of the CTV1 center of mass with CT-to-CT fusion of the stereotaxic IR reflecting metallic body markers and with a CT-to-CT registration of the pelvic bony structures, allowed to assess the weekly repositioning reproducibility

Table 7 Late Rectal Toxicity According to Boost Dose (RTOG Score)

Dose (Gy)	G-0	G-1	G-2
5	5	1	0
6	5	1	1
7	4	3	0
8	16	5	2

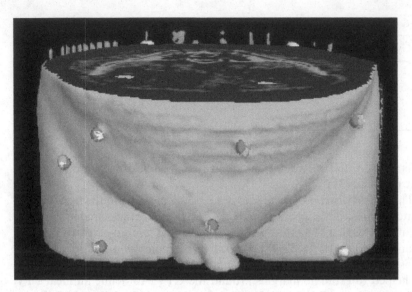

Figure 5 Digital volumetric reconstruction to simulate the setup reproducibility with ExacTrac. Infrared marker based registration between the CT at simulation (*red*) and the CT while on treatment (*green*) performed to assess target repositioning quality. (*See color insert.*)

and to estimate the PTV1 margin width for these 11 patients. These results were compared with the repositioning reproducibility and the estimated PTV2 margin width for the 22 patients assessed during the CTV2 treatment period (boost), treated with identical immobilization conditions but with an endorectal balloon to optimally reduce the internal organ motion.

The estimated PTV margins around the prostate, for the 22 patients evaluated under optimal setup conditions (i.e., bone registration and endorectal balloon), were 2.4, 4.3, and 6.4 mm in the latero-lateral, antero-posterior, and cranio-caudal dimensions, respectively. According to the same model, the estimated PTV1 margins around de CTV1 for the 11 patients evaluated under setup conditions involving exclusively bone registration, but not a rectal balloon, were 1.9, 7.6, and 7.4 mm in the latero-lateral, antero-posterior, and cranio-caudal dimensions, respectively. Thus, an optimally positioned rectal balloon significantly reduced the estimated antero-posterior PTV margins around the target from 7.6 mm (without balloon) to 4.3 mm (with balloon), an improvement factor of 1.77.

FINAL COMMENTS AND CONCLUSIONS

Dose escalation above 70 Gy is necessary to improve curative treatment of localized prostate cancer with RT. This is a challenge for radiation oncologists in their search for an optimal treatment of a movable, centrally located, almost spherical target surrounded by dose-limiting critical organs (the rectum, the bladder, and the femoral heads).

Optimal repositioning reproducibility is crucial if the goal is to deliver, via external RT, the highest dose to the tumor while optimally decreasing the treatment volume (i.e., reducing the safety margins around the target). This may reduce the dose to the organs at risk and improve normal tissue tolerance. In the present study, under optimal setup conditions (i.e., bone registration and rectal balloon), estimated PTV safety margins around the CTV were roughly 2, 4, and 6 mm in the latero-lateral, antero-posterior, and cranio-caudal directions, respectively. This is a significant reduction compared to the usually recommended margins of >10 mm, with standard immobilization approaches based on skin markers or tattoos. Furthermore, even after optimal setup with bone registration, the use of a rectal balloon improved repositioning in the antero-posterior axis by a factor of 1.77.

Significant treatment volume reduction in the present study (compared to more standard radiotherapy approaches for prostate cancer) may explain the relative low incidence of acute or late toxicity at the urinary and/or lower GI levels. Among the 43 patients fully evaluable for late lower GI tolerance, 13 patients (30%) presented moderate grades 1–2 late toxicity. This contrasts with a worse tolerance among 175 patients treated in Geneva since 1999 with 74–78.4 Gy standard fractionated conformal external RT and with a minimum of eight-month follow-up. A 45% incidence of grades 1–2 late rectal toxicity was observed among those patients (unpublished data).

The highest dose may be preferentially delivered in areas of the prostate with the largest number of tumor cells (e.g., the prostatic peripheral zone). Thus, a non-uniform dose distribution within the prostate may well be a treatment optimization tool if the highest dose is delivered to areas at highest risk for failure. Progress in imaging (e.g., endorectal MRI with or without spectroscopy and PET with C11 acetate or F18 choline) may help to better define these areas at risk within the prostate and improve targeting strategies in the future. Furthermore, reducing the prostatic treatment volume by purposely underdosing areas of potentially lower tumor burden (e.g., transitional zone of the prostate) allows the risk of potential urethral damage to be kept to a minimum level during the delivery of the hypofractionated boost.

Prostate cancer cells may have more chance of surviving low-dose fractions (i.e., 2 Gy or less) than high-dose fractions (i.e., 4 Gy or more). Thus, if fractionation schedules in prostate cancer are to be adapted to take into account radiobiological considerations, large fractions are likely to play a role in more effective curative strategies. Some, however, cautiously question this approach by suggesting that the benefit derived from reoxygenation of hypoxic cancer foci between fractions may be lost if few large-dose fractions are used (33). In the present study, the administration of the first 64–64.4 Gy in 32–35 daily fractions of 1.8–2 Gy, preceded in the less favorable cases with androgen blockade, might have helped to decrease the problem of hypoxia by reducing significantly the tumor volume before the delivery of the final hypofractionated boost.

Although all patients in the present study have their disease under biochemical control, longer follow-up will be required before cure rates can be evaluated. Caution is called for, especially considering the tight PTV boost margins used, that may have underdosed part of the CTV2 volume. Only time will tell whether or not this underdosage has a negative influence on local control. The choice of the tight 3 mm margins, however, was based on the need to protect the urethra, which might not have always been possible with larger margins. The present quality assessment indicates that margins of 4 mm minimum in the transverse plane are needed under optimal setup conditions.

THE AZ-VUB EXPERIENCE

INTRODUCTION AND RATIONALE

Radiotherapy is one of the major treatment modalities for cancer of the prostate. Increased dose levels are known to significantly improve treatment outcome but require specialized techniques to avoid important and sometimes permanent side effects to bladder and rectum. The AZ-VUB has adopted three distinctive measures to avoid these complications with the introduction of the Novalis system (BrainLAB, A.G., Heimstetten, Germany) for stereotactic body radiation therapy (SBRT). Application of laparoscopic lymphadenectomy allows for omission of prophylactic irradiation of the pelvic nodes for the majority of cases. Application of conformal radiation therapy (CRT) techniques, such as dynamic field shaping arc or IMRT and accurate target positioning by image-guided radiation therapy (IGRT) techniques, allow for a dose delivery with the highest possible precision (34–37). A preliminary follow-up based on the first 100 patients treated showed an almost complete absence of acute digestive complications. The use of reduced treatment volumes does not seem to compromise outcome as illustrated by the two-year biochemical control rate of 96%.

TREATMENT PROTOCOL AND IRRADIATION TECHNIQUE

The current protocol is limited to patients that present with a localized curative disease (T1-3N0M0) (38). For this patient cohort three prognostic factors are important for the appropriate choice of treatment modality: T-stage, PSA, and Gleason score (39–42). Based on these criteria a classification into three groups is possible. Based on somewhat differing data from literature (2,3,7,43,44), these classes have been defined as follows at the AZ-VUB: good prognosis (combination of PSA ≤ 10 ng/mL, stage T1-2 and Gleason score 2-6), bad prognosis (PSA ≥ 20 ng/mL combined with stage T3-4 or Gleason score ≥ 7), and intermediate prognosis (all other cases). For the cohort with good prognosis, local treatment, or in case of elderly patients, a wait-and-see approach are considered adequate after discussion with the patient provided a close follow-up schedule is applied. Those patients from the intermediate cohort (in particular those with life expectancy of 10 years or more) will be proposed for a local treatment with curative intent. Patients with bad prognosis are treated with loco-regional RT. T3-4 patients from the intermediate and bad prognosis groups will additionally receive hormone therapy (45–47). Local treatment usually consists of surgery or (external) RT at the AZ-VUB. Surgery has the psychological advantage of removal of the tumor, but a recent meta-analysis showed 75% occurrence of impotence (50). Radiotherapy has the advantage of being non-invasive, yet suffers from other disadvantages. Acute complications might occur such as irritation of bladder, and (depending on the irradiate bowel volume) abdominal cramps and diarrhea. In the long term, RT might be the cause of chronic radiocystitis, erectile disfunction, and chronic radiorectitis. In recent years it has been shown that with radiation doses of up to 78 Gy a higher biochemical control can be achieved compared to conventional dose levels of 70 Gy, especially for the intermediate prognosis cohort (3,43,48–50). Needless to say that with these higher doses limitation of the irradiated volume of healthy tissue becomes more important (3,51–53).

With the introduction of CRT, and IGRT, the AZ-VUB has attempted to optimize the irradiation technique for a complication-free prostate treatment with curative intent. Based on the above rationale the low-risk (PSA ≤ 10 and T1-2 and Gleason 2–6) and high–risk (PSA > 20 and T3-4 or Gleason 7–10) patients will be treated with 70 Gy, whereas the intermediate cohort receives 78 Gy. Three distinctive measures can be identified: limitation of the irradiated volume, application of CRT or IMRT, and high accurate target positioning or IGRT.

a. *Limitation of the irradiated volume.* Previously, most patients received a 50 Gy prophylactic irradiation of the pelvic nodes, with known problems such as abdominal pain and diarrhea. Additionally, a 20 Gy boost was administered to the prostate and seminal vesicles. Currently, based on the threefold classification T-PSA-Gleason, the probability of microscopic disease of pelvic nodes and seminal vesicles can be assessed (54,55). For those patients that present a low risk (i.e., ≤10% for the AZ-VUB) prophylactic irradiation will be omitted. A laparoscopic lymphadenectomy will be suggested for those patients with a risk that exceeds 10%. When the "No" status is confirmed, the prophylactic pelvic irradiation is omitted and the seminal vesicles are not included in the irradiated volume when the risk of microscopic involvement is lower than 10%. When the latter is not the case, only the proximal half of the seminal vesicles will be included in the CTV most patients present with T1-2 tumors of which is known that the possible involvement is limited to this area (56).

b. *IGRT*. Based on a three-step positioning study with the Exac-Trac/Novalis BODY system (see previous chapter), the PTV margins have been adapted to the precision that can be realized with the different positioning techniques. All prostate patients are positioned with the stereoscopic X-ray system and based on the previous studies (34,35,37) the following margins are being applied: (1) For patient positioning on bony structures (fusion of X-ray images and DRRs) a 6 mm margin latero-lateral, and 10 mm antero-posterior and cranio-caudal. (2) For patients with implanted radio-opaque markers a 5 mm margin is applied in the antero-posterior and cranio-caudal direction, whereas a 3 mm margin in left–right direction is used. Again, the IGRT will help to reduce the irradiated volume.

c. *Irradiation technique*. To obtain a dose distribution true to the shape of the PTV, two techniques possible with the Novalis system are applied at the AZ-VUB. Depending on the absence or presence of concavities, respectively, dynamic field shaping arc or IMRT are used (37). The former consists of one coplanar arc of which the leaves dynamically adapt to the shape of the PTV during rotation of the arc. In many cases the leaves showing over-lap with the rectum at gantry position 90° and 270° are manually retracted to the border of the rectum using beams-eye-view to fulfill the dose limitations to the rectum. The IMRT technique consisting of five non-opposing beams is explained in more detail in a previous chapter on Novalis. In the AZ-VUB experience (actual 180 patients treated, October 2003) only five required IMRT to meet the requirements with respect to toxic rectum dose. The rectal dose constraints are a maximum of 74 Gy to the entire volume of the rectum, less than 70 Gy to one-quarter and less than 65 Gy to half of the rectum.

CLINICAL FOLLOW-UP

Presented are preliminary data on the first 100 patients treated with dynamic field shaping arc and IGRT (based on fusion of bony structures, ExacTrac 2.0/Novalis BODY) from May 2000 to October 2002. Follow-up is still short: median follow-up of 12 months (3–29 months). The patient cohort consisted of patients with relative good prognosis (90% T1-2, 73% Gleason

Table 8 Characteristics of the First 100 Patients Treated on the Novalis System at the AZ-VUB

T-stage		Gleason score		PSA (ng/mL)	
1	46	2–6	73	0–4	10
2	44	7	16	>4–10	51
3	8	8–10	6	>10–20	29
4	0			>20	9
Unknown	2	Unknown	5	Unknown	1

2–6) (Table 8). Thirty-four patients underwent lymphadenectomy prior to treatment. For 69 patients, radiotherapy was the unique treatment modality and the 31 remaining cases received (neo-)adjuvant hormonal therapy (27) or presented local recurrence after prostatectomy (4). Sixty-five patients received a 70 Gy total dose, whereas 35 patients (intermediate prognosis) were treated with a 78 Gy total dose. Acute toxicity (occurring the first three months from the treatment start with radiotherapy) was scored using the RTOG/EORTC classification (57). The questionnaire was presented to the patient on the last treatment day, one and four months after treatment. Even unique intake of symptomatic medication was classified as being grade 2. The biochemical control was based on the ASTRO (American Association for Therapeutic Radiology and Oncology) consensus panel (58), which classifies recurrence after three consecutive PSA rises. Due to applicability of this definition for RT patients only, the biochemical analysis was limited to this cohort only (69 patients), whereas the entire group was analyzed for toxicity.

A biochemical control of disease was observed for 96% of the patients treated with radiotherapy alone for two years. PSA dropped from 8.9 ± 4.8 ng/mL (1 SD) preradiotherapy to 1.0 ± 0.5 ng/mL (1 SD) 18 months after finalizing RT. Only a low number of acute digestive complications have been observed and the 12 grade 1 toxicities observed might have been attributed to other causes such as a period of enteritis in the family of the patient or simultaneous use of potential diarrhea stimulating medicaments (Table 9). Three cases of anal pain were observed in this group of 12 patients (a side effect that is not included explicitly in the RTOG.EORTC scoring system). Acute urinary complaints have been reported by 54% of the patients, yet medication was needed for a minority only. All acute side effects had disappeared at control consult four months after termination of RT. No causal relationship has been found between acute side effects and treatment dose. The preliminary nature of the present data does not allow for late side effects and a long-term follow-up is needed. So far, one patient developed a chronic side effect: radiocystitis with macroscopic hematuria. This patient received coagulation and is currently free of complaints.

Table 9 Acute Toxicity Observed on 100 Patients Treated
on the Novalis System at the AZ-VUB

Grade	Digestive	Urinary
0	88	46
1	12	39
2	0	15
3	0	0
4	0	0

Although currently no clear causal relationship between biochemical control and survival has been proven the predictive value with respect to local control and metastasis has been shown (22,59), and PSA allows for an early predictive evaluation of treatment for prostate carcinoma. The 96% biochemical control obtained in this study has to be interpreted as a preliminary result and indeed it has been shown that with increasing follow-up time these figures have a tendency to decrease (60). Typically a slow decreasing progression of the PSA is observed where the nadir is reached after one year or later (61). No consensus has been reached as to which nadir corresponds to disease-free status and values between 0.6 and 1.4 ng/mL have been suggested (62). Nonetheless, a PSA value < 0.5 ng/mL five-year postradiotherapy may not warrant absolute cure (63). Concerning late side effects follow-up is again too short to allow for valid conclusions. Side effects in radiotherapy are generally related to dose and irradiate volume of healthy tissue (64), comorbidity, and an increased risk seems to occur after surgery for diabetics (65,66). Grade 2 acute toxicity (i.e., in need of medication) has been observed in 45–60% of the patients treated conventionally with prophylactic pelvic irradiation, whereas this fraction decreases to 25–30% with conformal irradiation techniques (48,67). Patients at the AZ-VUB have not only been irradiated using CRT techniques but also IGRT has been routinely applied on all patients, which might explain the reported low figure of 15% acute grade 2 side effects. The use of implanted radio-opaque markers for increased image-guided target localization (including internal organ movement) is being investigated at the AZ-VUB of which clinical follow-up is currently on-going.

REFERENCES

1. Hanks GE, Martz KL, Diamond JJ. The effect of dose on local control of prostate cancer. Int J Radiat Oncol Biol Phys 1988; 15:1299–1306.
2. Zelefsky MJ, Leibel SA, Gaudin PB, Kutcher GJ, Fleshner NE, Venkatramen ES, Reuter VE, Fair WR, Ling CC, Fuks Z. Dose escalation with three-dimensional conformal radiation therapy affects the outcome in prostate cancer. Int J Radiat Oncol Biol Phys 1998; 41:491–500.

3. Pollack A, Zagars GK, Starkschall G, Antolak JA, Lee JJ, Huang E, von Eschenbach AC, Kuban DA, Rosen I. Prostate cancer radiation dose response: results of the M.D. Anderson phase III randomized trial. Int J Radiat Oncol Biol Phys 2002; 53:1097–1105.

4. Fiveash JB, Hanks G, Roach M, Wang S, Vigneault E, McLaughlin PW, Sandler HM. 3D conformal radiation therapy (3DCRT) for high grade prostate cancer: a multi-institutional review. Int J Radiat Oncol Biol Phys 2000; 47: 335–342.

5. Vicini FA, Abner A, Baglan KL, Kestin LL, Martinez AA. Defining a dose-response relationship with radiotherapy for prostate cancer: is more really better? Int J Radiat Oncol Biol Phys 2001; 51:1200–1208.

6. Cheung R, Tucker SL, Dong L, Kuban D. Dose-response for biochemical control among high-risk prostate cancer patients after external beam radiotherapy. Int J Radiat Oncol Biol Phys 2003; 56:1234–1240.

7. Zelefsky MJ, Hollister T, Raben A, Matthews S, Wallner KE. Five-year biochemical outcome and toxicity with transperineal CT-planned permanent 1–125 prostate implantation for patients with localized prostate cancer. Int J Radiat Oncol Biol Phys 2000; 47:1261–1266.

8. Lebesque JV, Bruce AM, Kroes APG, Touw A, Shouman T, van Herk M. Variation in volumes, dose-volume histograms, and estimated normal tissue complication probabilities of rectum and bladder: implications for treatment planning. Int J Radiat Oncol Biol Phys 1995; 33:1109–1119.

9. Roeske JC, Forman JD, Mesina CF, He T, Pelizzari CA, Fontenla E, Vijayakumar S, Chen GTY. Evaluation of changes in the size and location of the prostate, seminal vesicles, bladder, and rectum during a course of external beam radiation therapy. Int J Radiat Oncol Biol Phys 1995; 33:1321–1329.

10. Rudat V, Schraube P, Oetzel D, Zierhuit D, Flentje M, Wannenmacher M. Combined error of patient positioning variability and prostate motion uncertainty in 3D conformal radiotherapy of localized prostate cancer. Int J Radiat Oncol Biol Phys 1996; 35:1027–1034.

11. Dawson LA, Man K, Franssen E, Morton G. Target position variability throughout prostate radiotherapy. Int J Radiat Oncol Biol Phys 1998; 42: 1155–1161.

12. Miralbell R, Özsoy O, Pugliesi A, et al. Weekly CT-control in 3-D conformal radiotherapy of prostate cancer: dosimetric implications of changes in repositioning and organ motion. Radiother Oncol 2003; 66:197–202.

13. Chen ME, Johnston DA, Tang K, Babaian RJ, Troncoso P. Detailed mapping of prostate carcinoma foci. Biopsy strategy implications. Cancer 2000; 89: 1800–1809.

14. Coakley FV, Kurhanewicz J, Lu Y, Jones KD, Swanson MG, Chang SD, Carroll PR, Hricak H. Prostate cancer tumor volume: measurement with endorectal MR and MR spectroscopic imaging. Radiology 2002; 223:91–97.

15. Hara T, Kosaka N, Kishi H. PET imaging of prostate cancer using carbon-11 choline. J Nucl Med 1998; 39:990–995.

16. Oyama N, Akino H, Kanamaru H, Suzuki Y, Muramoto S, Yonekura Y, Sadato N, Yamamoto K, Okada K. [11]C Acetate PET imaging of prostate cancer. J Nucl Med 2002; 43:181–186.

17. Price DT, Coleman E, Liao RP, Robertson CN, Polascik TJ, de Grado TR. Comparison of 18F Fluorocholine and 18F Fluorodeoxyglucose for positron emission tomography of androgen dependents and androgen independent prostate cancer. J Urol 2002; 168:273–280.
18. Fowler J, Chappell R, Ritter M. Is alfa/beta for prostate tumors really low? Int J Radiat Oncol Biol Phys 2001; 50:1021–1031.
19. Brenner DJ, Martinez AA, Edmundson GK, Mitchell C, Thames HD, Armour EP. Direct evidence that prostate tumors show high sensitivity to fractionation (low DD ratio) similar to late-responding normal tissue. Int J Radiat Oncol Biol Phys 2002; 52:6–13.
20. Brenner DJ. Hypofractionation for prostate cancer radiotherapy—what are the issues. Int J Radiat Oncol Biol Phys 2003; 57:912–914.
21. Logue JP, Hendry JH. Hypofractionation for prostate cancer. Int J Radiat Oncol Biol Phys 2001; 49:152.
22. Kupelian PA, Reddy CA, Klein EA, Willouughby TR. Short-course intensity-modulated radiotherapy (70 Gy at 2.5 Gy per fraction) for localized prostate cancer: preliminary results on late toxicity and quality of life. Int J Radiat Oncol Biol Phys 2001; 51:998–993.
23. Yeoh EEK, Fraser RJ, McGowan RE, Botten RJ, Di Matteo AC, Roos DE, Penniment MG, Borg MF. Evidence for efficacy without increased toxicity of hypofractionated radiotherapy for prostate carcinoma: early results of a phase III randomized trial. Int J Radiat Oncol Biol Phys 2003; 55:943–955.
24. Parker C, Warde P, Catton C. Salvage radiotherapy for PSA failure after radical prostatectomy. Radiother Oncol 2001; 61:107–116.
25. Popowski Y, Kebdani T, Taussky D, Rouzaud M, Nouet P, Miralbell R. Dose escalation with high-dose rate (HDR) brachytherapy boost in prostate cancer: preliminary results. 7th Annual Meeting of the Scientific Association of Swiss Radiation Oncology, Geneva, Switzerland, Apr 3–7, 2003.
26. Roach M, Marquez C, Yuo H-S, Narayan P, Coleman L, Nseyo UO, Navvab Z, Carroll PR. Predicting the risk of lymph node involvement using the pre-treatment prostate specific antigen and Gleason score in men with clinically localized prostate cancer. Int J Radiat Oncol Biol Phys 1993; 28:33–37.
27. Low A, Harms W, Mutic S, Purdy J. A technique for the quantitative evaluation of dose distributions. Med Phys 1998; 25(5):656–661.
28. Depuydt T, Van Esch A, Huyskens DP. A qualitative evaluation of IMRT distributions: refinement and clinical assessment of the gamma evaluation. Radiother Oncol 2002; 62:309–319.
29. Perez CA, Brady LW. Overview. Quantification of treatment toxicity. In: Perez CA, Brady LW, eds. Principles and Practice of Radiation Oncology. Philadelphia: Lippincott, 1992:51–55.
30. Pavy J-J, Denekamp J, Letschert J, Littbrand B, Mornex F, Bernier J, González-González D,Horiot J-C, Bola M, Bartelink H. Late effects toxicity scoring: the SOMA scale. Int J Radiat Oncol Biol Phys 1995; 31:1043–1047.
31. Miralbell R, Mollá M, Arnalte R, Canales S, Vargas E, Linero D, Waters S, Nouet P, Rouzaud M, Escudé L. Target repositioning optimization in prostate cancer: is intensity modulation radiotherapy under stereotactic conditions feasible? Int J Radiat Oncol Biol Phys 2004; 59:366–371.

32. McKenzie AL, van Herk M, Mijnheer B. The width of margins in radiotherapy treatment plans. Phys Med Biol 2000; 45:3331–3342.
33. Nahun AE, Movsas B, Horwitz EM, Stobbe CC, Chapman JD. Incorporating clinical measurements of hypoxia into tumor local control modeling of prostate cancer: implications for the a/b ratio. Int J Radiat Oncol Biol Phys 2003; 53:391–401.
34. Soete G, Van de Steene J, Verellen D, et al. Initial clinical experience with infrared reflecting skin markers in the positioning of patients treated by conformal radiotherapy for prostate cancer. Int J Radiat Oncol Biol Phys 2002; 52(3): 694–698.
35. Soete G, Verellen D, Michielsen D, et al. Clinical use of stereoscopic X-ray positioning of patients treated with conformal radiotherapy for prostate cancer. Int J Radiat Oncol Biol Phys 2002; 54:948–952.
36. Verellen D, Linthout N, Soete G, et al. Considerations on treatment efficiency of different conformal radiation therapy techniques for prostate cancer. Radiother Oncol 2002; 63:27–36.
37. Verellen D, Soete G, Linthout N, et al. Quality assurance of a system for improved target localization and patient set-up that combines real-time infrared tracking and stereoscopic X-ray imaging. Radiother Oncol 2003; 67: 129–141.
38. UICC International Union Against Cancer. TNM Classification of Malignant Tumours. New York: Wiley-Liss, 1997.
39. D'Amico AV, Whittington R, Malkowicz SB. Pretreatment nomogram for prostate-specific antigen recurrence after radical prostatectomy or external beam radiation therapy for clinically localized prostate cancer. J Clin Oncol 1999; 17:168–172.
40. Gleason DF. Classification of prostatic carcinomas. Cancer Chemother Rep 1966; 50:125.
41. Kattan MW, Zelefsky MJ, Kupelian PA, et al. Pretreatment nomogram for predicting the outcome of three-dimensional conformal radiotherapy in prostate cancer. J Clin Oncol 2000; 18:3352–3359.
42. Shipley WU, Thames HD, Sandler HM, et al. Radiation therapy for clinically localized prostate cancer. A multi-institutional pooled analysis. JAMA 1999; 281:1598–1604.
43. Lyons JA, Kupelian PA, Mohan DS, et al. Importance of high radiation doses (72 Gy or greater) in the treatment of stage T1–T3 adenocarcinoma of the prostate. Urology 2000; 55:85–90.
44. Hanks GE, Schultheiss TE, Hunt MA, et al. Factors influencing incidence of acute grade 2 morbidity in conformal and standard radiation treatment of prostate cancer. Int J Radiat Oncol Biol Phys 1995; 31:25–29.
45. Bolla M, Collette L, Blank L, et al. Long-term results with immediate androgen suppression and external irradiation in patients with locally advanced prostate cancer (an EORTC study): a phase III randomised trial. Lancet 2002; 360: 103–106.
46. Lawton CA, Winter K, Murray K, et al. Updated results of the phase III radiation therapy oncology group (RTOG) trial 85–31 evaluating the potential benefit of androgen suppression following standard radiation therapy for unfavorable

prognosis carcinoma of the prostate. Int J Radiat Oncol Biol Phys 2001; 49: 937–946.

47. Pilepich MV, Winter K, John MJ, et al. Phase III radiation therapy oncology group (RTOG) trial 86–10 of androgen deprivation adjuvant to definitive radiotherapy in locally advanced carcinoma of the prostate. Int J Radiat Oncol Biol Phys 2001; 50:1243–1252.

48. Hanks GE, Hanlon AL, Pinover WH, et al. Dose selection for prostate cancer patients based on dose comparison and dose response studies. Int J Radiat Oncol Biol Phys 2000; 46:823–832.

49. Pollack A, Smith LG, von Eschenbach AC. External beam radiotherapy dose response characteristics of 1127 men with prostate cancer treated in the PSA era. Int J Radiat Oncol Biol Phys 2000; 48:507–512.

50. Zelefsky MJ, Hollister T, Raben A, Matthews S, Wallner KE. Five-year biochemical outcome and toxicity with transperineal CT-planned permanent 1–125 prostate implantation for patients with localized prostate cancer. Int J Radiat Oncol Biol Phys 2000; 47:1261–1266.

51. Boersma LJ, van den Brink M, Bruce AM, et al. Estimation of the incidence of late bladder and rectum complications after high-dose (70–78 Gy) conformal for prostate cancer, using dose–volume histograms. Int J Radiat Oncol Biol Phys 1998; 41:83–92.

52. Schultheiss TE, Lee WR, Hunt MA, et al. Late GI and GU complications in the treatment of prostate cancer. Int J Radiat Oncol Biol Phys 1997; 37:3–11.

53. Storey MR, Pollack A, Zagars G, et al. Complications from radiotherapy dose-escalation in prostate cancer: preliminary results of a randomized trial. Int J Radiat Oncol Biol Phys 2000; 48:635–642.

54. Pisansky TM, Zincke H, Suman VJ, et al. Correlation of pretherapy prostate cancer characteristics with histologic findings from pelvic lymphadenectomy specimens. Int J Radiat Oncol Biol Phys 1996; 34:33–39.

55. Pisansky TM, Blute ML, Suman VJ, et al. Correlation of pretherapy prostate cancer characteristics with seminal vesicle invasion in radical prostatectomy specimens. Int J Radiat Oncol Biol Phys 1995; 36:585–591.

56. Kestin L, Goldstein N, Vicini F, et al. Treatment of prostate cancer with radiotherapy: should the entire seminal vesicles be included in the clinical target volume? Int J Radiat Oncol Biol Phys 2002; 54:686–697.

57. Cox JD, Stetz J, Pajak TF, et al. Toxicity criteria of the Radiation Therapy Oncology Group (RTOG) and the European Organization for Research and Treatment of Cancer (EORTC). Int J Radiat Oncol Biol Phys 1995; 31(5): 1341–1346.

58. ASTRO Consensus Panel. Consensus statement: guidelines for PSA following radiation therapy. Int J Radiat Oncol Biol Phys 1997; 37:1035–1041.

59. Horwitz EM, Vicini FA, Ziaja EL, et al. The correlation between the ASTRO consensus panel definition of biochemical failure and clinical outcome for patients with prostate cancer treated with external beam irradiation. Int J Radiat Oncol Biol Phys 1998; 41:267–272.

60. Vicini FA, Kestin LL, Martinez AA. The importance of adequate follow-up in defining treatment success after external beam irradiation for prostate cancer. Int J Radiat Oncol Biol Phys 1999; 45:553–561.
61. Kabalin JN, Hodge KK, McNeal JE, et al. Identification of residual cancer in prostate following radiation therapy: role of transrectal ultrasound guided biopsy and prostate specific antigen. J Urol 1989; 142:326–331.
62. Van Cangh PJ, Richard FJ. Prostate-specific antigen after definitive radiation therapy. Curr Opin Urology 1994; 4:256.
63. Yock TI, Zietman AL, Shipley WU, et al. Long-term durability of PSA failure-free survival after radiotherapy for localized prostate cancer. Int J Radiat Oncol Biol Phys 2002; 54:420–426.
64. Emami B, Lyman J, Brown A, et al. Tolerance of normal tissue to therapeutic irradiation. Int J Radiat Oncol Biol Phys 1991; 21:109–122.
65. Douchez J, Allain YM, Cellier P, et al. Cancer de la prostate: intolerance et morbidite de la radiotherapie externe. Bull Cancer 1985; 72:573–577.
66. Herold DM, Hanlon AL, Hanks GE. Diabetes mellitus: a predictor for late radiation morbidity. Int J Radiat Oncol Biol Phys 1999; 43:475–479.
67. Vijayakumar S, Awan A, Karrison T, et al. Acute toxicity during external-beam radiotherapy for localized prostate cancer: comparison of different techniques. Int J Radiat Oncol Biol Phys 1993; 25:359–371.

11

ECSRT for Spinal Tumors

Samuel Ryu

*Department of Radiation Oncology and Neurosurgery, Henry Ford Hospital,
Detroit, Michigan, U.S.A.*

Fang-Fang Yin

*Department of Radiation Oncology, Duke Medical Center, Detroit,
Michigan, U.S.A.*

INTRODUCTION AND CLINICAL INDICATIONS

Tumors of the Spine and the Spinal Cord

Primary tumors of the spine and the spinal cord are rare, and these include the tumors arising from the vertebral bone, hematopoietic tumors like myeloma, or tumors arising from the cord itself. Metastatic tumors are the most common involving the spine or spinal cord. Metastatic disease is a common complication of cancer during the course of the disease in the majority of cancer patients. Among these, the vertebral bones are the most common site and may be involved in about 40% of the cancer patients (1). Up to 20% of patients with neoplastic involvement of the vertebral column develop spinal cord compression (2). It is estimated that more than 20,000 cancer patients per year in the United States develop spinal cord or root compression as a manifestation of their metastatic disease (3–5). Compression of the spinal cord or nerve roots is second only to brain metastasis as the most frequent neurologic complication of cancer (6,7). Usually, vertebral bone metastasis occurs prior to developing compression to the spinal cord. The estimated number of patients diagnosed with spinal metastases has increased with the use of CT and MRI scans (3,4). The common presenting symptoms of spine metastasis are back pain and spinal cord compression with weakness and numbness below the level of spinal involvement. Many patients, if not treated, become paraplegic or lose control of bowel and bladder, which results in significant morbidity and poor quality of life. Early treatment prior to the development of significant neurologic deficits improves the chance for patients to remain ambulatory (8). Because cancer patients are now experiencing longer survival, quality of life has become an important factor in making the treatment decision and offering palliative treatment. This is particularly true in the treatment of spine metastasis since pain and neurologic symptoms further reduce the quality of life.

Treatment for spinal metastasis and/or cord compression has been external beam radiotherapy and/or decompressive surgery. External beam radiation therapy is offered, initially combined with steroids, in the vast majority of patients. The effectiveness of external beam radiotherapy has been well established. Varying degrees of pain relief were seen in two-thirds of patients by three months after radiation (9,10). Surgery is usually offered for a rapid neurologic change, spinal instability, or for tissue diagnosis (11,12). Surgery has also been used for more aggressive and radioresistant tumors, combined with radiation. Chemotherapy is offered for chemosensitive tumors such as small cell carcinomas or lymphomas. Whatever treatment is chosen, the intent of treatment for spine metastasis or cord compression has been palliative. The main goals of the treatment are relief or reduction of pain, improvement of neurological function, or to limit tumor progression, if possible. Although there have been many efforts to improve the treatment of these tumors by using multimodality treatments, the clinical outcome of the available treatment for spinal tumors is still limited compared to the progress of treatments for the other tumor sites.

Radiosurgery of the Spine

Radiosurgery delivers a highly conformal large radiation dose to a localized tumor by a stereotactic approach. This requires accurate targeting and immobilization of the target organ during irradiation. The difficulty of applying radiosurgery to the extracranial site is mainly due to organ motion associated with breathing and/or lack of immobilization techniques. Among the extracranial organs, the spinal cord and vertebrae are the organs with the least breathing-related organ movement. This makes the spinal cord and vertebrae particularly suitable for stereotactic radiosurgery.

Stereotaxis has been used exclusively for cranial applications for several decades. However, interestingly, the first attempt of stereotactic localization began, long before brain stereotaxy, with experimental sites of the spinal cord by Dittmar and Worosciloff in the late 19th century, although these systems were not based on a true coordinate system (13). The history of the spinal stereotaxy is summarized in Table 1. The first stereotactic instrument using Cartesian coordinate system for the spinal cord was reported by Clarke in 1920 (14). Rand et al. performed the first stereotactic procedure on the human spinal cord for percutaneous cordotomy and cryosurgery in 1965 (15). All the spinal stereotaxy was limited to the cervicomedullary

Table 1 History of Spine Stereotaxy

1873	Dittmar	Device for directing probes to the spinal cord
1874	Woroschiloff	Myelotome using clamps for skeletal fixation in animal
1920	Clarke	First spinal stereotactic device using Cartesian coordinate system
1947	Spiegel	First cranial stereotactic frame
1951	Leksell	First stereotactic radiosurgery for brain
1965	Rand	First clinical stereotactic cryosurgery of cervical cord
1972	Nadvornik	First spinal radiosurgery for lumbar vertebrae with skeletal fixation
1982	Betti	Linear accelerator modified for radiosurgery of brain
1994	Lax	Body frame with contour mold fixation
1995	Hamilton	Skeletal fixation frame with bone-screw fixation
2000		Frameless spinal radiosurgery

region because the device was fixed to the skull and open surgery was needed to anchor the cradles to the bony structures of the spine. In 1972, Nadvornik et al. expanded its clinical usefulness with an apparatus designed for lumbar region (16). It also required fixation to the vertebral arch in an open laminectomy wound. Since then, spinal radiosurgery has been used in limited numbers of cancer patients (17). The method used by Takacs and Hamilton (18) and Hamilton et al. (19) was also an invasive procedure that required anchoring of the stereotactic frame to the spinous process under general anesthesia. Despite its invasiveness, the clinical outcome was encouraging.

More recently, image-guided frameless stereotactic technology of the spine has been developed and used in the clinic to treat the patients with spinal tumors. There are basically two different methods to achieve stereotaxy without frames by using the implanted seed as a point fiducial, or using the internal rigid bony structure (such as vertebral bone or target tumor itself) as a volume fiducial. The former system is used in CyberKnife® unit (Accuray, Sunnyvale, California, U.S.A.), in which mean total radial error was 1.6 mm and the positioning error along each axis was ±0.9 mm in the phantom (20). This also has an invasive component with implantation of a few metal markers in the patient to help determine the target. The later system of frameless stereotaxy is the Novalis® shaped beam radiosurgery unit (BrainLAB, AG, Heimstetten, Germany). This system utilizes image fusion of anatomical structures such as vertebral bone and infrared marker technology for tumor localization and patient positioning. This procedure is entirely non-invasive. The volume of the fixed bony structure is registered at the time of simulation and used for image fusion. The precision of this system was reported with less than 2 mm of isocenter variation for intensity-modulated spinal radiosurgery (21). This radiosurgery procedure and clinical experience with encouraging clinical results will be discussed in this chapter.

TECHNIQUES FOR SPINAL RADIOSURGERY

The challenge for spinal radiosurgery is how to accurately localize the treatment target and deliver the prescribed dose to the treatment target while keeping the dose to the normal tissues within the tolerances. The success of stereotactic radiosurgery for brain tumors is mainly attributed to its precision in patient immobilization, target localization, and conformal dose delivery. Less than 1 mm positioning error for the head fixation is technically achievable because the head could be treated as a quasi-rigid body with negligible organ motion (22). However, some of techniques used for the brain radiosurgery will not be feasible for spinal tumors due to difficulties in immobilizing non-rigid patient body, localizing targets associated with organ motion, and mechanical limits associated with allowable gantry and couch rotations. Traditional arc techniques used for brain radiosurgery may not be suitable to spinal radiosurgery. For spinal tumors, critical organs such as spinal cord, kidney, and lung are always adjacent to the targets and present technical challenges for protection. Therefore, different techniques should be adopted for spinal radiosurgery, including new approaches for patient immobilization, target localization, and treatment planning and delivery. The procedures developed at Henry Ford Hospital are schematically illustrated in Figure 1.

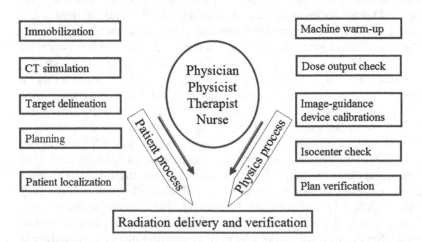

Figure 1   Schematic illustration of clinical procedures for spinal radiosurgery.

Immobilization and Simulation

Immobilization involves patient immobilization and organ/structure immobilization. Patient immobilization during spinal radiosurgery is the first but critical step, because a single or a few fractional high doses of radiation will be delivered to spinal or para-spinal tumors surrounded by critical normal organs such as the spine. Radiosurgery typically takes more time than conventional treatment and therefore requires the patient to be rigid and stable throughout the treatment. Any patient movement during the treatment could lead to the failure of the radiosurgery. Traditional immobilization devices, such as alpha cradle and vacuum bags, may not be sufficient for patient immobilization because they do not have constraints to limit patient movement. The ideal immobilization devices should be able to provide some type of constraints to the patient but also be feasible for all kinds of patients to stay at the same position for a period of time up to 1 hr. Several approaches have been used for immobilization during spinal radiosurgery. The early approach used a metal frame to fix the vertebral bodies because of the relatively fixed relationship among spinal tumors, spinal cord, and vertebral bodies (19). Therefore, accurate localization of vertebral bodies is equivalent to the accurate localization of the target region. Although reasonable accuracy is achievable in terms of patient immobilization, it is an invasive surgical procedure with anesthetic involvement. Several alternative non-invasive immobilization devices are now available such as BodyFIX® (Medical Intelligence, Schwabmünchen, Germany) and Stereotactic Body Frame (ELEKTA AB, Stockholm, Sweden). The BodyFIX device combines a vacuum cushion and a piece of special plastic foil (21,23). The vacuum cushion is used to stabilize the patient in a comfortable position while the plastic foil is used to constrain the patient by evacuating the region between the patient and plastic foil so that the patient is constrained between the vacuum cushion and plastic foil. The Body Frame uses a vacuum cushion to stabilize the patient in the supine position inside a body frame and adds a diaphragm control to the patient's chest to minimize respiratory movement (24). Figure 2 illustrates immobilization setups using the BodyFIX and Body Frame devices.

The effect of organ motion is relatively minimal for spinal radiosurgery because the spinal tumors are typically located very close to vertebral bodies. When the patient is in the supine position, the vertebral body motion is limited to within 1 mm (21). This effect could be documented by fluoroscopic imaging using a conventional simulator. However, if the patient is in the prone position, the vertebral body motion could be more than 5 mm due to breathing. Therefore, it is ideal to position the patient supinely for spinal radiosurgery.

CT simulation has been the gold standard for conventional radiosurgery for brain tumors. It provides not only accurate patient geometry but also three-dimensional (3D) anatomical information for dose calculation.

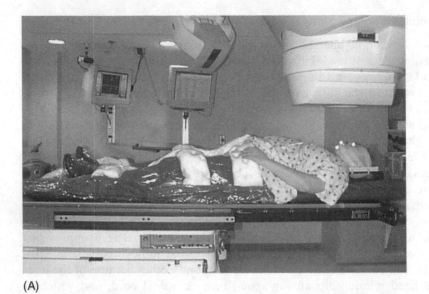

(A)

(B)

Figure 2 Illustration of (**A**) BodyFIX® and (**B**) Body Frame® immobilization devices.

Similarly, CT simulation should be used for spinal radiosurgery. To accommodate complicated immobilization devices and variety of patient sizes, a large bore CT simulator as supplied by both Philips Medical Systems (Andover, Maryland U.S.A.) and GE Healthcare Technologies (Waukesha, Wesconius, U.S.A.) would be preferable. Any localization markers should be placed on or implanted in the patient prior to CT imaging. For example, if infrared markers are used for patient setup and localization, infrared sensitive radiopaque markers should be placed on the patient skin so that they are shown in the CT images for patient localization in the process of treatment planning (21). The relative location between the localization markers and the planned isocenter could be established in the treatment planning system using this technique.

Contrast agents such as Optiray 200 mg/mL organically bound iodine are typically used to enhance tumors in the CT images. Enough patient body portions should be scanned in simulation to assist accurate identification of vertebral bodies and to provide sufficient anatomy for the use of non-coplanar planning beams. A slice thickness of 3 mm or less without spacing should be selected for scanning. When slice thickness is larger than 5 mm, the quality of digitally reconstructed image (DRR) as calculated from CT images is shown to be not good enough for accurate image fusion between DRRs and kV X-ray images which are taken for the localization of isocenter in the treatment room (25). To minimize the data transfer burden and potential errors, the simulation DICOM 3.0 CT images should be electronically sent to the dedicated treatment planning system through the internal network (26).

Treatment Planning

Treatment prescription involves both volume and dose. In addition to the gross target volume (GTV), critical organs such as the spinal cord, kidneys, and lungs are identified in CT images so that the radiation dose to these organs can be minimized. The majority of GTVs involved one or two segments of the vertebral column. To accurately delineate the GTV for each disease site, multiple imaging information is often referenced, especially contrast-enhanced MR images. Image fusion between CT and MR images needs special caution and is often done manually to ensure the accurate anatomical matching. Depending on the immobilization device used, proper margin should be added to the GTV to generate the planning target volume (PTV). When a BodyFIX device is used for immobilization, a margin of 2–3 mm would be sufficient to accommodate patient positioning and target localization variations (21). Typically, this expansion is not extended into the critical organs, especially not the spinal cord. Note that the dose distributions at the joints between the target and the critical organs in an inverse plan are determined by their relative beam weights given in the prescription. Radiosurgery dose is usually prescribed to the isodose line that encompasses the PTV.

Treatment planning involves the construction of radiation beams to deliver a conformal dose distribution. The treatment planning method is influenced by the delivery technique used. Non-coplanar beams are usually used for treatment planning when a CyberKnife® unit (Accuray, Sunnyvale, California, U.S.A.) is applied for treatment. Coplanar beams are usually applied for any tomotherapy treatment devices (NOMOS Corporation Chatsworth, California, U.S.A., and TomoTherapy Inc., Madison, Wisconsin, U.S.A.). When a conventional linac-based treatment unit such as Novalis Shaped Beam unit (BrainLAB Inc., Westchester, Illinois, AG, Heimstetten, Germany) or Varian Trilogy (Varian Medical Systems, Palo Alto, California, U.S.A.) is used, the majority of treatment plans for the spinal radiosurgery use multiple intensity-modulated beams to minimize the dose to critical organs. Sometimes, dynamic shaped conformal arcs may be used when the avoidance of critical organs is not a high priority, such as intra-spinal tumors and tumors involving the sacral portion of the vertebral column. Both coplanar and non-coplanar intensity-modulated beams are used for spinal radiosurgery. Typically, coplanar beams are used for tumors located close to the thoracic, lumbar, and sacral sections of the vertebral column while non-coplanar beams are sometime used for tumors near the cervical vertebral bodies.

Intensity-modulated beams are commonly used for spinal radiosurgery and are generated using an inverse treatment-planning algorithm, such as the dynamically penalized likelihood method and a pencil beam dose calculation algorithm by BrainLAB (27,28). Dose–volume histograms (DVHs) are traditionally used to specify the dose constraints for both target volumes and critical organs. The DVH is also used to evaluate treatment plans. For a given set of dose constraints specified by DVHs, the outcome of the planning results is influenced by the setting of priority weights for both the target and the critical organs. Typically, the higher the priority weight, the better the dose coverage to each structure. An additional parameter, the conformity index (C), may be used to evaluate treatment plans. Here, the conformity index could be defined as $C = 1 + (Vn/Vt)$. Vn is the volume of the normal tissue and Vt is the volume of the target receiving the indicated dose (21,29). An acceptable plan is judged by the reasonable compromise between the doses to the target and critical organs. This compromise is determined by the setting of DVH constraints and priority weights.

When an inverse treatment plan is delivered using a multileaf collimator (MLC) during intensity-modulated radiosurgery (IMRS), the beam number ranges from 5 to 9, with the majority being seven beams. The beam orientation of a typical seven-coplanar intensity-modulated beam arrangement involves nearly equal gantry angles such as 150°, 100°, 50°, 0°, 310°, 260°, and 210° with 0° at the anterior direction. Sometime, when the target is not located too deeply, 5 to 6 IMRS beams could be set within a fan range between 120° and 150° to avoid excessive dose to normal tissues. An example of an intensity-modulated treatment plan with seven equally spaced beams is

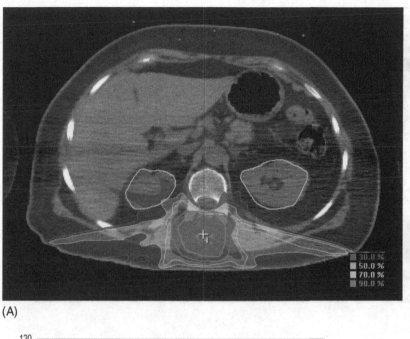

(A)

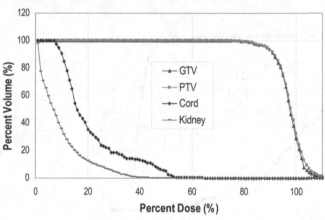

(B)

Figure 3 (**A**) An inverse plan using equally distributed seven beams and (**B**) corresponding DVHs. (*See color insert.*)

shown in Figure 3A and its corresponding dose–volume histogram is shown in Figure 3B. An example of an intensity-modulated treatment plan with six equally spaced fan beams is shown in Figure 4A and its corresponding dose–volume histogram is shown in Figure 4B, where the dose is normalized

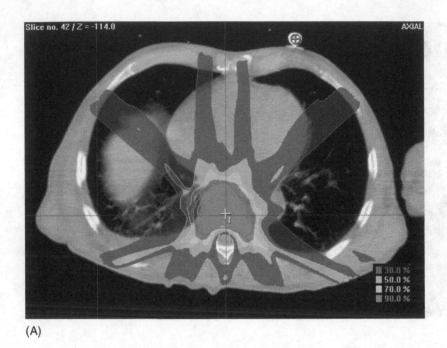

(A)

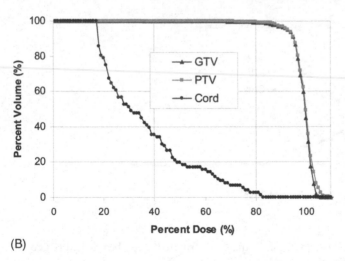

(B)

Figure 4 (**A**) An inverse plan using five beams and (**B**) corresponding DVHs. (*See color insert.*)

to the isocenter and the dose is prescribed to the volume included by the 90% isodose line. The inhomogeneity corrections are included in dose calculation for all treatment plans using IMRT. The number of the IMRT beams in a treatment plan affects the dose distribution to the target as well as to the normal tissues. Typically, dose distribution improves as beam number increases. However, this trend becomes less obvious when the beam number is greater than nine.

After the radiation oncologist selects a suitable inverse treatment plan, all treatment data should be electronically transferred to the treatment unit. An electronic verification system, such as Varis, record-and-verify system (Varian Oncology Systems) in the treatment unit will help to secure the delivery accuracy. Similarly, when an image–guided system is used for patient localization, such as Novalis Body system, the patient positioning information could be electronically exported to the controlling system for patient setup and target (or isocenter) localization (21,26).

Patient Setup and Target Localization

Accurate patient positioning and target localization are the keys for the success of spinal radiosurgery. After the treatment plan is completed, the next step for spinal radiosurgery is to reposition the patient in the treatment room as in the simulation room and to align the planned isocenter to the treatment machine isocenter. Since traditional methods such as skin marks are not quite capable of providing high precision patient setup and target localization, various image-guided techniques have been developed for patient setup, target localization, treatment monitoring, and verification. Among them are ultrasound guided techniques, infrared camera imaging techniques, and kV X-ray imaging techniques (30,21,31). In-room kV X-ray imaging appears to be a very promising approach for spinal radiosurgery. Some of the image-guided localization devices are the use of orthogonal dual kV imaging technique in the CyberKnife unit (31) and a dual kV X-ray imaging system which is called Novalis Body system in the Novalis unit (21). Differing from the CyberKnife unit (as shown in Fig. 5A) in which the radiation beam orientation as controlled by the robotic arm modifies as the isocenter shifts as detected by kV X-ray imaging, the Novalis unit (as shown in Fig. 5B) uses an image-guided system to adjust patient positioning by moving the treatment couch.

The Novalis Body system as shown in Figure 5B consists of infrared and video cameras and kV X-ray imaging system. The major functions for infrared cameras are to detect infrared sensitive markers placed on the patient skin, to automatically compare marker locations to the stored reference information, and to instruct the treatment machine to move the patient to the preplanned position by moving the treatment couch. A dedicated video camera system is coupled to the infrared camera system to provide a visual check of patient positioning. The two kV X-ray tubes and two amorphous silicon (aSi) flat panel digital detectors are controlled by an integrated computer

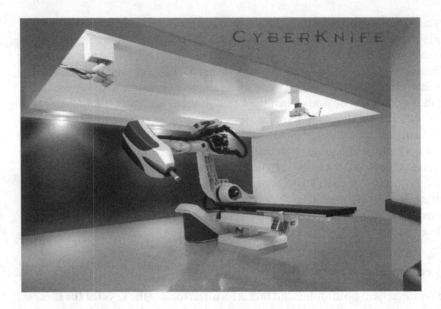

(A)

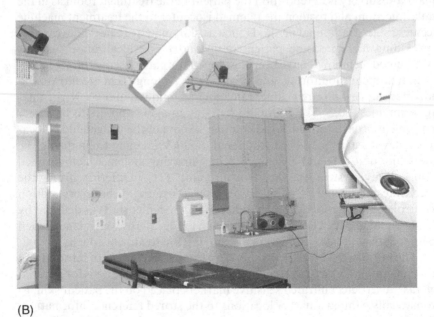

(B)

Figure 5 Image-guided target localization systems in (**A**) CyberKnife® system and in (**B**) Novalis® treatment unit.

system with some image analysis software. Two digitally reconstructed radiographs (DRRs) could be generated from the planning CT images at the same orientations at which two kV X-ray images are taken. The system automatically compares internal structures such as vertebral bodies or implanted markers, in the kV X-ray images to those in the DRR images and indicates the potential isocenter deviations between the DRRs and the X-ray images for the patient setup. The deviations are evaluated by the radiation oncologist and forwarded to the computer control system for recommended adjustment of the isocenter position. It is an automated process because the Novalis Body system is integrated with the treatment machine. This procedure could be repeated during the treatment. Both anatomical structures and implanted markers could be used for image fusion using either a manual or an automated image fusion algorithm. Patient shift and rotational information could be identified using a rigid body 3D to 2D image fusion technique in which DRRs are generated iteratively with different angulations to simulate potential patient deviations in all directions (32). Note that the accuracy of image fusion based on anatomical markers using a rigid body 3D to 2D image fusion technique depends on liability of those structures used for matching in both types of images. Regarding contrast, the image fusion based on the implanted markers is often more accurate and reliable (25,32). A cone-beam technology (33) will allow three-dimensional comparison of treatment anatomy and should be a very promising method for patient localization and treatment verification.

After the patient is immobilized on the treatment couch, the infrared camera system guides the patient's setup to the initial treatment position based on the localization infrared sensitive markers placed on the patient skin. Since the infrared markers only reflect the patient surface information and do not guarantee the accuracy of the planned isocenter, two kV X-ray images are required to check the isocenter position. The internal structures such as the vertebral bodies displayed in two X-ray images and those displayed in two corresponding DRRs are compared to indicate the relative isocenter deviations from the planned isocenter position. After reviewing the comparison result, the radiation oncologist decides whether an adjustment of the isocenter position is necessary. If so, the infrared camera system will guide the patient to the adjusted position. With this image-guided patient localization technique, accuracy of 1 mm is achievable as shown in a study using a rigid-body phantom (25). However, depending on the immobilization technique used for the actual patient treatment, the localization accuracy of 3 mm or less isocenter deviation is achievable. This accuracy is considered to be acceptable if proper margin can be added.

Treatment Delivery

Accurate delivery of conformal dose as planned is another challenging step for spinal radiosurgery. Traditional devices and arc techniques used for brain radiosurgery are not quite feasible for the majority of spinal radiosurgeries. Various new delivery techniques are now available for stereotactic radiosurgery of localized spinal tumors such as the use of a CyberKnife technology (31), the use of a Novalis shaped beam surgery unit (21), and the use of a linac with fine MLC (23). Other technologies such as tomotherapy units may also be used for such treatment (34,35). The Cyber-Knife unit uses multiple circular cone beams and others use fine MLCs to deliver intensity-modulated beams. For inverse plans delivered using different MLCs, the leaf width may potentially affect the dosimetry. However, the dosimetric difference of intensity-modulated beams delivered using the MLC leaf width of 5 mm or less is negligible (29).

The Novalis shaped beam unit is used for spinal radiosurgery at Henry Ford Hospital and it is equipped with a built-in micromultileaf collimator (mMLC) with a single 6 MV photon energy (36,37). There are 26 pairs of leaves (14 pairs with a leaf width of 3 mm, six pairs with a leaf width of 4.5 mm, and six pairs with a leaf width of 5.5 mm) which form a maximum field size of 10 × 10 cm. It is capable of delivering radiation through circular cone arcs, fixed-shape conformal beams using mMLC, fixed-shape conformal arcs using mMLC, dynamic shape conformal arcs using mMLC, and fixed-gantry with static and dynamic intensity-modulation beams. The dosimetric characteristics of this treatment unit are discussed in a separate report (36). Intensity-modulated radiosurgery is capable of delivering conformal dose distribution to minimize radiation damage to the critical organs. Typically, only a single isocenter is required for any kind of target shape. Multiple isocenters may be required if the target size is larger than the maximal field size (for example, 10 cm × 10 cm in the Novalis unit). Since the entire process could be completed within a few hours, the procedure is non-invasive, frameless, accurate, and efficient.

Either a sliding window (or dynamic MLC) or step-and-shoot technique is used to deliver the intensity-modulated beams through the mMLC. Typically, there is no substantial difference between these two techniques if the number of segments using the step-and-shoot technique is over 20 (21). Typically, a dose rate of 480 MU/min is used for delivery. The overall root-mean square (RMS) of the leaf traveling accuracy by the use of this dose rate is relatively, but not substantially, smaller than that by use of a dose rate of 800 MU/min. The analysis of RMS values in the MLC log files recorded in the MLC workstation for a few typical IMRS plans shows this trend.

Precision delivery of high-dose radiation could be also achieved by other means. The earlier reported spinal radiosurgery procedure combined the surgical fixation of patients with high-dose irradiation (19). In that study, the procedure of surgically implanting the stereotactic fixation device to the vertebral body was necessary for both patient immobilization and localization because the patient was positioned in the prone position. High-dose radiation was planned and delivered based on the conventional techniques instead of IMRT. In an attempt to reduce the invasiveness of spinal radiosurgery, the CyberKnife unit (31,38) uses a robotic arm to deliver 6 MV photon beam in a wide range of beam orientations, except at the posterior region where the two X-ray detectors are located. The use of a different acceleration technique makes its treatment head much smaller than the conventional accelerator gantry and, therefore, its head movement is much more feasible using a robotic arm. The beam orientation is modified and guided by two real-time imaging systems and the isocenter is modified at any time when the imaging system indicates a deviation from the planned isocenter. Therefore, delivery accuracy is largely dependent on the accuracy of the detected signals and the accuracy of robotic arm movements. To improve the accuracy, a few metal markers are implanted in the patient so that the treatment target can be easily determined based on the markers in X-ray images. This, however, adds an invasion component to this procedure. Since the treatment unit delivers radiation through various circular cones, multiple isocenters and/or cones with different diameters have to be used for irregular target volumes in a single treatment. Instead of using intensity-modulated beams, the conformal dose distribution is delivered by the use of numerous circular beams with variable isocenters.

Treatment Verification and Quality Assurance

Treatment verification involves verification of treatment plan, patient setup, treatment isocenter, and dose calculation and delivery. Quality assurance (QA) involves machine specific-QA and patient-specific QA. In the case of intensity-modulated radiosurgery using MLCs, machine-specific QA involves examination of MLC leaf sequence, leaf position, dosimetry, etc. Patient-specific QA involves isodose measurement, intensity spectrum distribution, etc. The detail procedures of these methods are described in several previous publications (39,40) and chapter 3. The imaging devices used for patient setup and target localization should be properly calibrated based on the requirements specified by the manufacturers (25,41).

Careful verification of the treatment plan involves verification of treatment parameters, such as isocenter position, beam geometry, monitor unit calculation, beam intensity spectrum, and dose measurements. An independent dose calculation algorithm, based on traditional dose calculation methods such as modified Clarkson method (42) or Monte Carlo method (43), may be used to calculate the isocenter dose contributed by each mMLC segment and its corresponding MUs for all segments of each intensity-modulated beam given by the planning system. Independent patient positioning verification could be achieved by taking orthogonal images and compareing them to simulation images. A pair of orthogonal portal films could also be used to document the final patient positioning accuracy. Alternatively, this documentation could also be accomplished by comparing the two kV X-ray images to the corresponding DRRs.

The intensity-modulated beams are delivered through the complicated precalculated leaf sequences. Each intensity map needs to be checked by delivering a given amount of radiation to a film such as Kodak EDR2 (44), an electronic imaging device such as Varian aSi500 portal imager (45), and a gantry mounted device (46). The resulting intensity distribution should be compared to the planned intensity map. To verify the absolute point dose, the planned intensity maps are usually exported to a verification phantom and the isocenter or any other point dose in the phantom is calculated. The phantom is then irradiated with all planned intensity-modulated beams. The point dose in the phantom is measured using a micro ion-chamber such as Exradin® T14 by Standard Imaging, Inc. (Middleton, Wisconsin, U.S.A.) and is compared to the planned point dose. Under normal conditions, the deviation between two is less than 3%. Sometimes, the detector may not be able to accurately measure the dose when the field is very small due to the partial volume effect of the detector.

The accuracy of dose delivery could be examined by a phantom study (21). An example of such procedure is described below. A hypothetical spinal tumor, a section of vertebral column, and the corresponding critical structure, spinal cord, in the Rando phantom are identified as the PTV and critical organ for treatment planning. To verify the dose distribution, a special film dosimeter (for example, GAFCHROMIC™ Dosimetry Type MD 55) is placed at the isocenter slice and a 12 Gy dose is delivered to the isocenter. For the purpose of calibration, a range of doses from 2 to 14 Gy is delivered to a set of films at the calibration distance. To minimize the effect of non-uniform dispersal of the sensor medium of the films, a double-exposure measurement technique proposed by Zhu et al. (47) can be used for this experiment. All films are digitized using a microdensitometer so that the film density could be converted to the dose. The resulting dose image is compared to the planned isodose distributions. The original CT image is shown in Figure 6A (the target and the spinal cord are shown with solid contours) and the planned dose distributions (90%, 50%, and 30% normalized to the isocenter) are shown in Figure 6B. Figure 7A illustrates the planned isodose distributions in the region where the film is inserted. Solid curves represent planned isodose lines labeled 90%, 50%, and 30% relative to the isocenter. Figure 7B shows the original film dose image with three corresponding isodose curves. The planned and the corresponding measured isodose distributions are then overlaid on the original CT image as shown in Figure 7C. Results indicate that isodoses between the calculated and measured results match well up to the 50% isodose line. The discrepancies between two 90% isodose lines are negligible. The majority of 50% isodose lines are matched within 1 mm discrepancy, except some portions between the lung/soft tissue interfaces where the

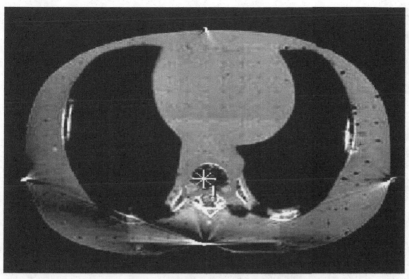

(A)

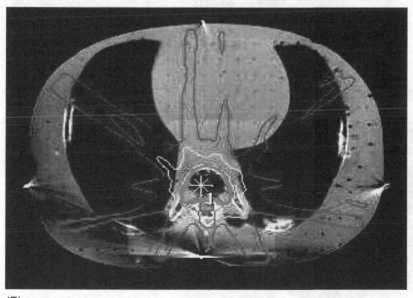

(B)

Figure 6 Phantom study images. (**A**) The original CT image with target and spinal cord indicated. (**B**) The planned dose distributions for 90%, 50%, and 30% isodose curves normalized to the isocenter. (*See color insert.*)

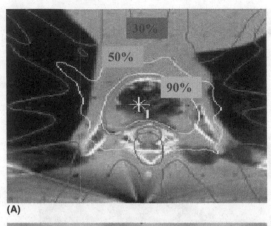

(A)

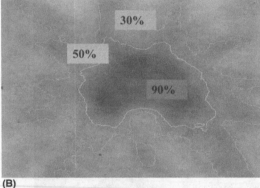

(B)

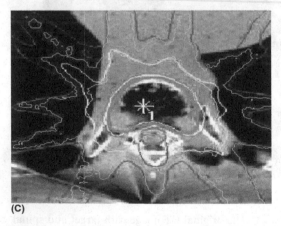

(C)

Figure 7 Phantom study results. (**A**) The planned isodose distributions in the region where the film was inserted. Solid curves represent planned isodose lines labeled 90%, 50%, and 30% relative to the isocenter. (**B**) The original film dose image with three corresponding isodose curves. (**C**) Both planned and corresponding measured iso-dose distributions are overlaid on the original CT image. (*See color insert.*)

discrepancy is up to 5%. This discrepancy is mainly related to the dose calculation and display accuracy.

CLINICAL APPLICATIONS AND OUTCOMES

Clinical Feasibility Study

The first clinical study was carried out to determine the precision and accuracy of the spinal radiosurgery. This is particularly important because the spinal cord is always the critical organ that is located in close contact with the vertebral column. Ten patients were enrolled at Henry Ford Hospital between April 2001 and December 2001. All patients had pathologically proven primary malignant neoplasm and had single or two contiguous vertebral metastasis with or without spinal cord compression that was seen on CT or MRI. To test the accuracy of radiosurgery and to achieve the desired palliation, standard external beam radiation therapy (25 Gy in 10 fractions) was given first and then radiosurgery boost (6–8 Gy single dose) to the site of the spine involvement or spinal cord compression. External beam radiotherapy was given based on conventional method including two vertebral bodies above and below the radiographic lesion. Following the external beam radiotherapy, the patients received intensity-modulated radiosurgery boost to the most involved site. During radiosurgery, orthogonal portal films were obtained for the final verification and to determine the accuracy of the isocenter. The endpoint of the study was to measure the isocenter variation in order to determine the accuracy and precision of the spinal radiosurgery. It was measured by image fusion of simulation and orthogonal portal films taken during radiosurgery.

The accuracy of the spinal radiosurgery was defined as the degree of variation (by distance) between the isocenters of the CT simulation and of the portal films at the time of radiation delivery. The deviation between the simulation and actual treatment isocenter was 1.36 ± 0.11 mm (48). We also measured the radiation dose at the isocenter using the same positioning parameters of the individual patients in a phantom with a micro ionization-chamber. The average deviation of the measured dose from the estimated dose was 2%. This level of precision of the isocenter obtained in this study was clinically acceptable for spinal radiosurgery.

Dosimetric Consideration of Spinal Cord Dose

The radiosurgery dose was invariably prescribed to the periphery of target tumor volume encompassed by the 90% isodose line. The radiation dose to the adjacent normal spinal cord was calculated using the computerized isodose calculation program. Average distance between the 90% and 50% isodose line at the spinal cord is 5.2 ± 0.9 mm (as shown in Figs. 3A and 4A). This represents the rapid dose fall-off of spinal radiosurgery. In a

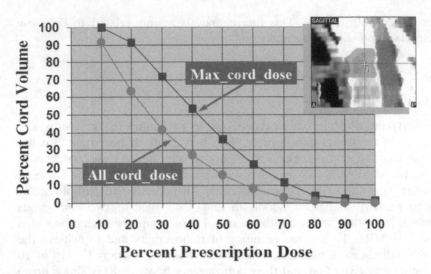

Figure 8 Dose–volume histograms (DVHs) for cord doses. (*See color insert.*)

transverse section at the isocenter level, 20% of the spinal cord volume immediately adjacent to the diseased vertebra received higher than 50% of the prescribed radiation dose (48). Figure 8 illustrates the average DVH for spinal cord dose in 50 cases. In this figure, only the portion of the spinal cord closer to the GTV is used for calculation. Also plotted in the figure is the average maximum cord dose DVH in which only two slices with the maximal cord dose were used for DVH calculation. The insert illustrated the types of cord anatomy.

To determine the factors that may affect the dose to the spinal cord, correlative analyses were performed from the dosimetry of 51 patients who received 10–16 Gy radiosurgery. The factors tested were target volume, length and width of target, spinal cord volume, and the number of the intensity-modulated beams. Average tumor volume was 57.0 ± 34.1 cc (range 3.4–217.0 cc). Average tumor length was 49.1 ± 15.3 mm (range 16.1–85.1 mm), and average tumor width was 45.5 ± 10.7 mm (range 12.9–89.5 mm). Average spinal cord volume at the corresponding level of the treatment was 5.9 ± 2.2 cc (range 2.4–14.7 cc). In the lumbar and sacral treatment, the vertebral canal was considered as spinal cord for volume analysis purpose. Dose–volume histograms were plotted and also the spinal cord volumes that received 20%, 40%, 60%, 80%, and 100% of the prescribed dose. Then, the best-fit correlation curves were obtained. From this analysis, total dose (above 14 Gy) and the number of intensity-modulated beams (less than seven beams) appear to be the most important factors affecting the spinal cord dose. The tumor volume and length did not affect the higher (>60%) isodose regions of the spinal cord. However, the dose to peripheral regions (lower than 60% isodose lines) was influenced by target volume greater than 100 cc and tumor length greater than 6 cm (49). This is in contrast to the experience of brain radiosurgery where the target volume is a major determinant for radiosurgery dose selection. We believe that the independence of the cord dose from the target volume or length is mainly due to the use of intensity modulation that limited the dose to the critical organ at risk.

Clinical Outcome in Single Spinal Metastasis

Encouraged by the level of accuracy for spinal radiosurgery and the acceptable spinal cord dose, a subsequent study was carried out to determine the dose and the clinical efficacy of radiosurgery for spine metastasis with or without cord compression. A total of 49 patients (24 males and 25 females) with 61 lesions were treated with radiosurgery alone from May 2002 to May 2003. All patients had diagnosis of pathologically confirmed malignant neoplasm and had either synchronous or metachronous metastasis to a single spine. Spinal metastases were diagnosed by radiologic studies with CT or MRI scans. Primary tumor sites were: breast 29.5%, lung 19.7%, prostate 9.8%, kidney 8.2%, and others 32.8%. The involved spines were: cervical 13.1%, thoracic 54.1%, lumbar 29.5%, and sacral 3.3% lesions. Patients had no previous radiotherapy to the involved spinal lesion. Radiosurgery dose was a single dose in the range of 10–16 Gy to the involved spine. The dose was prescribed to the periphery of target tumor volume encompassed by the 90% isodose line. The majority of patients (70% of the lesions) experienced moderate to severe pain. Karnofsky's status was above 70 in 75%. Since the goals of treatment for spinal metastasis are pain control and preservation of neurologic function, the endpoints of evaluation were the assessment of pain, neurologic status, and radiologic studies for tumor control.

Pain Control

Pain was scored by using verbal/visual analogue scale; from 0 (no pain) to 10 (the worst imaginable pain). The scoring was performed before radiosurgery, four weeks, and eight weeks following radiosurgery. During the first four weeks the patients were evaluated by telephone for assessment of pain status. Complete relief was defined as a complete absence of pain and no need of analgesics. Partial relief was defined as a decrease of at least three levels of the pain score or significant reduction of analgesic medication such as elimination of narcotics or breakthrough medication. The time to achieve pain relief was recorded as the time span of pain relief/reduction from the day of radiosurgery. The duration of pain relief was measured as lack of progression of pain or without an increase in analgesic medication. Pain progression was defined as an increase in the pain score by three levels and/or increased pain medication.

Rapid pain relief was achieved with the median time of 14 days (range 1–69 days). The earliest pain relief was seen within 24 hr. The change of pain scores before and after radiosurgery showed a clear shift toward lower pain scale following radiosurgery treatment. Four weeks after radiosurgery, complete pain relief was achieved in 37.7% of cases involving pain, and partial pain relief in 47.6% of cases. At 8 weeks, complete relief was seen in 46%, partial relief in 18.9%, and stable levels in 16.2% of cases. The estimated median duration of pain relief was 16.6 months. Overall pain control rate for one year was 84% (50).

Factors that may affect the pain relief were analyzed. Uni- and multivariate analyses did not reach statistical significance with age, Karnofsky's performance status, primary tumor type, presence of neurologic symptoms systemic metastases other than the spine, number of spinal lesions, dose of radiosurgery, and chemotherapy. However, there was a strong trend of increased pain control with higher radiation dose $\geq$14 Gy (50).

Neurological Improvement

There were 18 patients who presented either neurologic signs of motor weakness and sensory changes of the extremities or radiologic epidural cord compression. Twelve patients were treated with decompression surgery followed by postoperative radiosurgery. There were six patients with spinal cord compression that were treated by radiosurgery alone. Follow-up clinical and radiological examination was performed before radiosurgery, one month, and then every 2–3 months following radiosurgery in patients who were able to make the follow-up visits. Five of these patients continued to be ambulatory or to have the full range of arm and finger motion (50). Due to the small number of patients treated so far, dose response analysis could not be established for neurologic and radiologic tumor control.

Treatment Failure and Complications

Four lesions (6.5%) had progressive pain at the treated site and required stronger analgesic medication. All these patients had progressive systemic metastases. Radiologic progression to the immediately adjacent vertebral bodies was seen in three patients (4.9%) at six and nine months after radiosurgery. The status of the treated spine were stable (51). These patients had progressive paraspinal soft tissue mass along the vertebral involvement.

Overall one-year survival rate was 74.3%. During this period, there were no clinically detectable neurological signs that could be attributable to the acute or subacute radiation-induced cord damage for a maximum follow-up of 24 months. The radiologic studies of six patients who have been followed up for more than one year did not reveal any sign that was suggestive of spinal cord injury. No patient was admitted to the hospital as a result of complications due to the radiosurgery treatment.

Treatment of Recurrent Spinal Metastasis

The outcome of the radiosurgery for recurrent spinal metastasis that was previously treated with external beam radiotherapy was similar to the new spinal metastasis as described above. The radiosurgery dose was somewhat limited due to the previous radiotherapy. Dose selection was individualized based on the previous radiation dose, interval between the treatments, and the patient's general condition. In the interim analysis, complete pain relief was also achieved in 40% of the patients and partial relief in 26%. The rapidity of the pain relief was also rapid within two weeks from radiosurgery. Complete and partial neurological recovery was also noted in six out of eight patients

Radiosurgery of Primary Spinal Tumors

Stereotactic radiosurgery is effective in the treatment of benign lesions of the brain and the head and neck, as well as malignant tumors (52,53). The role of radiosurgery for the treatment of benign and malignant spinal tumors has been also defined (51,54). Spinal radiosurgery allows the use of a higher dose needed to destroy the neoplastic tissue. Benign and malignant primary spinal tumors were treated with a single dose or fractionated radiosurgery. The primary spinal cord tumors include glioblastoma, anaplastic ependymoma, gliomas, chordoma, neurofibroma, etc. The results show excellent tumor response and these results are being analyzed. The primary osseous tumors arising from the spine were also treated successfully (55).

Current Practice at Henry Ford Hospital

The spinal radiosurgery program at Henry Ford Hospital (HFH) is being carried out in a multi-disciplinary effort for spinal metastasis and primary spinal tumors at the weekly spine tumor board. For metastatic disease, patients are

Table 2 HFH Spinal Radiosurgery for Spinal Metastasis

Group 1	Focal disease with minimal neurologic deficit
	Radiosurgery alone to the involved spine
Group 2	Focal disease with significant neurologic deficit and spinal cord compression
	Surgical decompression/stabilization followed by radiosurgery
Group 3	Diffuse metastatic disease with minimal neurologic deficit or symptoms
	Radiosurgery alone to the most symptomatic site
Group 4	Widespread metastatic disease
	External beam radiation therapy ± boost radiosurgery

placed into one of four cohorts as shown in Table 2. All patients are pre-screened for evidence of spinal instability. Following treatment, the follow-up program includes questionnaires and clinical and radiologic tests. Follow-up clinical evaluation and neurologic examination are performed every two months. A baseline MRI prior to radiosurgical treatment is followed by repeat MRI examination at 2, 6, and 12 months. Patient questionnaires consist of entry demographic information and monthly quality of life assessments (completed by the patient or a family member). The endpoints for clinical investigation are patient quality of life, neurologic and pain status, and radiographic spinal cord abnormality and tumor control.

The use of spinal radiosurgery is not limited as a single modality to new or recurrent lesions. It is also effective as an adjuvant to decompression surgery, or in combination with vertebroplasty, or as the boost treatment to external beam radiotherapy, or in combination with ongoing chemotherapy. Multidisciplinary treatment efforts can improve the patient's quality of life and are, therefore, a significant addition to the armamentarium for the management of spinal tumors. Our extracranial radiosurgery program was also extended to other organ sites such as head and neck cancers with excellent tumor control (56).

REFERENCES

1. Wong DA, Fornasier VL, MacNab I. Spinal metastasis: the obvious, the occult, the imposters. Spine 1990; 15:1–4.
2. Siegal T, Siegal T. Current considerations in the management of neoplastic spinal cord compression. Spine 1989; 14:223.
3. Young JM, Funk FJ Jr. Incidence of tumor metastases to the lumbar spine. A comparative study of roentgenographic changes and gross lesions. J Bone Joint Surg Am 1953; 35:55–64.
4. Lada R, Kaminski HJ, Ruff RL. Metastatic spinal cord compression. In: Vecht C, ed. Neuro-oncology, Part III. Neurological disorders in systemic cancer. Amsterdam: Elsevier Biomedical Publishers, 1997:167–189.
5. Black P. Spinal metastases: current status and recommended guidelines for management. Neurosurgery 1979; 5:726–746.
6. Posner JB. Management of central nervous system metastasis. Semin Oncol 1997; 4:81.
7. Barron KD, Hirano A, Haraki S, Terry RD. Experiences with metastatic neoplasms involving the spinal cord. Neurology 1959; 9:91.
8. Helweg-Larsen S. Clinical outcome in metastatic spinal cord compression: a prospective study of 153 patients. Acta Neurol Scand 1996; 94:269–275.
9. Gilbert RW, Kim JH, Posner JB. Epidural spinal cord compression from metastatic tumor: diagnosis and treatment. Ann Neurol 1978; 3:40–51.
10. Greenberg HS, Kim JH, Posner JB. Epidural spinal cord compression from metastatic tumor: results with a new treatment protocol. Ann Neurol 1980; 8:361–366.

11. Loblaw DA, Laperriere NJ. Emergency treatment of malignant extradural spinal cord compression: an evidence-based guideline. J Clin Oncol 1998; 16:1613–1624.

12. Siegal T, Siegal T. Surgical decompression of anterior and posterior malignant epidural tumors compressing the spinal cord: a prospective study. Neurosurgery 1985; 17:424–432.

13. Al-Rodham NR, Kelly PJ. Pioneers of stereotactic neurosurgery. Stereotact Funct Neurosurg 1992; 58:60–66.

14. Clarke RH. The Johns Hopkins Hopsital Reports. In: Investigation of Central Nervous System, Part I. Methods and Instruments. Baltimore: The Johns Hopkins Press, 1920:11121–11124.

15. Rand RW, Bauer RO, Smart CR, et al. Experiences with percutaneous stereotactic cryocordotomy. Bull LA Neurol Soc 1965; 30:142–147.

16. Nadvomik P, Frolich J, Jezek V, et al. New apparatus for spinal cord stereotaxis and its use in the microsurgery of lumbar enlargement. Confin Neurol 1972; 34:311–314.

17. Gabriel EM, Nashold BS. History of spinal cord stereotaxy. J Neurosurg 1996; 85:725–731.

18. Takacs I, Hamilton AJ. Extracranial stereotactic radiosurgery. Neurosurg Clin N Am 1999; 10:257–269.

19. Hamilton AJ, Lulu BA, Fosmire H, Stea B, Cassady JR. Preliminary clinical experience with linear accelerator-based spinal stereotactic radiosurgery. Neurosurgery 1995; 36:311–319.

20. Murphy MJ, Cox RS. The accuracy of dose localization for an image-guided frameless radiosurgery system. Med Phys 1996; 23:2043–2049.

21. Yin FF, Ryu S, Ajlouni M, Zhu J, Yan H, Guan H, Faber K, Rock J, Abdulhak M, Rogers L, Rosenblum M, Kim J. A technique of intensity-modulated radiosurgery (IMRS) for spinal tumors. Med Phys 2002; 29:2815–2822.

22. Schell MC, Bova FJ, Larson DA, et al. Stereotactic Radiosurgery: Report of Task Group 42 Radiation Therapy Committee. College Park, MD: American Institute of Physics, 1995:6–8.

23. Shiu AS, Change EL, Ye JS, Lii M, Rhines LD, Mendel E, Weinberg J, Singh S, Maor M, Mohan R, Cox JD. Near simultaneous computed tomography image-guided stereotactic spinal radiosurgery: an emerging paradigm for achieving true stereotaxy. Int J Radiat Oncol Biol Phys 2003; 57:605–613.

24. Lax I, Blomgren H, Naslund I, Svanstrom R. Stereotactic radiotherapy of extracranial targets. Z Med Phys 1994; 4:112–113.

25. Yan H, Yin FF, Kim JH. A phantom study on the positioning accuracy of the Novalis Body system. Med Phys 2003; 30:3052–3060.

26. Yin FF, Rubin P. Imaging for radiation oncology treatment process. In: Bragg DG, Rubin P, Hricak H, eds. Chapter 8 in Oncologic Imaging. 2nd edn. Philadelphia: WB Saunders Company, 2002.

27. Llacer J. Inverse radiation treatment planning using the dynamically penalized likelihood method. Med Phys 1997; 24:1751–1764.

28. Llacer J, Solberg TD, Promberger C. Comparative behavior of the dynamically penalized likelihood algorithm in inverse radiation therapy planning. Phys Med Biol 2001; 46:2637–2663.

29. Fiveash JB, Murshed H, Duan J, Hyatt M, Caranto J, Bonner JA, Popple RA. Effect of multileaf collimator leaf width on physical dose distributions in the treatment of CNS and head and neck neoplasms with intensity modulated radiation therapy. Med Phys 2002; 29:1116–1119.

30. Timothy CR, Meeks SL, Traynelis V, Haller J, Bouchet LG, Bova F, Pennington EC, Buatti JM. Ultrasonographic guidance for spinal extracranial radiosurgery; technique and application for metastatic spinal lesions. Neuiosurg Focus 2001; 11(6).

31. Murphy MJ, Change S, Gibbs L, Le QT, Martin D, Kim D. Image-guided radiosurgery in the treatment of spinal metastases. Neurosurg Focus 2003:11.

32. Kim JK, Yin FF, Kim JH. Characteristics of a CT/Dual X-ray image registration method using 2D texture map based DRR, gradient ascent, and mutual information. ICCR 2004.

33. Jaffray DA, Siewerdsen JH, et al. Flat-panel cone-beam computed tomography for image-guided radiation therapy. Int J Radiat Oncol Biol Phys 2002; 53: 1337–1349.

34. Mackie TR, Balog J, Ruchala K, Shepard D, Aldridge S, Fitchard E, Reckwerdt P, Olivera G, McNutt T, Mehta M. Tomotherapy. Semin Radiat Oncol 1999; 9:108–117.

35. Kuo JV, Cabebe E, Al-Ghazi M, Yakoob I, Ramsinghani NS, Sanford R. Intensity-modulated radiation therapy for the spine at the University of California, Irvine. Med Dosim 2002; 27:137–145.

36. Yin FF, Zhu JH, Yan H, Guan H, Hammoud R, Ryu S, Kim JH. Dosimetric characteristics of Novalis shaped beam surgery unit. Med Phys 2002; 29: 1729–1738.

37. Cosgrove VP, Jahn U, Pfaender M, Bauer S, Budach V, Wurm R. Commissioning of a micro multi-leaf collimator and planning system for stereotactic radiosurgery. Radiother Oncol 1999; 50:325–336.

38. Ryu SI, Chang SD, Kim DH, Murphy MJ, Le QT, Martin DP, Adler JR. Image-guided hypo-fractionated stereotactic radiosurgery to spinal lesions. Neurosurgery 2001; 49:838–846.

39. LoSasso T, Chui CS, Ling CC. Physical and dosimetric aspects of a multileaf collimation system used in the dynamic mode for implementing intensity modulated radiotherapy. Med Phys 1998; 25:1919–1927.

40. LoSasso T, Chui CS, Ling CC. Comprehensive quality assurance for the delivery of intensity-modulated radiotherapy with a multileaf collimator used in the dynamic mode. Med Phys 2001; 28:2209–2219.

41. Phillips MH, Singer K, Miller E, Stelzer K. Commissioning in image-guided localization system for radiotherapy. Int J Radia Oncol Biol Phys 2000; 48:267–276.

42. Zhu J, Yin FF, Kim JH. Point dose verification for intensity-modulated radiosurgery using Clarkson's method. Med Phys 2003; 30:2218–2221.

43. Siebers VJ, Mohan R, Monte Carlo. Intensity-modulated radiation therapy: the state of the art. In: Jatinder R Palta, Rockwell Mackie T, AAPM, eds. 2003.

44. Zhu XR, Jursinic PA, Grimm DF, Lopez F, Rownd JJ, Gillin MT. Evaluation of Kodak EDR2 film for dose verification of intensity modulated radiation therapy delivered by a static multileaf collimator. Med Phys 2002; 29:1687–1692.

45. Warkentin B, Steciw S, Rathee S, Fallone BG. Dosimetric IMRT verification with a flat-panel EPID. Med Phys 2003; 30:3143–3155.
46. Ma L, Phaisangittisakul N, Yu CX, Sarfaraz M. A quality assurance method for analyzing and verifying intensity-modulated fields. Med Phys 2003; 30:2082–2088.
47. Zhu Y, Sirov AS, Mishra V, Meigoomi AS, Williamson IF. Quantitative evaluation of radiochromic film response for two-dimensional dosimetry. Med Phys 1997; 24:223–229.
48. Ryu S, Yin FF, Rock J, Zhu J, Chu A, Kagan E, Rogers L, Ajlouni M, Rosemblum M, Kim J. Image-guided and intensity-modulated radiosurgery for patients with spinal metastases. Cancer 2003; 97:2013–2018.
49. Ryu S, Sharif A, Yin FF, Ajlouni M, Kim JH. Tolerance of human spinal cord to single dose radiosurgery. Proceedings of International Congress of Radiation Research, 2003.
50. Ryu S, Rock J, Yin FF, Ajlouni M, Rosenblum M, Kim JH. Image-guided single dose radiosurgery for single spinal metastasis. Proceeding of American Society of Clinical Oncology (ASCO) 2004.
51. Ryu S, Rock J, Rosenblum M, Kim JH. Pattern of failure after single dose radiosurgery for single spinal metastasis. Journal of Neurosurgery 2004; 101: 402–405.
52. Chin LS, Szerlip NJ, Regine WF. Stereotactic radiosurgery for meningiomas. Neurosurg Focus 2003; 14:1.
53. Foote RL, Pollock BE, Gorman DA, et al. Glomus jugulare tumor: tumor control and complications after stereotactic radiosurgery. Head Neck 2002; 24:332–338.
54. Gertzen PC, Ozhasoglu C, Burton SA, Vogel WJ, Atkins BA, Kalnicki S, Welch WC. Cyberknife frameless single-fraction stereotactic radiosurgery for benignm tumors of the spine. Neurosurg Focus 2003; 14:1–5.
55. Rock J, Kole M, Yin FF, Ryu S, Guittierez J, Rosenblum M. Radiosurgical treatment for Ewing's sarcoma of the lumbar spine. Spine 2002; 27:471–475.
56. Ryu S, Khan M, Yin FF, Ajlouni M, Concus A, Benninger MS, Kim JH. Image-guided Radiosurgery of Head and Neck cancers. Otolaryngology Head and Neck Surg 2004; 130:690–697.

12

Stereotactic Radiotherapy of Head and Neck Tumors

Robert Smee

*Department of Radiation Oncology, Prince of Wales Hospital, Randwick,
New South Wales, Australia*

Reinhard Würm

Abteilurg Strahlentherapie, Universität Klinikum, Charite, Berlin, Germany

INTRODUCTION

Highly conformal radiotherapy is now becoming the norm for treatment delivery. This principle has added significance for head and neck (HN) sites because more typically we are dealing with malignancies (typically carcinomas) that require higher doses for control in the context of nearby dose-sensitive normal structures. The latter ranges from critical structures, such as the ocular apparatus and the spinal cord, to dose important organs such as the major salivary glands. The latter structures impact very much upon the quality of life of those treated, importantly the long-term survivors. The three-dimensional (3D) conformal treatment approach including intensity modulated radiotherapy (IMRT) is able to set particular structures as a dose-defining structure, and using either forward or inverse planning to limit the dose to these structures. It is important obviously that the adequate dose be given to the tumor being treated. This can create a circumstance of competing priorities, with concern that the large areas of intervening normal tissue may receive a higher dose. In the above example of sparing normal tissues, the major salivary glands may receive an acceptable dose for maintenance of salivary function, but the minor salivary glands more typically excluded in the parallel-opposed technique may receive a high dose that could significantly impair their function. The end result may thus be that the patient experiences the same side effect but caused by a different end organ.

Stereotactic irradiation offers many possibilities for HN tumors. This may be used as definitive treatment for the primary lesion, as a boost after prior wide field treatment, or for recurrence. These listed situations apply equally to stereotactic radiosurgery (SRS), as well as to fractionated stereotactic treatment. The impetus for this consideration relates to the necessity to give higher doses for local control in a circumstance of adjacent dose critical structures. The concept of making this dose delivery stereotactic relates to an extra dimension of treatment delivery accuracy over and above that achievable by some form of conventional setup.

Broadly, stereotactic irradiation is divided into two: single-dose SRS and stereotactic fractionated treatment. Machine limitations and tumor location will influence the treatment method chosen for those with available technology. The literature, however, supports both methods with acceptable outcomes in disease-specific circumstances. The aim of this chapter is thus to bring to reader's attention the techniques available, how they have been used, their value, and thus whether the results justify continuing with this approach. In addition, the treatment approach utilized at Prince of Wales Hospital will be demonstrated; a number of case histories are used to demonstrate the capabilities of these treatment methods.

BACKGROUND

Stereotactic Radiosurgery

This approach was the genesis of all stereotactic irradiation procedures. It involves the fixed attachment of a head ring device for coordinate localization purposes and delivery of the irradiation on the same day. Given that a high single dose is delivered, there is a limit on the size of the lesion that can be treated. As the head ring is typically attached to the frontal bone (some publications have raised the concept of the needle insertion into the maxilla for lower ring placement) the conditions treated are limited to those at the base of skull or nasopharynx.

Three methods available are:

- GammaKnife
- Linear accelerator (linac)
- Charged particles

The radiobiological effect in tissue of each of these methods is very similar. Typically, a high dose is given to a small target using the conformality of the treatment approach to limit the dose to adjacent structures. It was first used in recurrent malignancies and as its value was demonstrated, an expanded role saw SRS being used as boost treatment in primary management of malignancies, and for more localized relatively radioresistant tumors. Table 1A (1–7) demonstrates the role that this approach has had for nasopharyngeal carcinomas in the context of recurrent disease. Although the patient numbers are small, a reasonably consistent local control figure of 50–70% is apparent, where radiosurgery is given either alone or combined with fractionated radiotherapy, for recurrent malignancies. This is for a low overall complication rate. It is recognized that this is a highly select group with relatively short follow-up. However, for patients who do receive this approach, it is likely that an improved and meaningful survival is obtained.

Chordoma is another skull base tumor treated by SRS. While histologically benign, this tumor assumes a locally progressive nature, which would limit responsiveness to conventional radiotherapy. Its typical site involves the clivus, which makes it surgically irresectable. Conventional dose radiotherapy with up to 60 Gy being delivered reports low local control rates of 20–30% (8). Hence, a reasonable approach was to consider giving a high single dose. Muthukumar published the University of Pittsburgh (9) experience of 15 patients (13 of whom had SRS plus surgery, two SRS alone). A mean marginal dose of 18 Gy was given, with only one patient having an in-field failure. Two patients progressed outside the treatment volume with a mean follow-up of four-year post-SRS. Whilst this is relatively short follow-up for this tumor, high local control rates are apparent for a single-dose procedure. It is sufficient that such treatment should be considered for localized tumors postsurgery, or indeed even de novo for small tumors.

Chemodectomas, principally, are a benign tumor arising from neuroendocrine tissue in the HN area, in the temporal bone, and in the carotid artery wall. This rare tumor is a slowly growing lesion with its presentation relating to its proximity to the neurovascular bundle. Pulsatile tinnitus is a common presenting event for temporal bone lesions, and a palpable mass being apparent for carotid lesions. A number of the lower cranial nerves (including the vagus) are adjacent to these tumors, hence surgical resection of these tumors places these nerves at high risk of being resected with subsequent deficit. As can be seen in Table 2 (10–16), with moderate single-dose radiosurgery very high local control rates can be achieved, within six of seven series there were no long-term complications. Patients rarely die from these tumors although their site can cause significant morbidity. Thus, the treatment that has high local control, low morbidity, and can be done on an outpatient basis should be regarded as a treatment of choice. It should be noted that these lesions need to be of a size suitable for SRS and it may thus be a selection criterion for these lesions. A fractionated radiotherapy approach needs to be considered for the larger lesions.

Only one other HN site has been reported for SRS with Habermann noting its use as a boost after surgical resection of nasal cavity and/or paranasal sinus carcinomas (17). Eight patients were so treated with the

GammaKnife, with seven patients being locally controlled with no adverse effects attributable to the SRS. Given that, this was combination treatment, it is difficult to define the true impact of the SRS in achieving local control. Its use, however, indicates that it can be considered for small volume residual macroscopic or microscopic disease.

Stereotactic Radiotherapy—Fractionated

While smaller tumors may be suitable for SRS, within the HN area there are a number of tumors, which either on the basis of the size of the macroscopic component or the necessity to include a significant volume of normal tissue for microscopic disease, dictate that if the treatment is to be delivered stereotactically, it has to be fractionated. This behooves the use of some form of relocatable fixation device. This device should allow extension of the treatment volume down into the neck. The GammaKnife would be excluded in this treatment device (on the basis of being a single-dose procedure, plus the inability to extend the treated area well down into the neck), and the common approach would be with a linear accelerator (Linac), although some centers have used charged particles particularly for skull base chordomas.

Whilst re-irradiation is an accepted method of managing locally recurrent nasopharyngeal carcinoma (18–21), only two centers have reported any results for fractionated stereotactic radiotherapy in this setting. Ahn reported 19 patients (4) utilizing the Gill Thomas Cosman (GTC) relocatable head ring, delivering 45–50 Gy in 18–20 fractions, to the radiologically abnormal area—Table 1B (4,22,23). Three patients died soon after, of distant disease with no local recurrence. Follow-up time was too short following this treatment to know whether long-term benefit would have been achieved, or indeed to report any complication. Dhanachai reported on 19 patients (22), using a similar approach, treated over a 30-month time frame. For 11 patients, this was for persistent/recurrent disease, for eight it was a boost. Doses delivered varied between the two situations, with the boost patients typically receiving only 4–6 fractions of 4–7 Gy each, whereas the retreated patients received up to 55 Gy in up to 28 fractions. In terms of results, only 5 of 11 retreated patients are alive with local control at the time of reporting, while all eight boost patients are alive, median follow-up of eight months, with local control. No complications were reported.

For both series, follow-up is short; however, it would be reasonable to consider SRT as a means of safe dose escalation in definitive management. Recurrent malignancy is still a major challenge for any treatment approach.

Irresectable chordomas have long been a radiotherapy challenge, predominantly because of the necessity to give higher doses with radiotherapy sensitive normal structures adjacent. Hence, charged particles have been used with the Bragg peak effect giving a dose distribution advantage. Utilizing either carbon ions or protons, local control rates at five years are a very respectable 70–90% (24,25). However, from the Harvard experience (26), it would seem that these results drop off to provide only 44% non-progression at 10 years. Against this background, Debus (27) reported on 45 patients treated postoperatively with median doses at the isocenter of 66 Gy for both chordomas and chondrosarcomas, with stereotactically delivered photons, and a local control of 82% at two years. However, similar to the Harvard experience this dropped to 50% at five years. The greatest success rate with SRS was almost certainly a reflection of the size factor, with much better local control (90%) in the proton series for smaller tumors.

Conventional radiotherapy has been used as part of the treatment approach for paranasal sinus carcinomas for many years. Treatment results with radiotherapy alone have been disappointing, but given postsurgery, high local control rates are evident (28). However, there has been no series reporting this approach with a stereotactic methodology.

Similarly with chemodectomas, despite the very good local control figures reported for the use of conventional radiotherapy alone with Hinerman (29) reporting 94% local control rate with many years of follow-up, there are no series reporting the use of fractionated stereotactic radiotherapy. It should be noted that the dose initially used (45–50 Gy) is the one tolerated by surrounding structures with low likelihood of morbidity (30), thus there may be less need for a highly conformal approach. It is the tumor, however, that does lend itself to this method, being usually well defined on imaging, without a need to consider covering microscopic disease.

The Prince of Wales Hospital approach has been to consider a stereotactic technique for appropriate situations. This has been to include both benign and malignant lesions, with the necessary volume expansion to encompass both macroscopic and microscopic components for the malignant lesions. Conditions treated are listed in Table 3. Fractionated stereotactic treatment became available in 1995, with, up to mid-2003, 380 patients treated, 51 being for extracranial or extra-intracranial location.

TECHNIQUE AND INDICATIONS

Fractionated Stereotactic Radiotherapy

All treatments have been with the LINC (Siemens MD2, and Primus; Seemens AE, Berlen, Germany) with a couch-mounted attachment. From 1995 to mid-2000, all treatments were delivered with cone-type collimation The cone size and number of isocenters used were heavily dependent upon the lesions size. The largest cone has a 4.5 cm diameter with gradations of cone size of 0.25 cm down to 0.5 cm in diameter. Thus, the shape of the lesion to be treated was covered by:

- varying the size of the cone,
- using multiple isocenters,

- preferential weighting of any of the arcs to give a more elliptical shape,
- using the primary jaws of the linac collimator system from either (or both) sides for a large lesion to "flatten" the spherical dose shape of the cone.

Once the 4-mm leaf width Radionics (Burlington, Massachetts, U.S.A.) MMLC became available, this became the main means of beam shaping. This is an add-on device to our linac fitting into the shadow-tray position. Attachment takes 15–20 min, which needs to be programmed into the machine timetable each day, with removal taking 10 min. Consequently, all patients are treated in one time block, usually the middle of the day, the start time being dependent upon whether there are any children having general anesthetics for this treatment. At any one time, there are 8–10 patients having this therapy. Thus, the dominant lesion for this technique remains intracranial tumors.

The MMLC weighs 20 kg and the attachment to the head of the machine needs to be considered in terms of gantry movement. Counterbalancing this weight was considered but after considerable testing, since the machine is not used in arc mode, this was not felt necessary. After three years of use, the linac gantry remains quite stable for stereotactic and non-stereotactic use. The field size of the MMLC is 10×12 cm; thus no stereotactic treatment is possible to lesions larger than this. Clearance of the MMLC from the patient is 45 cm, with the collimator set at 90° to avoid collisions. Thus, gantry angles of 0–360% are possible for beam entry.

Planning for all fractionated stereotactic treatments is done on the Radionics X-Plan Planning System (Version 4). The process involves, as with any 3D conformal technique critical structure outlining (both volumes to be treated, and avoided or minimized), evaluation of which beam entry portals are to be used and beam's eye view (BEV) used to select the beam portals with consideration given to target coverage for the coverage of critical structures. For fixed field treatment, evaluation of dose–volume histogram (DVH) is used to make the final assessment of the volume to be covered and structures to be avoided. A plan is then generated, printed, and evaluated. If accepted, as part of the QA process, the physics staff verifies all beam and dose parameters, and treatment characteristics are incorporated into the linac Record and Verify System (RVS).

For the IMRT patients, the inverse planning system (Konrad) requires particular dose characteristics to be set including maximum and minimum dose for the tumor to be treated as well as for any nominated critical structure. Priorities and penalties are set for exceeding the specified dose for any of these structures. Thus, after the outlining component and nomination of beam numbers and entry direction, as for the fixed field treatment, all the material is imported into Konrad and the IMRT planning begins. Generation of DVHs require export back into XPlan where the fluence maps are generated. This process takes only a few minutes and thus any change can be incorporated and evaluated quickly. Prior to the actual treatment, the whole treatment process is delivered to X-ray film, and the developed fluence maps are compared qualitatively and quantitatively with the planned fluence maps.

Head and neck fixation was done initially by the Radionics GTC fixation device for awake patients and the Radionics TLC device for anesthetized children. The GTC fixation is a bite block-based device using maxillary dental attachment, to which is then attached the stereotactic ring, which also serves for attachment and fixation, to the couch mount system. Edentulous patients can be accommodated by adding more bulk to the dental plate. Velcro-backed strips are then pulled upwards across the side of the head applying upward pressure against the gum margins. A depth helmet is then attached to the ring, and initially 20 depth measurements were taken for each treatment with a variation of no greater than 2 mm allowed before continuing with treatment. After thousands of measurements were taken it was apparent that the only variation was in six of the sites, and thus measuring all sites was unnecessary. The QA process could thus be shortened without reducing its effect, by dispensing with redundant parts of the process. A similar concept is used for the HN localizer (HNL). The base board is attached at fixed points to the treatment couch, and to this is then attached the stereotactic localizer, and depth readings are done to make sure the patient is being setup in the same position. Skin marks are used as a final verification process for patient setup.

Prior to the first treatment, the actual treatment process is simulated with the gantry and couch position for each treatment position verified to ensure no potential collision. An isocenter phantom is used for GTC setup. The treatment sequence is then delivered, with the head ring or HNL fixed in position on to the couch, to ensure that all leaf sequences proceed as determined by the planning computer and loaded into the R and V system. For the actual treatment, the patient is lying on the couch with the head ring attached, which is then "docked" to the fixation device on the couch. The patient is made comfortable, and a final QA process begins. With a clear Perspex box attached to the head ring, and clear paper sheets placed on each of three surfaces (anterior and two laterals) the machine laser lights are used to verify centering of the head ring or HNL, and the entry portal for each beam direction is set accurately. Once all these steps are complete, treatment can take place. All gantry positions can be set at the linac console, and movement of the gantry takes place from there. Couch movements are done inside the room. The total treatment time each day, including the QA steps for the first session is less than the time it takes to treat a 4-field breast patient. For the IMRT procedures, treatment time is about 30 min, this however being dependent upon the number of segments treated. This includes head ring application, with QA about 5 min longer than for multiple fixed fields with the MMLC. No treatments are done with the native 1-cm leaf width MLC.

The advantage of this is that a better-collimated treatment is delivered but the disadvantage is the limited field size (10 × 12 cm).

The practice for HN cancers requiring large field irradiation has been to use conventional wide field coverage, to say 50–56 Gy. The stereotactic approach can then be used to take the primary up to the specified dose (70–74 Gy) with any neck nodes boosted to the required doses. Those malignancies in which the pattern of failure is more predominantly local have all their treatment delivered stereotactically.

For the benign tumors (e.g., chemodectoma), all treatment is delivered stereotactically.

Nasopharyngeal Carcinoma

Ample evidence now exists to indicate that to achieve optimum local control for T2-4 carcinomas, doses of 70–80 Gy are required, even with concurrent chemotherapy. These doses are beyond the tolerance of adjacent mandible, temporal lobes, and brain stem, if delivered with conventional radiotherapy. For this treatment, a typical 3-field non-salivary gland sparing approach was given to 50–56 Gy, with electrons to the posterior neck after the spinal cord received 40 Gy. The neck was boosted with electrons as required, dependent upon the bulk of the nodal disease. The primary site, typically all of the nasopharynx and adjacent paranasopharyngeal area, was then boosted stereotactically with a minimum of 20 Gy. The contralateral paranasopharyngeal was excluded if the carcinoma was lateralized. Throughout the treatment 2 Gy fractions were used. Limits on the dose to the temporal lobes and mandible were set at a maximum of 10 Gy over that given by phase 1 treatment.

Three case histories represent the capabilities of this approach.

Patient 1—A 14-year-old teenager, who presented with left neck disease with presumed nasopharyngeal primary, was given conventional field treatment to 26 Gy, and then stereotactic IMRT with the 1-cm leaf width MLC to 66 Gy with major salivary gland sparing (Fig. 1). This particular patient, whilst satisfactorily treated, raised concern regarding our QA process for the larger width MLC to such an extent that we did not continue with that approach. All this treatment was thus done as one field with the primary site receiving a dose of 1.8 Gy per fraction, while the neck was treated bilaterally at 1.4 Gy per fraction over the same number of fractions using the intensity-modulated component to decrease the dose per fraction to areas of lower risk disease.

Patient 2—An Asian male aged 45 years presented a 12-month history of intermittent epistaxis and neck pain. As Figure 2A indicates, there was extensive spread of his carcinoma through the base of skull into sphenoid sinus and clivus, resulting in a significant parasellar and prepontine mass,

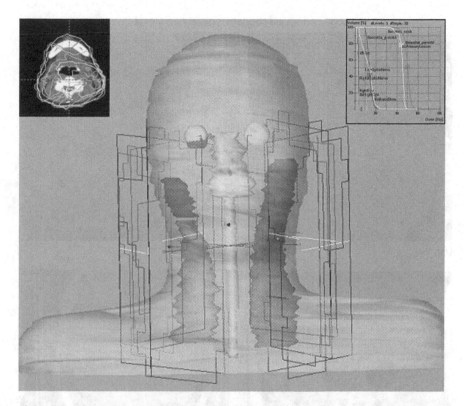

Figure 1 Fourteen-year-old teenager with nasopharyngeal carcinoma and involved left neck nodes. Stereotactic MLC treatment. DVHs demonstrate dose separation between malignancy and adjacent critical structures.

the latter encircling the basal artery and displacing the pons posteriorly. In addition, there was a dural plaque of carcinoma extending along the clival surface to the foramen magnum. Superiorly, its extension was up toward the optic chiasm although there was 3 mm separation between these two structures. Thus, in this situation the dose-limiting structures were: temporal lobes, optic chiasm, and brain stem, with the maximum of 50 Gy set for both phases 1 and 2. Despite the bulk of the primary there was no nodal disease, and thus phase 1 with a conventional 3-field technique went to 46 Gy, the remainder was taken to 70 Gy, this being the extensive primary site and bilateral nasopharyngeal areas, delivered with concurrent cis-platinum and 5FU. The stereotactic component of his treatment was given with multiple fixed fields using the MLC for beam shaping. The pituitary was enveloped by the primary mass and could not be spared receiving full dose.

In terms of outcome, two-year post-treatment, this patient remains disease free with a normal functioning pituitary, mild xerostomia, and

Locally Advanced Nasopharyngeal Carcinoma

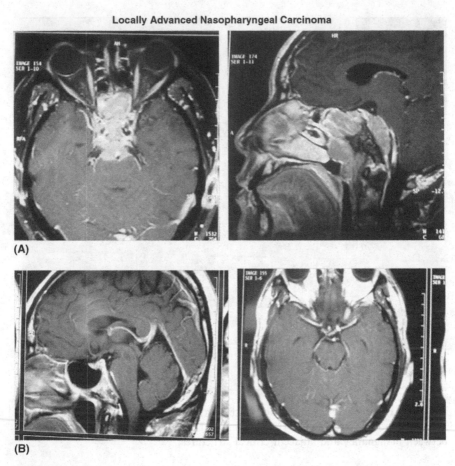

Figure 2 (A) MRI: Extensive nasopharyngeal carcinoma extending through the sphenoid sinus and clivus to pre-pontine location with dural plaque of malignancy extending to foramen magnum. (B) MRI 18-months post-treatment: No evident malignancy.

normal taste (Fig. 2C). The only area of fibrosis is in the left neck, where he received 46 Gy the right neck, which received the same dose, has minimal long-term effect.

Patient 3—A 65-year-old male presented a right nasopharyngeal primary on a background of 10 years previously having had a laryngectomy and postoperative radiotherapy to bilateral neck and pharyngeal areas to 50 Gy for an advanced larynx cancer. This new primary was thus his second significant cancer. His neck had considerable fibrosis and thus would not tolerate any significant extra dose. The primary site (whole nasopharynx and right paranasopharyngeal area up to and including the base of skull) was thus treated with stereotactic IMRT abutting up to the top edge of the previous treatment field. The typical dose-limiting structures within the field such as brain stem and chiasm could be regarded as untreated structures. Total dose was 66 Gy in 33 fractions at 2 Gy per fraction. In this circumstance, however, the intensity modulation was used to increase the dose per fraction to the radiologically evident abnormality (GTV) such that this area was receiving 2.4 Gy per fraction as a concurrent relative hypofrac-tionated boost. There was significant acute mucositis associated with this. Unfortunately, this patient had two adverse outcomes. First, he failed in the contralateral neck with nodal disease, and second he developed a radio-necrotic ulcer at the site of the boost area. Subsequent investigations indicated markedly abnormal bilateral carotid vasculature, probably subse-quent to his initial radiotherapy plus the predisposing history of cigarette smoking prior to his laryngectomy. In this circumstance presumably the mucosa could not cope with the further radiotherapy from a vascular healing effect. The increased dose per fraction, be it to malignancy, resulted in a non-healing situation. Thus, this patient's subsequent quality and quan-tity of life was mainly influenced by the constraints of his previous disease and treatment. Hyperbaric oxygen, the appropriate treatment for his radio-necrotic ulcer, would have been inappropriate in the circumstance of progressive malignancy.

Chemodectoma

This is a benign lesion readily identifiable on imaging (best with MRI—not all patients today would have angiography) either at the skull base or projecting into the neck. The significance of it being benign is that there is no necessity to add a margin for microscopic disease. Thus what is defined on scans is all that needs to be treated. Given that there can be significant cranial/caudal growth, it is unlikely that a head base fixation and the stereotactic coordinate system would suffice for the majority of lesions. The smaller glomus tympanicum lesions can be adequately treated by SRS by ensuring that the head ring is placed as low as possible with marginal doses of 14–16 Gy sufficing.

With the larger glomus tympanicum, and certainly all of the glomus jugulare lesions a fractionated approach is more reasonable, the standard being 1.8–2.0 Gy fractions to 45–50 Gy. This follows the outstanding results so far demonstrated for conventional radiotherapy. The purpose in delivering this treatment stereotactically is the ability to mainly lower the dose to surrounding normal structures.

The neck fixation system is either by bite block or customized mask attachment to a carbon fiber backboard around which fits the stereotactic coordinate system. Both components fit on to a diagnostic CT couch top and the treatment couch. Accurate positioning of this board in relationship

Fixed Beams, Arcs or IMRT - Glomus Tumor

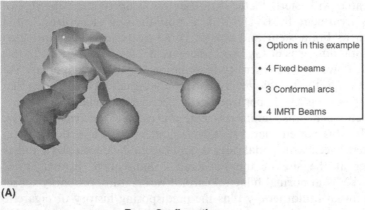

- Options in this example
- 4 Fixed beams
- 3 Conformal arcs
- 4 IMRT Beams

(A)

Beam Configurations

4 Beams - Fixed or IMRT   3 Arcs (14 fixed beams)

(B)

Isodose Comparison

4 Fixed fields   4 IMRT   3 Conformal Arcs

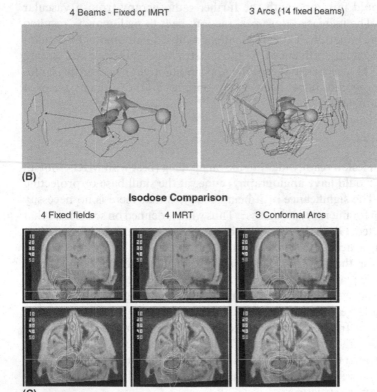

(C)

Figure 3 Chemodectoma—glomus tympanicum. (**A**) Volume rendered structures—treatment options. (**B**) Field arrangement—14 fixed beams simulating three conformal arcs. (**C**) Isodose display demonstrating conformality of various options, with IMRT as the best option.

to the isocenter is important to ensure the day-to-day reproducibility of the stereotactic reference system. This component of each patient's treatment is longer, although the treatment times with multiple fixed fields may not vary, compared to the GTC head fixation system. In addition adjacent normal structures, although important, are less critical, particularly given the doses being used so there is little advantage to using IMRT. Multiple fixed fields usually give adequate coverage. Entry and exit directions can be defined using BEV, with MMLC leaf placement used to shape the field to the lesion margins allowing a 3-mm expansion around the tumor as a PTV (Fig. 3A). Although there can be some organ movement within the pharynx and larynx (with swallowing and breathing, respectively), given the lateral location for these lesions this is unlikely to have much effect. Hypofractionating the dose has the advantage of convenience, but with an uncertain track record. Conventional fractionation for the larger lesions would seem to be the current standard of care.

Figure 3B demonstrates the dose shell display, field arrangement, and DVH for a large glomus jugulare tumor with multiple static fields using the MMLC. The criteria of benefit, as with most benign tumors, are lack of progression (achieved in about 90% of cases) with most patients enjoying considerable improvement in symptoms.

Paranasal Sinus Carcinomas

Although a number of centers have reported the use of radiotherapy alone for these malignancies, this is also usually inferior to the figures generated where major surgical resection and postoperative radiotherapy are delivered. Nodal spread is uncommon unless there is local extension through the anterior wall of the maxilla into the skin of the cheek. Thus, for the majority of patients, local control relates very much to the cancer-specific survival. In the postoperative setting, it is typically microscopic disease that is being addressed. Adjacent critical structures include bilateral globes (unilateral if an orbital exenteration has been performed), optic nerves, optic chiasm, frontal lobes, and brain stem. Typical postoperative doses of 56 Gy plus are required, this being above the tolerance of these structures even with the conventional fractionation. Published series report significant ocular and neurological morbidity rates using these types of doses. Two of the cases treated with chondrosarcomas required higher doses (70 Gy). There are a number of unique circumstances with these types of cancers·

- Use of the GTC head ring needs modification to allow most if not all of the maxilla to be included in the CTV. A spacer can be added to the dental plate to allow for an extra margin of inferior extension.
- In the postoperative setting (except where orbital exenteration is done in combination with a craniofacial resection and a large

microvascular free flap is used to fill in the defect), a large air cavity is created leading to some dose uncertainty due to the "build up" and "build down" effect on the residual sinus walls. It is important that the dose algorithm in the planning system be able to cope with this.

Given the above critical structures, malignancies in this site lend themselves appropriately to the use of IMRT. Figure 4 depicts the dose display,

Paranasal Chondrosarcoma - Treatment of a Cavity

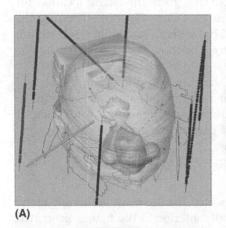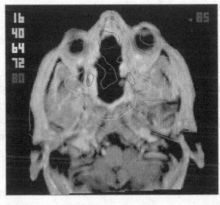

(A)

Paranasal Chondrosarcoma - Organs at Risk-DVH

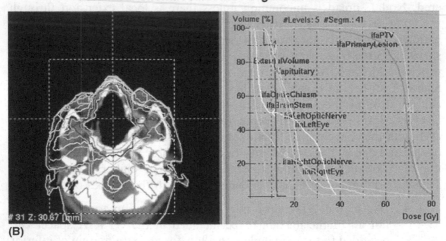

(B)

Figure 4 (A) Paranasal chondrosarcoma demonstrating postsurgical air cavity. Field arrangement and dose display on axial MRI. (B) DVH display of comparative dose to tumor and adjacent structures.

and DVH for a patient treated postoperatively for a chondrosarcoma where the mean dose delivered was 70 Gy at 2 Gy per fraction. Head fixation was via the GTC head ring.

Skin Carcinoma—Perineural Spread

Skin carcinomas are the commonest malignancy affecting the Australian population. A small proportion has perineural spread (this can occur with both basal and squamous cell carcinomas), more typically this is evident histologically and is usually an indication for postoperative radiotherapy. Some patients present overt features of perineural spread, typically as a consequence of involvement of nerves within the cavernous sinus. Thus, diplopia or altered facial sensation is a typical presenting feature. Figure 5A demonstrates the extent of spread for one patient there was extension back along the maxillary branch of the trigeminal nerve centripetally to involve the nerve within the cavernous sinus, trigeminal ganglion, and then along the main trunk toward the brain stem (MRI was not possible as this patient had a cardiac pacemaker in situ).

In this situation, a high dose of 60–66 Gy at 2 Gy fractions is necessary to provide reasonable chance of control of the macroscopic component (surgery and/or chemotherapy are not viable options) with brain stem being the dose critical structure. This dose has significant risk of damage to those areas within the cavernous sinus, as well as to the carotid artery. However, with informed consent this risk is acceptable as the alternative of giving a lower (and safer) dose would be a far higher risk of failure. Microscopic

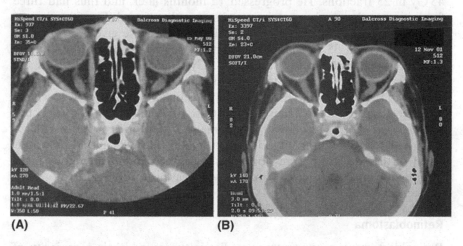

(A)   **(B)**

Figure 5 (A) Axial CT indicates enlarged right cavernous sinus and enhancing mass with central necrosis adjacent to brainstem. (B) Axial CT two-years post-treatment indicating complete resolution of disease.

extension into the brain stem toward the trigeminal nerve nucleus cannot be excluded.

Thus, a dose limit of 50 Gy was set on the brain stem for the treatment given via multiple fixed fields. Although IMRT was considered, the alternative plan is quite acceptable. Eighteen months after treatment, while the patient still had altered facial sensation a subsequent CT scan (Fig. 5B) indicates complete clearance of macroscopic tumor, without any additional neurological deficit.

For all the situations an IMRT plan has to be clearly superior to a fixed field plan to be preferred; for this patient there was no added advantage.

Chordomas

These are regarded as being radioresistant, although some conventionally fractionated series do report reasonable results, be it with short-term follow-up. The charged particle series, however, demonstrate that at least 5–10-year post-treatment control rates of 50% can be achieved. The advantage of charged particles is the Bragg–Peek effect whereby the dose to adjacent structures can be significantly reduced allowing dose escalation to the tumor, in this situation delivering 70 Gy. There is no major radiobiological advantage to protons versus photons.

A 45-year-old male, engaged in active sport, had presented three years prior to his stereotactic treatment a 3 to 4-month history of altered sensation down both arms and bilateral shoulder weakness. Investigations indicated the presence of a C3 chordoma. Debulking surgery was done and he was given postoperative radiotherapy via a parallel-opposed technique receiving 45 Gy in 25 fractions. He progressed 12 months later, and thus had three further surgical procedures and was subsequently referred (Fig. 6A). Stereotactic IMRT using the MMLC was delivered; the dose given was a mean dose of 69 Gy in 35 fractions. His spinal cord was set as a dose-limiting structure as it had already received 45 Gy. Figure 6B demonstrates the DVH for the dose-defining structures noting that the curve for the spinal cord is shifted well to the left, with only a small volume of cord receiving a higher dose. The fluence map demonstrates that all field angles were chosen to avoid chord. In follow-up, he remained well for 21 months with no treatment-related abnormality, but unfortunately his MRI at that time indicated further disease progression. This outcome demonstrates that high-dose treatment can be given, even as a retreatment, although it does not ensure success.

Retinoblastoma

Retinoblastoma is an uncommon pediatric tumor, which in a majority of circumstances is a local disease. It, typically manifests in infants, is usually sporadic and it unilateral, but in at least 30% of cases there is a family

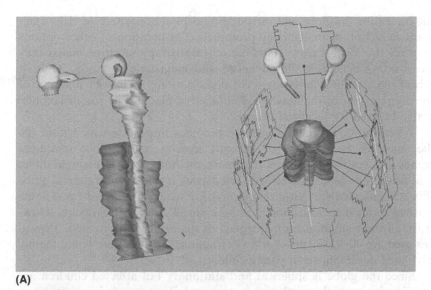

Figure 6 (A) Volume display of target volume wrapping around dose critical structure, the spinal cord. (B) Dose display, DVH, and fluence maps indicating the sparing of the spinal cord and high dose to chordoma.

history and it is bilateral. Enucleation is the preferred method of addressing the unilateral case, and it is appropriate for the bilateral cases to the worse affected eye. For many years, radiotherapy to the affected eye was a frequent event with high local control rates; however, its effect upon normal tissue (including the globe and surrounding orbital bone) and the risk of significant induction of malignancy prompted consideration of other options to control the local disease. This is a chemotherapy-sensitive malignancy demonstrating benefit in the advanced and metastatic situation. Thus, it has been utilized in infants for local disease along with laser ablation of more discrete foci of malignancy. Radioactive plaques, as for melanoma, can also be used for localized disease.

When, however, the malignancy becomes more extensive within the globe, such as the presence of vitreous seeding, whole globe treatment becomes a necessity. Published treatment methods include a single direct lateral field for unilateral disease (directed away from the contralateral globe if this is unaffected) or parallel opposed for bilateral affected eyes. Some published series have also looked at specialized electron treatments. However, in all these situations a major part of the orbit is still treated. Typical doses used are 40–45 Gy at 1.5–1.8 Gy fractions—a dose that would mainly retard bone development in young children.

Since the globe is spherical and stationary (all affected children are treated under general anesthetic), a stereotactic approach is appropriate. Head fixation and stereotactic localization is via the TLC head ring, allowing free access to the anesthetist for all anesthetic procedures. All treatment methods can be considered (arcing with cones, fixed MMLC shape field, and IMRT with an MMLC), depending upon dose coverage of all relevant structures. In this circumstance, adjacent bone becomes a dose-defining structure. These children are at increased genetic risk of developing a second malignancy, with sarcomas in adjacent bone being a reported event occurring because of the susceptibility plus the known long-term effects of radiotherapy. Sparing of the lens would be a desired goal; however, since the cases now treated have extensive local disease this is usually not possible.

Our treatment approach has evolved with initially only cones available. Figure 7A demonstrates a 15-month-old female with bilateral disease in which the malignancy was progressing in one eye only, thus unilateral treatment was given, the contralateral orbit and globe dose being kept very low (as a principle in a young child, plus also in case contralateral treatment was required). This treatment cleared the vitreous component and most of the retinal disease, although laser oblation was required to a small residual focus; functioning vision remained. Eighteen months later, malignancy progressed in the opposite globe by which stage the MMLC was being used for routine treatment. While a comparable dose was given to the globe, a lower dose was possible on adjacent bone. Similarly, good tumor control was achieved with seemingly good vision initially. In the second eye, there was more extensive anterior globe disease and thus the lens dose was higher resulting in cataract formation at two-year post-treatment. Intra-ocular lens replacement significantly improved vision. Both eyes and the child remained well controlled of malignancy with adequate vision preservation.

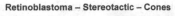

Retinoblastoma – Stereotactic – Cones

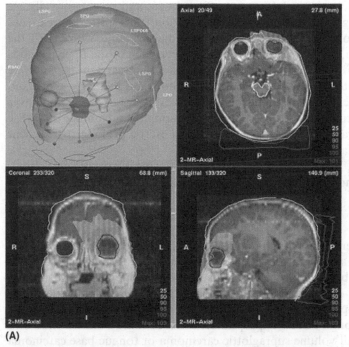

(A)

Retinoblastoma Stereotactic Development Arc vs. Fixed field vs. IMRT

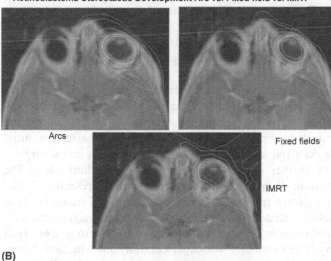

(B)

Figure 7 (A) MRI: Axial, coronal, and sagittal display of dose distribution using cones for conformality. (B) MRI: Axial display of three different treatment methods: (i) arcs with cones, (ii) multiple fixed with MMLC, and (iii) IMRT with MMLC, the last one giving lower dose to adjacent bone.

Subsequently, a 15-month-old boy with bilateral disease was referred having had enucleation of the worst affected eye, and progressive disease in the remaining eye. IMRT was now an option, thus all three treatment methods were compared to evaluate dose on adjacent bone, with IMRT the preferred option, although the difference between each of the three methods was not great (Fig. 7B). For an anesthetized child, the treatment time may be a significant factor. Fortunately, all three methods are relatively short, and thus the final decision rests on the therapeutic advantage of one method over another. Unfortunately for this young boy, despite the advantage of IMRT progressive intra-ocular disease occurred because of prolonged treatment time due to social circumstances.

Currently, IMRT is the preferred option for locally progressive retinoblastoma. For more bulky disease, localized dose escalation is always possible.

HN Tumors

Most HN cancers require high dose (66–70 Gy) for the best chance of local control as well as coverage of adjacent lymph nodes to moderate doses if uninvolved for best regional control. There can also be considerable organ movement with swallowing during the time frame of each individual treatment. It is an option for more localized cancers such as a unilateral glottic carcinoma although not an appropriate choice. It could be considered as a boost for a small volume supraglottic carcinoma or tongue base carcinoma to try to avoid high dose to the arytenoids for voice maintenance. Although the stereotactic localization becomes less critical (given the organ movement) as a means of lateralizing treatment and compensating for organ movement within the CTV for infratemporal fossa diseases, a viable treatment approach thus becomes available. Figure 8 demonstrates such an approach.

For any malignancy involving the infratemporal fossa, stereotactic irradiation could be considered. A 65-year-old female presented an adenocarcinoma ex pleomorphic adenoma arising 20 years after initial superficial parotidectomy for a pleomorphic adenoma. Twelve months after the initial surgery, recurrence occurred secondary to capsule rupture at initial surgery. This was treated by further surgery and postoperative radiotherapy. The carcinoma arose from the deep lobe of the parotid, and thus presented a bulky local disease not surgically resectable. The laterally placed mandible thus became the dose-defining structure having already received a significant dose from the previous radiotherapy. The aim in this situation was to give 66 Gy at 2-Gy fractions. Very little morbidity was experienced in this situation. Nodal volumes were not included as the pattern of failure is either local or distant for adenocarcinoma. Perhaps a higher dose should have been given, for despite seemingly good initial control and radiological improvement, ultimately, local progression occurred.

Unilateral Larynx Cancer

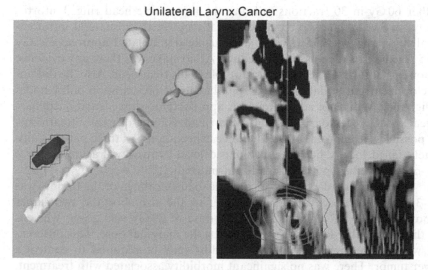

Figure 8 MRI: Axial slices demonstrating volume to be treated.

Stereotactic Radiosurgery

For smaller lesions (maximum diameter less than 3.5 cm) situated at the skull base, single-dose SRS is an appropriate treatment method. All treatments were delivered with head fixation and stereotactic localization via a BRW head ring. Frontal bone pin insertion was as low as possible to allow the ring to be placed below the defined lesion. Planning took place with XKnife® with the common theme being to individualize each patient's treatment. Cones were used with the linac in arc mode to deliver the treatment. Over a 12-year time frame, nine patients were treated, three with recurrent nasopharyngeal carcinoma, four glomus tympanicum as primary treatment, and two chordomas also as primary treatment. One of the patients with nasopharyngeal carcinoma demonstrates the utility of stereotactic treatment. He presented in June 1994 a T2N3 nasopharyngeal carcinoma and received conventional radiotherapy (prior to the availability of fractionated stereotactic treatment) to a dose of 68 Gy in 34 fractions obtaining a complete remission. Fifteen months later, he recurred on the right lateral nasopharyngeal wall as a localized area. This was treated with SRS receiving a dose of 20 Gy to the 100% isodose curve within the lesion. Once again, there was complete clearance of tumor only to recur at the same site 3.5 years later. Since this was still a localized disease, he had nasopharyngeal resection with microvascular free flap reconstruction. There were no untoward healing problems with this, given the vascularized graft. Surgical margins were very close, and thus he went on to have fractionated stereotactic radiotherapy receiving via a cone and arc technique a further 60 Gy in 30 fractions utilizing the relocatable head ring. Unfortunately, two years later he recurred laterally out in the ipsilateral infratemporal fossa and was given via a stereotactic fractionated approach 35 Gy in 15 fractions as a palliative procedure. At no stage was there any evidence of bone or soft tissue necrosis attributable to his treatment. Also, he did not develop recurrent nodal disease despite having at presentation bulky nodal malignancy. While not advocating this approach for all recurrent nasopharyngeal cases, it demonstrates that with small volume disease retreatments are possible with normal tissue tolerance expectation. All three patients ultimately failed locally however, prolonged local control was achieved for a day-only-procedure with no significant morbidity.

For the chemodectoma patients, the diameter range of the tumors was 1.8–3.2 cm with dose varying according to the size. For the two larger tumors (3.1 and 3.2 cm in diameter), a dose of 20 Gy was given, whereas for the two smaller lesions it was 14 Gy as the marginal dose. This differential was on the premise that a higher dose may be required to control a larger tumor. There was no significant morbidity associated with treatment, and all four patients had controlled tumor with the pulsatile tinnitus decreased in all four.

The two chordoma patients had relatively localized tumor (maximum diameter being 2.5 and 3.2 cm). Cones and arcs were used to deliver 20 and 18 Gy, respectively. The smaller lesion slightly increased in size, while the larger lesion that received a slightly lower dose remains controlled eight years after treatment.

The decision to use a stereotactic fractionated procedure is very much based on the clinical circumstances, age, and the proximity of dose-limiting structures. In a pediatric setting, there is an almost universal use of this approach provided it fits into a field size determinant. The necessity to limit the dose to adjacent growing normal brain with an anticipated many years of life is the driver for this approach. Although dose-escalation studies and thus dose–response relationships have not been done in many of the suitable pediatric tumors, intuitively, a safe increase of dose, particularly if there is macroscopic disease being treated, would seem to provide a greater likelihood of local control. It is worth noting that previous attempts at dose increase would have been mainly limited by the inability to deliver high doses with conventional treatment approaches safely. More wide field treatment, such as paranasal sinus malignancy or nasopharyngeal carcinoma in a child or teenager, can be performed using the stereotactic approach by using the native 1-cm leaf width MLC for the linac, or by abutting the fields—a traditional concept in conventional radiotherapy. In this approach, say to treat the neck, conventional radiotherapy can be used for this component and then the stereotactic approach for the local site (e.g., the sinus or nasopharynx). The limiting feature is going to be not having the neck treatment influenced by the stereotactic localizing device. The GTC head ring typically fits around the chin using a dental plate device for head ring application; this may then influence treatment of the neck disease. The alternative is the use of a plastic mask device through which treatment can be delivered although this may slightly compromise the precision of the stereotactic approach. The reproducible accuracy for the bite block fixation device is 1–2 mm (of error), with a mask device having an error rate of 2–3 mm. The planning approach has to be with co-planer fields for the stereotactic approach, thus placing some limitation upon beam direction and normal organ avoidance. Scatter off the leaves needs to be considered as a contributor to the abutted neck fields. The dosimetric aspects of this would need to be tested in a phantom situation during the QA process for dose verification.

Clinical circumstances dictating the stereotactic approach include those tumors for which there is a readily defined tumor, well demonstrated on imaging procedures, in which there is no necessity to encompass microscopic disease. Chemodectomas fit into this circumstance, although it could be argued, however, that since moderate dose treatment (50 Gy) provides 90% or greater chance of local control, conventional or even non-stereotactic 3D conformal approaches could be used. Other clinical circumstances include the requirements to dose escalation, such as for nasopharyngeal and paranasal sinus carcinomas. For nasopharyngeal carcinomas, numerous studies demonstrate a benefit in terms of local control with dose escalation. Shrinking fields provides the opportunity to encompass microscopic disease with sequential dose escalation. IMRT approaches allow the opportunity to simultaneously dose escalate, although the effect of a higher dose per fraction upon normal tissue contained within the malignancy needs to be considered.

Different normal tissues have varying tolerance levels. The most sensitive structure is hair, although this is not typically regarded as a dose-determining structure for treatment. A stereotactic approach even in this situation may provide an advantage. Multiple fields (even 6–10) can be used and thus the entry (and to lesser extent exit) dose for each beam portal will consequently be less. Thus patchy alopecia, rather than large volume hair loss may occur. More importantly, however, it is internal structures that define sensitivity. The optic structures, starting with the lens through to retina, optic nerve, and chiasm, are the dominant organs, progressing through to the brain stem, and increasingly the temporal lobe. These can be regarded as absolute determinants of dose and dose per fraction. The relative determinants are now salivary glands, with preservation of function impacting upon quality of life. Long-term follow-up has now demonstrated that cranial nerve dysfunction (e.g., hypoglossal) can develop even 10–15 years following treatment. As local control becomes a more achievable aim, factors such as this may influence how we address the neurovascular structures within or adjacent to treated tumors.

For SRS, given that a high single dose is used, the indications are more specific. Size is by far the greatest determinant, with this approach unable to deliver meaningful doses to lesions larger than 3.5 cm maximum diameter, even with multiple isocenters. This would exclude the opportunity to encompass microscopic disease around any malignancy. Organ movement can be important, and thus make this approach difficult to extend below the skull base even if a suitable stereotactic device were developed. Thus, the effect of laryngeal movement with breathing and swallowing would make it such that the high dose given as a single fraction with SRS would create significant risk of damage to normal tissues during the time frame the tumor moves out of the treatment beam and normal tissue into it. For skull base tumors, this is less of a problem as there is little to no organ movement at this site. There are few dose-limiting structures at this level other than the spinal cord. Most centers will use a separation of 3 mm from the optic chiasm for the treatment of suprasellar tumors, and it would seem reasonable to use the same approach for spinal cord, e.g., for foramen magnum lesions. Whilst frameless stereotactic systems are being developed that can be used for SRS, their definition of accuracy is of the order of 2–4 mm "error" allowable, compared to less than 1 mm for a fixed stereotactic system. Specific tumors that are likely to be treated include: meningiomas (more typically extending from intra to extracranial), chemodectomas, schwannomas, nasopharyngeal carcinomas (as a boost at primary presentation or a relapse), or other localized carcinomas (including in the pediatric age group).

INCIDENCE

The number and types of tumors that will be treated are very much influenced by the referral pattern for the particular department. Obviously, where a department has a relatively large referral practice for, say, nasopharyngeal carcinomas, this malignancy will feature prominently in the number of patients treated. Although infrequent, pediatric tumors typically require very conformal treatment approaches including dose escalation for optimum local control whilst limiting dose to adjacent structures. Thus, normal tissue sparing has an added dimension, given the impact of chemotherapy (typically used in all pediatric malignancies), and for the survivors the longevity of life that they are exposed to after their cure.

The type of tumors treated is reflected by a co-operative multi-disciplinary interaction with HN surgeons, neurosurgeons, and pediatricians. The typical HN cancers are unlikely to be treated in this fashion, except as a boost to macroscopic disease. With these cases excluded, it is the infrequent benign tumors that would be more likely appropriate for this approach as a definitive treatment. The number of these tumor types referred to any HN unit is always going to be few; hence, the tumor experience would be small.

Neurosurgical tumors may indeed constitute the majority of lesions treated in this region. The types of tumors treated by this approach could include:

- schwannomas
- neurofibromas
- cervical metastases
- chordomas
- hemangioblastomas

There is certainly evidence in the intracranial tumor population that stereotactic approaches (specifically SRS) have a track record of benefit for these types of lesions. While some altered movement would occur in the neck region, the proximity of these lesions to the vertebral bodies is going to limit that as a variable. Thus, a hypofractionated or even single-dose approach could be considered. There is evidence for intracranial vestibular schwannomas that hypofractionated methods have high control rates, and authors stated benefit in terms of hearing preservation. Although there is no literature evidence to support it, this philosophy could be applied in the cervical vertebral region where the dose-limiting structure, the spinal cord, is crucial. While conventional wisdom would see the use of 1.8–2.0-Gy fractions, the parallel of the vestibular schwannoma in apposition to the brain stem, in tolerating the hypofractionated approach, would make this method worth considering. This approach has certainly been used with the CyberKnife® and could be used for other systems that have an extracranial technique.

ORGAN SITE-SPECIFIC DIFFICULTIES

Recognition of the dose-limiting structures in any region of the body is the beginning to determining which tumor types can be treated in that region. Moving outside the head and considering relatively small volumes, the dominant structure in the neck is going to be the cervical spinal cord. This structure is going to have varying sensitivities depending upon whether single dose, hypofractionated, or conventionally fractionated approaches are used. From the experience of vertebral metastases, it is known that at least 2–3 vertebral segments of the cervical cord will tolerate a single dose of 8 Gy, 20 Gy in five fractions, and 30 Gy in 10 fractions. The limiting feature to carté blanche use of these doses is that the majority of so-treated patients do not survive many years after treatment. Thus, our current statement of tolerance may be an over statement. Certainly, the large worldwide experience with HN cancers would have 50 Gy conventionally fractionated as well tolerated by the spinal cord. The tolerance of laryngeal cartilages to large single doses or hypofractionated doses is not well known in the long-term situation. This should be considered cautiously, particularly if large volumes of the cartilage are to be included in the treatment fields.

The main sites of specific difficulty would then relate to specific tumors and their shape. Foramen magnum meningiomas adopting a "horse-shoe shape" that have intra- and extracranial components represent a specific challenge. At the beginning of this process, the fixation has to allow treatment across the skull base boundaries. This would exclude any head-orientated fixation device, since the ring-base system would not be able to be extended sufficiently down into the neck while maintaining the head attachment. The HNL fixation device copes with this application being able to be applied for coordinate referencing in the head and neck without altering patient position. This can be used with a bite block chin positioning system or thermoplastic mask. It must be recognized that both devices have reproducible "errors" of setup at best 1–2 mm, worst 2–4 mm.

For any fixation device in the neck to work well, a patient with a long neck is ideal. The patient of stocky build with very short neck can be taxing for any device. Tolerance of an extended neck posture for longer time can be difficult in this circumstance. This is obviously exacerbated for all patients by any degree of kyphosis. Providing extended support for the head may allow too much movement within the stereotactic fixation device such as to negate this as a treatment approach.

Those tumors adjacent to the spinal cord provide some challenge in terms of dose delivery. Fortunately, most of the benign tumors (e.g., meningiomas, schwannomas, etc.) have dose-control parameters that fit within tolerance levels of the spinal cord. As indicated above, however, for those tumors that abut up to the cord on multiple surfaces (such as a horse-shoe type shape), respecting cord tolerance in this situation is difficult. It is for this reason that parallel-opposed field arrangements are frequently used. This, however, regards the spinal cord as a target structure to the same extent as the tumor. This circumstance is handled well with stereotactic IMRT using the MMLC. Figure 9A demonstrates such a case with a foramen magnum meningioma, the DVH contrasting the dose received by the cord for 1-cm leaf width MLC (Fig. 9B) versus the 4-mm leaf width with MMLC (Fig. 9C). Although the differences are not large, the concept of lowering normal tissue dose is paramount.

There are malignancies arising within the cervical region for which control with radiotherapy can be expected; however, the doses required are those that would ordinarily exceed spinal cord tolerance. Cervical cord chordomas and neurofibrosarcomas (malignant schwannomas) are two such malignancies, fortunately quite rare. Doses of the order of 70 Gy are required for control. Conventionally planned treatment cannot provide this.

There are also situations in which retreatment is considered. This could apply to both benign and malignant lesions, provided reasonable benefit had been gained from the initial treatment. Any distance away from the cord makes sparing this structure easier. However, proximity to the cord does not exclude this option, particularly where there is no other treatment

(A)

(B)

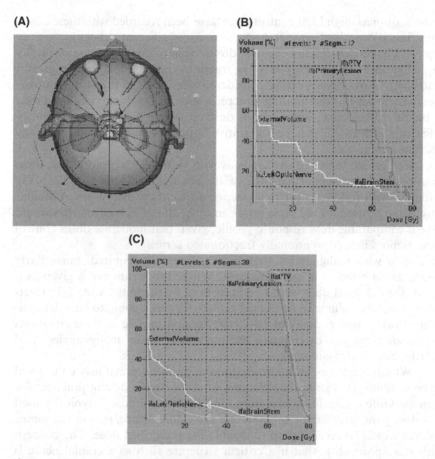

(C)

Figure 9 Foramen magnum meningeoma. (**A**) Volume "shell" demonstrating proximity of structures. (**B**) DVH for 1-cm leaf width MLC. (**C**) DVH for 4-mm leaf width MMLC.

method available. The cervical chordoma patient detailed above demonstrates that retreatment is still possible even for a relatively radio-resistant malignancy.

FRACTIONATED DOSE SELECTION

Results with conventional radiotherapy give us a background for determining appropriate doses. For most of the benign tumors (e.g., schwannomas, chemodectomas, etc.), doses of 45–50 Gy provide local control rates of 85–95%. A more sophisticated approach is unlikely to improve on this. Even for retinoblastomas, high local control rates have been recorded with these doses. Thus, initial consideration is going to be to avoid adjacent structures.

Malignancies require higher doses, macroscopic disease typically requiring doses of 60–70 Gy in 2-Gy fractions, microscopic disease greater than 55 Gy. Lower doses can be considered where the treatment is hypofractionated; however, dose-limiting structures such as the spinal cord need then to be duly considered. Simultaneous dose escalation within the malignancy is feasible with IMRT using comparative hypofractionation while normally treating a large area.

For benign tumor control such as with vestibular schwannomas, there is ample evidence supporting SRS, with that marginal doses of 12–14 Gy sufficing, with follow-up for many series up to about five years. A similar dose could be used for the same tumor in other sites. Chemodectomas would have a comparable dose response profile, given that moderate doses control these tumors in a conventionally fractionated series.

It is with malignancies that higher doses are required, particularly where this is given as a sole treatment. Where this treatment is given as a boost, the delivered dose would be influenced by the initial wide field treatment plan. The volume to be treated is also obviously going to be a determinant. Thus, marginal doses of 18–24 Gy are appropriate in these situations for nasopharyngeal carcinomas, infratemporal fossa malignancies, and chordoma/chondrosarcomas.

Within the tumor dose, heterogeneity has been previously considered to be a significant feature, a reflection of the different dosing practices for GammaKnife versus linac treatment. The 50–60% isodose is typically used as a dose parameter for a GammaKnife procedure, hence, part of the tumor volume would be receiving up to double the prescribed dose. The concern with this approach is that if a critical structure such as a cranial nerve is at the site of dose maximum, then this would increase the risk of treatment related side effects. This does not appear to be a problem with currently used doses for benign tumors as the cranial nerve deficit rate, say in treating vestibular schwannomas, is low. However, when higher marginal doses, 18–20 Gy, were used to treat these tumors, cranial nerve palsy rates of the order of 10–20% were encountered. There is no reason to believe that the same effect would not happen in the extracranial situation. The high local control rates of nasopharyngeal carcinoma with low morbidity indicates that these doses can be tolerated provided what is treated is the macroscopically evident malignancy, without allowing for microscopic extension. Unless some form of control can be achieved obviously, progressive malignancy will cause the same deficit with certainty.

There is less heterogeneity with the linac and charged particle treatment methods as the dosing is to the 80–100% isodose. Hence, the dose maximum is fortunately not that much greater than the prescribed dose. Although there are fewer published linac series, comparable results are reported suggesting that dose inhomogeneity may not be a fact or in achieving tumor control. As indicated above, it may have an impact, however, on complication rates.

TREATMENT DELIVERY

Stereotactic Radiosurgery

These patients are treated similar to any patient with an intracranial lesion who is having SRS. An MRI is performed on the day, or within a few days prior to the procedure, the BRW headring is applied, and then the non-contrast CT scan is performed. The two images sets are fused, and all outlining is performed on the MR images, and in whatever planes that are necessary— axial, coronal, or sagittal. Utilizing BEV various beam directions are chosen, and a beam shaping method selected. If the lesion is spherical/elliptical then cones are used; thus the planning process will require selection of appropriate arc start and stop points, each patient's treatment being individualized. There is no formal library of plans. An isocenter is thus determined. The dose contribution from each arc is evaluated with the accompanying number of monitor units for each arc. After approval of the best plan, a paper printout is then generated with all dose parameters being verified by an independent physicist. Once this step has been accepted, all treatment parameters are delivered to the linac control and Record and Verify System (RVS). The phantom base is attached to the couch mount system, and the isocenter location is further verified, and all arcs go through a dummy run to ensure there is no collision prospect. The patient is then placed on the couch, and the head ring "docked" to the couch mount system. A simple verification is then performed to ensure that there has been no movement of the head ring during the day, as all measurements are in relationship to the head ring, not the patient's head. A port film, AP and lateral, is taken with the angiogram localizer box attached. Subsequently, the fiducial points on this are digitized and a coordinate determined. This is a verification that the intended isocenter is in fact the point treated. The localizer box is removed and treatment proceeds. Gantry movements are directed from outside the room at the console, couch movements are done inside the room. Following this the head ring is removed and the patient goes home, all these treatment being done as an outpatient. For irregular shaped lesions, not suitable for treatment via cones, the MMLC can be used for field shaping, but the dose is delivered as a single fraction. In this situation, 10–15 different beam directions are usually used as static fields. This enables slightly larger lesions to be treated. The same planning process takes place with static field directions being the only differential. The MMLC is directly linked to the linac RVS and control system. Isocenter verification is performed in the same manner.

For neck lesions, a different fixation system is used with depth readings replacing the phantom localizer. Although single-dose treatments could be performed, the slightly greater "error" (2–3 mm) on setup would create concern about their use.

Fractionated Stereotactic

Irrespective of how many fractions are being used, a relocatable device is still required. The planning process is essentially the same, the same treatment being delivered each day, same amount of monitoring, same verification process, and input to the RVS. For all patients an isocenter verification port film is done with the localizer box, the fiducial points being digitized, and compared to the intended isocenter. For the patients having only a few treatments, only one port film (AP and lateral) is taken, but for those patients having many weeks of treatment this is done once per week.

For the first five years, this treatment was done with cones (if necessary multiple isocenters, and arcs, using the same fixation and setup devices). There were more restrictions on the amount of arc travel possible because of the shoulders compared to intracranial lesions. Hence to begin with, there were few patients treated for extracranial HN lesions during this time frame. However, with the MMLC multiple fixed fields became possible. Treatment planning was the same, as was delivery. In terms of scheduling, all MMLC patients were grouped together for convenience. Given the long background with fractionated stereotactic treatments, there is no real difference in delivery process for cone versus MMLC.

LOGISTICS

In terms of treatment delivery devices, this can be divided into dedicated and semidedicated. It can be argued that a cyclotron delivering charged particles is a dedicated device. Other than chordomas, there are few reports of extracranial tumors in the HN region being treated by protons. Thus, for the dedicated facilities, this can be further divided into GammaKnife and linac. Because of the limitation of extending the GammaKnife into the neck, its role is always going to be limited to the tumors at the immediate skull base and only to radiosurgery. Whilst a linac can be designed to function as a dedicated machine for stereotactic treatment, in most facilities it would work as a semidedicated device. BrainLAB has developed the Novalis® as a designated device capable of providing: single-dose and fractionated treatment, multiple fixed fields or arcing, and dynamic or segmental IMRT.

For the semidedicated facilities, many of the reported series have used 1-cm leaf width MLC for beam shaping for their treatment. Any of the three major manufacturers (Varian, Siemens, and ELEKTA) can provide this method. For smaller irregular field treatment, the smaller leaf width MMLC can provide greater dose conformality (Fig. 10). Varian has an accelerator model with a smaller leaf width capability at the middle of its MLC that

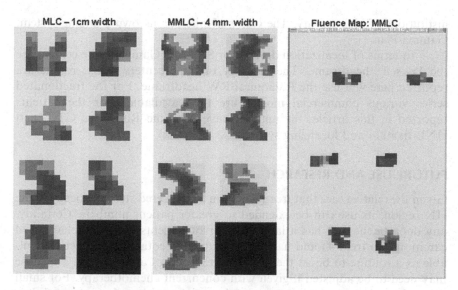

Figure 10 Fluence maps generated as part of IMRT quality assurance indicating better target shaping with the smaller leaf width MMLC. MLC: 1-cm leaf width; MMLC: 4-mm leaf width.

is capable of providing small and large field capability. Virtual MMLC treatment may be possible with MLC devices by rotating the gantry head through 90° for part of the treatment, and thus delivering the divided dose from 0° to 180° and 90° to 270° angulation. True MMLC treatment typically requires an "add-on" device, and in this situation the weight of the MMLC and its effect upon gantry rotation needs to be considered. BrainLAB has their own MMLC as an integral part of the Novalis. The Radionics MMLC can be added to both Varian and Siemens linac. Collimator clearance from the patient with Varian-may place some limitation with an add-on MMLC for particular gantry positions.

Helical tomotherapy using a small linac imbedded in a CT gantry can also be considered a dedicated facility although there are no reports of this being used stereotactically.

Treatment and planning systems require a suitable planning platform that provides both hardware and software. Usually a workstation is required for the former with the software having full 3D visualization processing, image fusion, and a fast inverse planning algorithm to allow for IMRT. Many of the commercially available planning systems that incorporate an IMRT component can be utilized in a stereotactic mode although not specifically designed for it. More dedicated software approaches exist with BRAINLAB and Radionics for stereotactic treatment. These modules also allow for SRS. There are also non-commercial packages developed by individual institutions of high quality. The GammaKnife has its own planning system, Gamma Plan.

In terms of localization devices for SRS, the GammaKnife centers use the Leksell® headframe. The majority of linac centers whose results are reported here will use the RadionicsBRW headframe. For the fractionated series various commercial models are now available. For the patients reported in this article, the authors have used the Radionics GTC, and HNL fixation and localizing systems.

FUTURE USE AND RESEARCH

Given the relative ease that treatments can be delivered stereotactically in the HN region, its use can be extended to greater patient numbers. Certainly, any department that has a large number of patients with nasopharyngeal carcinoma to treat should have fractionated stereotactic approaches available as a routine to boost the primary site to doses of 70–80 Gy. This dose may need to be adjusted if given with concurrent chemotherapy. For small primaries, or where significant regression of the primary has occurred during treatment, SRS may be an appropriate boost method. Stereotactic IMRT may become a preferred method for the total duration of the radiotherapy in the same context that many centers will now use IMRT as their standard approach for nasopharyngeal carcinoma. Retreat situations require high doses to be given to imaging evident lesions, an ideal situation for stereotactic treatment.

Other malignancies that can be considered for stereotactic approach are paranasal sinus carcinomas and chordomas. There would seem to be little role for SRS in the primary situation except as a boost. With the appropriate head fixation device this site lends itself to this approach with high doses required and critical normal structures immediately adjacent to at risk areas. Given the ability to dose escalate, it may be possible to consider definitive radiotherapy as an alternative to major surgery and postoperative radiotherapy. As there would not be an option for surgical salvage, this would require truly informed consent to have this as a standard method. An appropriate circumstance is obviously the patient with surgically resectable disease who has a medical contraindication to such a procedure.

Gating techniques are now being developed to enable higher dose delivery for lung cancers. A similar approach could be applied to laryngeal malignancies that are localized in nature. The clinical circumstance, however, is going to be limited, as it will only relate to those malignancies that have low likelihood of developing nodal disease. This relates to the fact that while the central larynx may move vertically with swallowing, the adjacent nodal areas remain stationary. There would have to be differential allowance for movement in larynx structure while another target remained stationary.

Salivary gland sparing is now a major challenge for radiotherapy techniques to improve the quality of life for the survivors. This has spawned the use of IMRT in the HN region particularly for nasopharyngeal carcinomas. Greater use of this approach is now possible with stereotactic fixation. A comparison of this method with non-stereotactic delivery is a worthy research project. It may come down to a difference only in the ease of reproducibility of patient setup.

The number of benign tumors available to be treated in this region is always going to be small, and since the doses required for control are usually well tolerated, demonstrating a clear advantage for a stereotactic approach may be difficult. There could be an advantage in hypofractionating the treatment, delivering the radiotherapy over 5–10 fractions. This would lead to less disruption to the patient in terms of treatment visits. For the larger lesions, a negative to this approach would be the length of the cranial nerve (usually the vagus) that would be exposed to the hypofractionated dose (e.g., $5 \times 4\,Gy$).

A crucial aspect of the process that makes all of this possible is the quality assurance program. For SRS, doses are being used that aim to damage the tissue being treated. It is the small size of the lesion being treated and the accuracy of delivery that makes this approach safe. While not compromising this aspect, streamlining the process may shorten overall treatment time, thus making it more comfortable for the patient. Similarly, with fractionated treatments evaluating the extent of the QA process may enable better use of departmental, including staff, resources.

REFERENCES

1. Dhanachai M, Kraiphibul P, Pochanugool L, Dangprasert S, Sitathanee C, Laothamatas J, Kulapraditharom B, Theerapancharoen V, Sirisinha T, Yongvithisatid P, Assavaprathuangkul P, Boonpitak K. Stereotactic radiotherapy in nasopharyngeal carcinoma—preliminary results. In: Kondziolka D, ed. Radiosurgery. Vol. 4. Basel: Karger, 2002:162–166.
2. Len Gyel E, Baricza K, Somo Gyi A, Olajos J, Papai Z, Godney M, Nemett G, Esik O. Reirradiation of locally recurrent nasopharyngeal carcinoma. Strahlenther Onkel 2003; 179(5):298–305.
3. Lee AW, Foo W, Law SC, Peters LJ, Poon YF, Chapell R, Sze WM, Tu SY, Lau WH, Ho JH. Total biological effect on late reactive tissues following reirradiation for recurrent nasopharyngeal carcinoma. Int J Radiat Oncol Biol Phys 2000; 46(4):865–872.
4. De Crevoisier R, Bourhis J, Domenge C, Wibault P, Koscielny S, Lusine A, Mamelle G, Janot F, Julieron M, Leridant AM, Marandas P, Armano JP, Schwaab G, Luboinski B, Eschwege F. Full-dose reirradiation for unresectable head and neck carcinoma: experience at the Gustave-Roussy Institute in a series of 169 patients. J Clin Oncol 1998; 16(11):3556–3562.
5. Hwang JM, Fu KK, Phillips TL. Results and prognostic factors in the retreatment of locally recurrent nasopharyngeal carcinoma. Int J Radiat Oncol Biol Phys 1998; 41(5):1099–1111.

6. Chau DT, Sham JS, Kwong DL, Wei WI, Au GK, Choy D. Locally recurrent nasopharyngeal carcinoma: treatment results for patients with computed tomographyassessment. Int J Radiat Oncol Biol Phys 1998; 41(2):379–386.

7. Bari ME, Kemeny AA, Forster DM, Radatz MW. Radiosurgery for the control of glomus jugulare tumors. J Pak Med Assoc 2003; 53(4):147–151.

8. Maarouf M, Voges J, Landwehr P, Bramer R, Treuer H, Kocher M, Muller RP, Sturm V. Stereotactic linear accelerator-based radiosurgery for the treatment of patients with glomus jugulare tumors. Cancer 2003; 97(4):1093–1098.

9. Eustacchio S, Trummer M, Unger F, Schrottner O, Sutter B, Pendl G. The role of Gamma Knife radiosurgery in the management of glomus jugular tumors. Acta Neurochir Suppl 2002; 84:91–97.

10. Elshakkh MA, Mahmoud-Ahmed AS, Kinney SE, Wood BG, Lee JH, Barnett GH, Suh JH. Recurrent head-and-neck chemodectomas: a comparison of surgical and radiotherapeutic results. Int J Radiat Oncol Biol Phys 2002; 52(4):953–956.

11. Foote RL, Pollock BE, Gorman DA, Schomberg PJ, Stafford SL, Link M, Kline RW, Strome SE, Kasperbauer JL, Olsen KD. Glomus jugulare tumor: tumor control and complications after stereotactic radiosurgery. Head Neck 2002; 24(4):332–328; discussion 338–339.

12. Leber KA, Eustacchio S, Pendl G. Radiosurgery of glomus tumors: midterm results. Stereotact Funct Neurosurg 1999; 72(suppl 1):53–59.

13. Jordan JA, Roland PS, McManus C, Weiner RL, Giller CA. Stereotactic radiosurgery for glomus jugulare tumors. Laryngoscope 2000; 110(1):35–38.

14. Liscak R, Vladyka V, Wowra B, Kemeny A, Forster D, Burzaco JA, Martinex R, Eustacchio S, Pendl G, Regis J, Pellet W. Gamma Knife radiosurgery of the glomus jugulare tumor—a multicentre experience. Acta Neurochir (Wien) 1999; 141(11):1141–1146.

15. Liscak R, Vladyka V, Simonova G, Vymazal J, Janouskova L. Leksell Gamma Knife radiosurgery of the tumor glomus jugulare and tympanicum. Stereotact Funct Neurosurg 1998; 70(suppl 1):152–160.

16. Zorlu F, Gurkaynak M, Yildiz F, Oge K, Atahan IL. Conventional external radiotherapy in the management of clivus chordomas with overt residual disease. Neurol Sci 2000; 21(4):203–207.

17. Debus J, Schulz-Ertner D, Schad L, Essig M, Rhein B, Thillmann CO, Wannenmacher M. Stereotactic fractionated radiotherapy for chordomas and chondrosarcomas of the skull base. Int J Radiat Oncol Biol Phys 2000; 47(3): 591–596.

18. Crockard A, Macaulay E, Plowman PN. Stereotactic radiosurgery. VI. Posterior displacement of the brainstem facilitates safer high dose radiosurgery for clival chordoma. Br J Neurosurg 1999; 13(1):65–70.

19. Muthukumar N, Kondziolka D, Lunsford LD, Flickinger JC. Stereotactic radiosurgery tor chordoma and chondrosarcoma: further experiences. Int J Radiat Oncol Biol Phys 1998; 41(2):387–392.

20. Kocher M, Voges J, Staar S, Treuer H, Sturm V, Mueller RP. Linear accelerator radiosurgery for recurrent malignant tumors of the skull base. Am J Clin Oncol 1998; 21(1):18–22.

21. Chua DT, Sham JS, Kwong PW, Hung KN, Leung LH. Linear accelerator-based stereotactic radiosurgery for limited, locally persistent, and recurrent nasopharyngeal carcinoma: efficacy and complications. Int J Radiat Oncol Biol Phys 2003; 56(1):177–183.
22. Ahn YC, Lee KC, Kim DY, Huh SJ, Yeo IH, Lim DH, Kim MK, Shin K, Park S, Chang SH. Fractionated stereotactic radiation therapy for extracranial head and neck tumors. Int J Radiat Oncol Biol Phys 2000; 489(2):501–505.
23. Chang JT, See LC, Liao CT, Ng SH, Wang CH, Chen IH, Tsand NM, Tseng CK, Tang SG, Hong JH. Locally recurrent nasopharyngeal carcinoma. Radiother Oncol 2000; 54(2):135–142.
24. Tate DJ, Adler JR Jr, Chang SD, Marquez S, Eulau SM, Fee WE, Pinto H, Goffinet OR. Stereotactic radiosurgical boost following radiotherapy in primary nasopharyngeal carcinoma. Int J Radiat Oncol Biol Phys 1999; 45: 915–921.
25. Kocher M, Voges J, Staar S, Treuer H, Sturm V, Mueller RP. Linear accelerator radiosurgery tor recurrent malignant tumors of the skull base. Am J Clin Oncol 1998; 21(1):18–22.
26. Cmelak AJ, Cos RS, Adler JR, Fee WE Jr, Goffinet OR. Radiosurgery tor skull base malignancies and nasopharyngeal carcinoma. Int J Radiat Oncol Biol Phys 1997; 37(5):997–1003.
27. Kondziolka D, Lunsford LD. Stereotactic radiosurgery for squamous cell carcinoma of the nasopharynx. Laryngoscope 1991; 101(5):519–22.
28. Habermann W, Aznarotti U, Groell R, Wolf G, Stammberger H, Sutter B , Pendl G. Combination of surgery and gamma knife radiosurgery—a therapeutic option for patients with tumors of nasal cavity or paranasal sinuses infiltrating the skull base. Acta Otorhinolaryngol Ital 2002; 22(2):74–79.
29. Schulz-Ertner D, Haberer T, Jakel O, Thilmann C, Kramer M, Enghardt W, Kraft G, Wannenmacher M, Debus J. Radiotherapy for chordomas and low-grade chondrosarcomas of the skull base with carbon ions. Int J Radiat Oncol Biol Phys 2002; 53(1):36–42.
30. Noel G, Habrand JL, Mammar H, Pontvert D, Hair-Meder C, Hasboun D, Moisson P, Ferrand R, Beaudre A, Boisserie G, Gaboriaud G, Mazal A, Kerody K, Schlienger M, Mazeron JJ. Combination of photon and proton radiation therapy for chordomas and chondrosarcomas of the skull base: the Centre d' Prontontherapie D'Orsay experience. Int J Radiat Oncol Biol Phys 2001; 51(2):392–398.
31. Debus J, Schulz-Ertner D, Schad L, Essig M, Rhein B, Thillmann CO, Wannenmacher M. Stereotactic fractionated radiotherapy for chordomas and chondrosarcomas of the skull base. Int J Radiat Oncol Biol Phys 2000; 47(3): 591–596.
32. Ahn YC, Lee KC, Kim DY, Huh SJ, Yeo IH, Lim DH, Kim MK. Fractionated stereotactic radiation therapy for extracranial head and neck tumors. Int J Radiat Oncol Biol Phys 2000; 48(2):501–505.
33. Lohr F, Debus J, Frank C, Herfarth K, Pastyr O, Rhein B, Bahner ML, Schlegel W, Wannenmacher M. Noninvasive patient fixation for extracranial stereotactic radiotherapy. Int J Radiat Oncol Biol Phys 1999; 45(2):521–527.

34. Pai PC, Chuang CC, Wei KC, Tsang NM, Tseng CK, Chang CN. Stereotactic radiosurgery for locally recurrent nasopharyngeal carcinoma. Head Neck 2002; 24(8):748–753.
35. Feigenberg SJ, Mendenhall WM, Hinerman RW, Amdur RJ, Friedman WA, Antonelli PJ. Radiosurgery for paraganglioma of the temporal bone. Head Neck 2002; 24(4):384–389.
36. Foote RL, Pollock BE, Gorman DA, Schomberg PJ, Stafford SL, Link MJ, Kline RW, Strome SE, Kasperbauer JL, Olsen KD. Glomus jugulare tumor: tumor control and complications after stereotactic radiosurgery. Head Neck 2002; 24(4):332–338; discussion 338–339.
37. Chau DT, Sham JS, Hung KN, Leung LH, Cheng PW, Kwong PW. Salvage treatment for persistent and recurrent T1-2 nasopharyngeal carcinoma by stereotactic radiosurgery. Head Neck 2001; 23(9):791–798.
38. Hinerman RW, Mendenhall WM, Amdur RJ, Stringer SP, Antonelli PJ, Cassisi NJ. Definitive radiotherapy in the management of chemodectomas arising in the temporal bone, carotid body, and glomus vagale. Head Neck 2001; 23(5):363–371.
39. Chau DT, Sham JS, Hung KN, Kwong DL, Dwong PW, Leung LH. Stereotactic radiosurgery as a salvage treatment for locally persistent and recurrent nasopharyngeal carcinoma. Head Neck 1999; 21(7):620–626.
40. Ahn YC, Kim DY, Huh SJ, Baek CH, Park K. Fractionated stereotactic radiation therapy for locally recurrent nasopharynx cancer: report of three cases. Head Neck 1999; 21(4):338–345.
41. Firlik KS, Kondziolka D, Lunstord LD, Janecka LP, Flickinger JC. Radiosurgery for recurrent cranial base cancer arising from the head and neck. Head Neck 1996; 18(2):160–165; discussion 166.
42. Buatti JM, Friedman WA, Bova FJ, Mendenhall WM. Linac radiosurgery for locally recurrent nasopharyngeal carcinoma: rationale and technique. Head Neck 1995; 17(1):14–19.

Index

Italics indicates pages with illustrations.

Printed in the United States
by Baker & Taylor Publisher Services